Teaching and Learning
in Physical Therapy

FROM CLASSROOM TO CLINIC

g

Teaching and Learning
in Physical Therapy

FROM CLASSROOM TO CLINIC

Margaret M. Plack, PT, EdD

Interim Senior Associate Dean for the Health Science Programs
School of Medicine and Health Sciences
The George Washington University
Washington, DC

Maryanne Driscoll, PhD

Educational Psychologist and Associate Professor
School of Health Sciences
Touro College
New York, New York

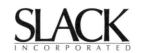

SLACK
INCORPORATED

www.slackbooks.com

ISBN: 978-1-55642-872-2

Teaching and Learning in Physical Therapy: From Classroom to Clinic Instructor's Manual is also available from SLACK Incorporated. Don't miss this important companion to *Teaching and Learning in Physical Therapy: From Classroom to Clinic.* To obtain the Instructor's Manual, please visit http://www.efacultylounge.com.

The procedures and practices described in this book should be implemented in a manner consistent with the professional standards set for the circumstances that apply in each specific situation. Every effort has been made to confirm the accuracy of the information presented and to correctly relate generally accepted practices. The authors, editor, and publisher cannot accept responsibility for errors or exclusions or for the outcome of the material presented herein. There is no expressed or implied warranty of this book or information imparted by it. Care has been taken to ensure that drug selection and dosages are in accordance with currently accepted/recommended practice. Due to continuing research, changes in government policy and regulations, and various effects of drug reactions and interactions, it is recommended that the reader carefully review all materials and literature provided for each drug, especially those that are new or not frequently used. Any review or mention of specific companies or products is not intended as an endorsement by the author or publisher.

SLACK Incorporated uses a review process to evaluate submitted material. Prior to publication, educators or clinicians provide important feedback on the content that we publish. We welcome feedback on this work.

Published by: SLACK Incorporated
                       6900 Grove Road
                       Thorofare, NJ 08086 USA
                       Telephone: 856-848-1000
                       Fax: 856-853-5991
                       www.slackbooks.com

Contact SLACK Incorporated for more information about other books in this field or about the availability of our books from distributors outside the United States.

Library of Congress Cataloging-in-Publication Data
Plack, Margaret.
  Teaching and learning in physical therapy: from classroom to clinic/Margaret Plack, Maryanne Driscoll.
      p. ; cm.
  Includes bibliographical references and index.
  ISBN 978-1-55642-872-2 (alk. paper)
 1. Physical therapy--Study and teaching. I. Driscoll, Maryanne. II. Title.
  [DNLM: 1. Physical Therapy Modalities--education. 2. Learning. 3. Teaching--methods. WB 18 P698t 2011]
  RM706.P48 2011
  615.8'2071--dc22
                         2010020711

Last digit is print number: 10 9 8 7 6 5 4 3 2 1

Dedication

I dedicate this book to my family, my ultimate community of practice. To my dad, who forever encouraged me to reach for the stars; to my mom, who was the strength behind us all; and to my in-laws, for their unending support in all things that mattered most. To my sister, Kathy, who never understood but always understood. To my children, John and Leigh-Ann, my loving cheering section, who supported me every step of the way, provided the motivation I needed to make this a reality, and who now have become my role models. To my husband and soul mate, Tom, who was always there and knew just what I needed, even if I did not, and without whom none of this would have been possible. And of course, to my coauthor, a very special person and good friend, who made the journey fun!

Margaret M. Plack, PT, EdD

I dedicate this book to my family, immediate and extended, for their love and support. Chuck, Meg, and Chad, educators in their own right, demonstrate daily the importance of being creative and seeking the best way to reach and teach the individuals in their charge. I am grateful to my colleagues and students for providing so many opportunities for me to learn and refine instructional strategies. I am indebted to Dr. Maya Frankfurt for her knowledge of neuroanatomy and her willingness to help me develop mine. And finally, I am thankful for the privilege of working, writing, and being friends with my coauthor, the most dedicated educator I know.

Maryanne Driscoll, PhD

Contents

Teaching and Learning in Physical Therapy: From Classroom to Clinic Instructor's Manual is also available from SLACK Incorporated. Don't miss this important companion to *Teaching and Learning in Physical Therapy: From Classroom to Clinic*. To obtain the Instructor's Manual, please visit http://www.efacultylounge.com.

Acknowledgments

Many individuals need to be acknowledged for their role in our learning experiences. First, to the many students we have taught over the years, we thank you for all you have taught us. The teaching-learning experience truly is a partnership, and this text is an outgrowth of all that we have learned in working with all of you. A special thanks to the many students and clinicians who provided their reflections and insights on learning in the classroom and clinic, as they participated in our research through interviews, focus groups, discussion board activities, and other written work. We would also like to acknowledge our faculties. It is an honor and privilege to work with faculty members who so willingly share their dedication and passion for teaching and for their profession as health care providers; again, we have learned so much. Finally, a special thank you to Joyce and Laurie. We have learned so much from this collaboration, and your contributions have significantly enhanced this text. This process has served to solidify our own teaching philosophies, and we want to thank all those who have touched our lives throughout this process.

About the Authors

Margaret M. Plack, PT, EdD, is an associate professor and Interim Senior Associate Dean for the Health Sciences Programs at The George Washington University, Washington, DC. Dr. Plack received her EdD in adult education from the AEGIS Program in the Department of Organization and Leadership at Teachers College, Columbia University, New York. Along with Dr. Driscoll, she has coauthored and taught a graduate course titled "Teaching in Physical Therapy Practice" in several academic institutions. She has also implemented the strategies to be discussed in this text in a number of teaching and learning venues including the American Physical Therapy Association's Combined Sections Meetings and Annual Conference and various other conferences on medical education. She has been involved in ongoing research related to adult learning principles, reflective practice, and educational outcomes and has published several manuscripts on topics related to this text. Dr. Plack has twice received the Stanford Award from the *Journal of Physical Therapy Education* for her writing.

Maryanne Driscoll, PhD, is an educational psychologist and associate professor in the Doctor of Physical Therapy Program at Touro College in New York. Dr. Driscoll received her PhD in educational psychology from Columbia University, New York. Dr. Driscoll consults with schools and hospitals throughout the metropolitan New York region on effective instruction. With Dr. Plack, she coauthored and taught a graduate course titled "Teaching in Physical Therapy Practice" for 2 postprofessional DPT programs, and she teaches similar content in 2 professional DPT programs. She has also implemented the strategies to be used in this text in a number of teaching and learning venues including the American Physical Therapy Association's Combined Sections Meetings and Annual Conference and various other conferences on medical education. Dr. Driscoll has been involved in ongoing research related to adult learning principles and educational outcomes and has published several manuscripts on topics related to this text.

Contributing Authors

Joyce R. Maring, PT, EdD
Associate Professor
School of Medicine and Health Sciences
The George Washington University
Washington, DC

Laurie J. Posey, EdD
Assistant Professor
School of Nursing
The George Washington University
Washington, DC

Foreword

At the forefront of health care are concepts related to quality, safety, effectiveness, and efficiency, all supported by the application of evidence to patient care. Health professionals are required to justify their care decisions based on evidence, whether supported by a single case study that may be the only available published evidence, application of clinical guidelines, or multicenter randomized controlled trials. Hallmarks of evidence-based practice, used by all health professionals when making care decisions, include the integration of the patient's goals and needs and the context in which these are to be applied, the expertise and judgment of the health professional, and available research.[1] Evidence-based practice has become common practice for health care professionals in providing optimal care for patients, clients, family, and caregivers and in supporting care decisions to third-party payers. Health care professionals are becoming more adept at accessing and applying evidence in their daily practice to benefit consumers and in response to the need for cost-effective and quality care. As consumers have become more sophisticated and adept at accessing information and research studies using available technologies, health care professionals are being asked increasingly more difficult questions and are being held accountable for a higher standard of care. Thus, evidence-based practice in health care has become an expected norm where all health care professionals are accountable.

Consider that if evidence-based practice has evolved as the standard of "best practice" across health care, then should teaching and learning be held to any different standard in health professions education and in practice when it comes to preparing future practitioners for clinical practice and educating patients? In the past, a model for learning was to "see one; do one; teach one" as a part of the apprenticeship process when learning to practice. Dr. Silberman notes that evidence for learning retention is greatest (about 90%) when one is able to teach concepts to another, demonstrating that the application and integration of concepts has occurred in order to teach another. In contrast, providing a lecture results in learners merely retaining about 5% of the concepts taught.[2] Likewise, our current knowledge of brain function and adaptation has dramatically altered understanding of how we learn as compared to 25 years ago. Thus, what we know about teaching and learning has evolved significantly based on research, neuroscience, and technology.

The concept of teaching as one was taught is far too common practice in higher education, where those demonstrating content and clinical expertise are presumed to be competent as teachers. Likewise, as society has become more technologically advanced, faculty are confronted with the dilemma of seeking evidence to judiciously select those instructional designs, technologies, and learning situations that have been shown to be effective in enhancing and supporting adult learning. As a learner, have you ever wondered how a faculty determines which technologies are most effective in augmenting teaching? Or how a faculty decides how to teach specific content, psychomotor skills, and professional behaviors to ensure learners are competent across all learning domains? How are faculty assured that learners are prepared as competent and safe health practitioners to provide consumers with optimal care? These are but a few of the many questions that teachers should consider when it comes to their instruction and students should wonder when it comes to their learning.

Thus, if an ideal textbook were to be written that would apply the principles of evidence-based practice to teaching and learning, we might expect that the authors would include information relevant to learners' and teachers' needs, goals, and the learning context, consider the expertise and judgment of faculty and their understanding of what learners bring to the situation, and incorporate and apply the research relevant to concepts associated with teaching and learning. Fortunately, the authors of *Teaching and Learning in Physical Therapy: From Classroom to Clinic* have achieved this desired outcome. This text is an excellent resource for the health professional that models evidence-based principles by being grounded in strong theoretical and evidence-based approaches to teaching and adult learning within the context of health care. The framework for this text considers the capabilities, needs, and goals of learners, patients, and educators with ample opportunities for readers to integrate and reinforce learned concepts through personal reflection, thought-provoking questions, and real-world case situations. It is not often that a book models and practices what it espouses. Every teacher, clinician, and learner could benefit from this practical resource and should have this book in his or her office library to provide strategies to promote effective learning experiences for students and patients with application across health professions education and various practice settings.

What makes this text such an excellent resource for teachers and learners in the health professions? The authors begin with an important premise that distinguishes teaching from learning and explains that how we teach is as important as what we teach. This distinction is critical for faculty to recognize that there are myriad factors that comprise the teaching and learning process that are amenable to theoretical constructs and evidence, analysis and assessment, and change. Likewise, when faculty are able to develop a systematic approach to their teaching by finding both proven and creative ways to assess how students learn, then the outcomes can be formidable in not only what students learn but also the degree to which new knowledge, skills, and professional behaviors are retained. The days of "pouring information" into learners' minds with an expectation of regurgitation is neither supported by evidence nor does it result in long-term retention and learning at higher cognitive levels. Thus, the authors provide a structure to facilitate the teaching and learning process that is easily understood and extremely applicable in many situations that are addressed in this text.

The systematic approach used by the authors is highly effective to design, implement, and evaluate teaching and learning and can be used by any health care professional involved in teaching others or when engaged as a learner. The authors provide both breadth and depth on teaching and learning by highlighting factors that may influence individual teaching and learning (ie, culture, gender, past experiences, generational factors, social roles, etc), the impact of contemporary brain research and its effect on teaching and learning processes, and the use of systematic processes to provide effective instruction in a variety of formats and for a variety of audiences to address learning across cognitive, psychomotor, and affective domains. In addition, the authors orient the reader to teaching and learning concepts that progress from an individual learner and teacher in the classroom, to teaching and learning in the clinical community, and to patient education and facilitating behavior change. Finally, the authors address the prudent use and application of various technologies (e-Learning products and resources, Web-based tools and technologies, social networking, etc) as resources in supporting and enhancing teaching, learning, and patient education.

The ability to make complex concepts more easily understood and readily applicable is an art unto itself. Each chapter in this book is systematically designed to address theoretical and evidence-based concepts while also being functional. More important, approaches used by the authors model the effective teaching and learning principles espoused in this text. Each chapter begins with a specific set of learning objectives that define what the reader will be able to do to at the end of the chapter as well as providing exemplars of well-written learning objectives. At the completion of each chapter, key summary points are provided to reinforce concepts and summarize the salient points. Content presented is supported by current evidence while also integrating active learning concepts. Periodically, the reader is asked to "Stop and Reflect," inviting a purposeful pause with time to think about questions, thereby discovering how new concepts can be integrated or adapted by the reader in his or her environment. Finally, "Critical Thinking Clinical Scenarios" promote the translation of knowledge into the real world by asking the reader to apply concepts to real-life situations that may parallel those that the reader encounters throughout his or her professional life.

Thus, the authors model and practice the lessons taught throughout this book and are to be commended for their effort. Evidence-based teaching and learning is powerful and can significantly contribute to the future of health professions education and practice. Often, teaching is portrayed as blending science with a craft. For some faculty, teaching may be an intuitive process that has led to successful outcomes by a combination of intention and happenstance. And yet, there are those wonderful times where the integration of evidence with engaging subject matter coupled with an artful performance results in magical moments for learners, so much so that we can long remember the learning experience and the teacher! Ultimately, if we chart a different course for how we teach and what we teach, learners will be more engaged in the process, and learning will change, which can influence how health professionals practice and educate patients. As health professions' standards have evolved with expectations of using evidence in their practice, so too should the same standards apply to teaching and learning in higher education and practice. This book will help health professionals change old paradigms in teaching and learning by applying and integrating the concepts presented by the authors using simple and elegant approaches.

Jody S. Gandy, PT, DPT, PhD
Director, Academic/Clinical Education Affairs
American Physical Therapy Association
Alexandria, Virginia

References

1. Straus SE, Richardson WS, Glasziou P, et al. *Evidence-Based Medicine.* 3rd ed. Philadelphia, PA: Elsevier Churchill Livingstone; 2005.

2. Silberman M. *Active Training: A Handbook of Techniques, Designs, Case Examples, and Tips.* 3rd ed. San Francisco, CA: John Wiley & Sons, Inc; 2006.

Introduction

"Learning and teaching are not inherently linked. Much learning takes place without teaching, and indeed much teaching takes place without learning." -Etienne Wenger, *Communities of Practices: Learning, Meaning, and Identity*

"Teaching, in my estimation, is a vastly over-rated function." -Carl Rogers, *Freedom to Learn*

Stop and Reflect

Consider the opening quotes:
- Why would we title this book *Teaching and Learning in Physical Therapy: From Classroom to Clinic?*
- Why, too, would we begin a book on teaching and learning with these quotes, which suggests that teaching is relatively unimportant and vastly overvalued?

As we prepared this text, a colleague asked us why we decided on the title *Teaching and Learning in Physical Therapy*. She asked, "Isn't it a book for educators; isn't it really about teaching? So why learning?" For us, teaching and learning are inseparable. Our goal in this text is to help you make that link between teaching and learning. In any teaching-learning situation, the goal is to ensure that learners learn. Whether we are in the formal setting of the classroom or the more informal community of clinic practice, learning is critical to professional development and quality patient care. In physical therapy, learning is a lifelong process, as is teaching. In practice, what was learned becomes more important than what or how something was taught. We would agree that teaching without learning is relatively unimportant and vastly overvalued!

To be effective instructors, it is important to understand who we are as learners, explore our learning styles, identify our strengths, and identify those areas in which we struggle. It is important to understand what we bring to the teaching-learning situation. We want to be certain that our teaching is linked to learning. For a long time, literature suggested that good teachers were born not made. More recently, the focus has shifted to identifying factors that lead to successful teaching. Teaching and learning are skills, and, like other physical therapy skills, they must be learned and perfected.

In physical therapy, knowledge is being generated at such an enormous rate that much of what we learn today may very well be obsolete within a few years. Unless we are helping our learners learn *how* to learn, we are only preparing them for today and not for the future. We want our learners to be prepared to learn without having to be taught; we want them to be prepared to identify their resources and to utilize their communities of practice to continue their process of lifelong learning. As a result, educators have moved from teaching to becoming facilitators of learning; from being the "Sage on the Stage" to being the "Guide on the Side." We no longer view our learners as blank slates or passive recipients of knowledge; rather, they are active participants in the learning process, in negotiating meaning, in developing identities, and in creating knowledge. Learning is not simply an accumulation of facts; it is a process of adapting information and transforming it into something useful.

Learning is about making connections and linking them to prior experiences so that we can learn from those experiences. Learning is a dynamic and complex process, and each new connection influences how we approach all future situations. As educators, our role is to identify and acknowledge the experiences our learners bring to the learning situation and to help them make those connections. It is important to recognize that as educators we too bring our own knowledge and past experiences to the teaching-learning situation and we learn and change with each experience. Even as authors of this text, we brought our personal histories and research to our writing and have learned from the process. So you see, for us, teaching and learning are inseparable, which is why we use the term *teaching-learning experience* throughout this text. Not only are they inseparable, they are integral to physical therapy practice.

Before you move on, we would like you to just take a minute and reflect on our role as educators in physical therapy.

Stop and Reflect

What do you think of when you think about "Teaching in Physical Therapy"?
- Who do we teach?
- What do we teach?
- Where do we teach?
- When do we teach?
- How do we teach?
- Why do we teach?

Teaching is a significant component of any clinical practice. In physical therapy, we continually teach patients, families, colleagues, students, community members, and other professionals, and as we teach, we learn. Teaching and learning are both formal and informal and happen on a daily basis (Figure I-1).

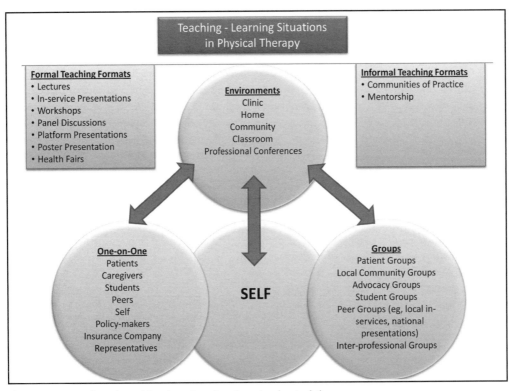

Figure I-1. Samples of teaching-learning situations in physical therapy.

Teaching and learning are dynamic skills that require both knowledge and practice to perfect. In this text, we will explore what it takes to be an effective teacher and learner in physical therapy and provide you with multiple opportunities to apply, adapt, and practice the skills required to ensure excellence in teaching and learning.

Aim and Audience

This book is designed for those looking to enhance their skills both as an educator and as a learner in physical therapy. Whether you are a student, clinician, first-time presenter, or faculty member, you will find this book useful. This book offers a systematic approach to designing, implementing, and evaluating effective teaching-learning experiences. Throughout, we offer practical strategies that can be adapted to a variety of teaching and learning situations. The concepts discussed are relevant for any health care provider, although given our experiences in physical therapy, the examples and activities relate specifically to physical therapy practice.

Content

This text is divided into 3 sections: (1) Who Are We as Learners and Teachers? (2) Designing, Implementing, and Assessing Effective Instruction; and (3) From Classroom to Clinic and Beyond. In Section I, we explore who we are as individuals, how that impacts the teaching-learning experience, and what that means for us as educators. We describe strategies to help us explore our own assumptions, to self-assess, and to become good critical thinkers essential to effective instruction.

In Chapter 1, "Filters: Individual Factors That Influence Us as Teachers and Learners," we begin by exploring different characteristics of learners and teachers. We use the terms *personal filters* or *lenses* to describe some of the factors that may impact how we teach and how we learn. We explore factors that influence our perceptions of any teaching-learning situation, including culture, gender, past experiences, generational differences, level of expertise, and current social roles (ie, family, work, community). We know these filters influence us as individuals, as learners, and as teachers; what we cannot know is the extent to which they may impact any given teaching-learning situation. This chapter highlights the importance of recognizing how designing effective instruction requires an appreciation of the dynamic interaction of all of these filters.

In Chapter 2, "Reflection and Action Learning: Keys to Self-Awareness, Problem Solving, and Continuous Improvement in Practice," we introduce reflection as a means of understanding ourselves and the assumptions we hold. We explore the reflective process, why it is important, and how to facilitate it. We describe how reflection is the basis for critical thinking, self-assessment, and continuous improvement, which are essential to the development of expertise in practice. Finally, we provide strategies to facilitate the process in ourselves, our learners, and others. We introduce the use of questions and action learning to facilitate reflection and critical thinking and examine how critical thinking is integral to clinical decision making. This chapter highlights how we can use the reflective process to better understand our learners and ourselves.

In Chapter 3, "The Brain: How Current Concepts in Brain Function May Inform Teaching and Learning," we begin to examine what we know about brain function and learning. We provide a brief overview of some of the major neuroanatomical structures of the brain involved in learning, memory formation, and memory retrieval. Recognizing the complexity of the human brain and how brain research is truly in its infancy, we explore the potential implications of brain research on teaching-learning. We explore concepts of emotion, attention, memory formation, and the use of prior knowledge to enhance learning and retention. Though direct links from current brain research to the classroom cannot be made (yet!), the goal of this chapter is to pique your interest in the potential applications of brain research to teaching and learning in the classroom and the clinic.

In Section II, we examine the design, implementation, and assessment of effective instruction. In Chapter 4, "Systematic Effective Instruction: Keys to Designing Effective Presentations," we present a comprehensive, systematic approach to instruction that includes assessing the needs of our learners, gaining their attention, and effectively presenting content to achieve the established objectives. We provide strategies to incorporate periodic motivational hooks, content boosters, formative assessments, practice opportunities, summaries, and summative assessments. We emphasize the importance of active learning, providing teaching strategies that are multidimensional and interactive. These concepts are reinforced in Section III, where you will see how these same concepts are important, not only for classroom or community presentations, but in planning effective patient education activities as well.

In Chapter 5, "Design Considerations: Adapting Instruction for Varied Audiences and Formats," we build on the principles presented in the previous chapter. The goal of this chapter is to help you adapt a presentation for different formats and different audiences. The concepts of systematic effective instruction are applied to a variety of formats common to physical therapy, including continuing education programs, platform presentations, panel discussions, health and wellness fairs, and the like. We discuss which components of systematic effective instruction are nonnegotiable, which can be modified or deleted depending on the situation, and what else we need to consider to meet the demands of these varied formats. We also problem solve challenging issues, such as what to do if you find that your audience is more knowledgeable than you anticipated, the room setup or learning environment is not what you expected, your presentation is taking much longer than planned, or you are faced with challenging audience behaviors.

In Chapter 6, "Strategies for Teaching and Learning Movement," we transition from to designing environments and conditions that encourage motor learning through active engagement and practice. Here, we focus on teaching movement, a topic integral to physical therapy patient care. We explore our role as movement educators and describe how theories of motor control and motor learning inform practice. We examine various types of movement, task characteristics, and movement taxonomies. Humans as information processors is discussed and linked to concepts such as attention, interference, response alternatives, and accuracy demands, all essential to helping our patients learn to move. We examine conditions of practice, types of practice, and practice schedules and how each can be used to optimize learning given the individual, the task, and the environment. Various forms of feedback are introduced and linked to effective learning. Finally, the chapter ends with a discussion of teaching and learning differences across the life span.

In Section III, we move from the classroom to the clinic and beyond. We focus here on how learning takes place in the clinical setting and how technology can be used to enhance learning for students, clinicians, and our patients and clients. In Chapter 7, "Communities of Practice: Learning and Professional Identity Development in the Clinical Setting," we explore the concepts of apprenticeship learning and learning within a community of practice. This chapter emphasizes the development of professional behaviors, including communication and interpersonal skills, because these are often the most challenging to teach and, for some, the most challenging to learn, yet they are critical to professional development and effective patient care. Though focused on the affective domain, the concepts we present can be generalized to all aspects of learning (psychomotor and cognitive) in the clinical environment. Throughout the chapter, you will see direct quotes from interviews with students and clinicians that illustrate and reinforce the concepts being discussed. Through the quotes, students and clinical instructors provide their perspectives on how they developed their own professional identity. The quotes also provide additional opportunities for you to apply the concepts presented throughout the chapter to real-world scenarios.

In Chapter 8, "The Learning Triad: Strategies for Optimizing Supports and Minimizing Barriers to Facilitate Learning in the Clinical Setting," we present the concept of a learning triad, which includes the learner, the instructor, and the clinical community. We examine the role of mentorship within the physical therapy community of practice and how mentorship in physical therapy moves beyond the one-to-one relationship of the student and clinical instructor to include the entire learning triad. We examine the role of the learning triad in supporting learning. We explore how the same components that support learning in the clinical environment can potentially hinder learning as well. Finally, we present a framework for learning that optimizes the supports and minimizes the barriers to learning in the clinical setting. As in the previous chapter, you will see direct quotes from students and clinicians that illustrate, reinforce, and provide opportunities to apply the concepts discussed. These quotes provide evidence of how learning in the physical therapy clinical environment is similar to, yet different from, a more traditional mentorship or apprenticeship model of learning.

In Chapter 9, "Patient Education: Facilitating Behavior Change," we examine the complexities of patient education. We explore the many factors to be considered in designing effective learning experiences for patients. We stress the importance of assessing patient's readiness to learn, both physically and emotionally. To do so, we link back to adult learning principles and motivation theory. We describe how you can use explanatory models to negotiate shared meaning and maintain your patients at the center of the decision-making process. We discuss strategies and processes to facilitate behavior change by understanding your patient's health beliefs. We explore the stages of change and suggest strategies to help move a patient along the continuum of behavior change. We examine some factors (including comorbid conditions) that may facilitate or hinder adherence and present a communities of practice framework to help you identify supports that may facilitate adherence in your patients. Given the prevalence of low literacy in the United States, we offer strategies to assess a patient's literacy level and provide mechanisms to design educational materials that will be optimally comprehensible by your patients. Finally, we offer a behavioral counseling strategy to facilitate long-term maintenance of behavior change in your patients.

The text concludes with Chapter 10, "Harnessing Technology: Tools to Enhance Learning in the Clinic and the Classroom." In this chapter, many of the concepts presented in earlier chapters are reinforced as they are applied to the design, development, implementation, and assessment of e-Learning products. From needs assessments and goal setting to the development of storyboards and e-Learning assessments, we provide strategies and resources to help you design effective educational offerings. Here, we present the basics of developing and incorporating digital images, audio, video, text, and interactivity in your e-Learning product to capture a diverse audience, including individuals with special needs. We provide examples of Web material including patient education, digital repositories, and clinical decision support tools along with criteria to evaluate online resources. Finally, the concepts of social networking and other Web 2.0 technologies are explored as possible sources of patient education and support strategies.

Format

Each chapter begins with a set of objectives that clearly delineate what you, the reader, will be prepared to do after completing the chapter and concludes with a summary of the major concepts presented in the chapter. Embedded throughout each chapter are opportunities for you to Stop and Reflect and actively engage with the content as you process the information presented. Additional information and activities are also included in the instructor's manual which can be found online at http://www.efacultylounge.com. Concepts are supported by research as well as clinical examples. You will have multiple opportunities to apply and adapt these concepts to real-world situations through Critical Thinking Clinical Scenarios. Finally, concepts are reinforced through frequent Key Points to Remember.

SECTION I

WHO ARE WE AS
TEACHERS AND LEARNERS?

Filters
Individual Factors That Influence Us
As Teachers and Learners

Chapter Objectives

After reading this chapter, you will be prepared to:
- Consider the influence of individual characteristics and experiences on us as teachers and learners in the classroom and the clinic.
- Describe the various factors or filters that influence who we are as teachers and as learners.
- Analyze how our cultural and generational experiences influence our role as teacher and learner.
- Describe how adult learning principles and learning styles influence us as teachers and learners.
- Recognize the influence of the dynamic interaction of these individual factors on our role as teacher and learner.
- Consider the implications of these dynamic interactions on designing effective teaching and learning experiences in the classroom and the clinic.

Individual Factors That Influence Us as Teachers and Learners

John Dewey is often considered the father of experiential learning. He believed that all learning is grounded in our experiences and our experiences very much influence how we learn and what we decide to learn.[1,2] Our past experiences influence how we view and react to the world around us, both as teachers and as learners. Before we can begin to think about how

to facilitate learning in others, we must first develop a better understanding of who we are and what we each bring to the learning situation. In this chapter, we will explore some of the factors that make us unique as individuals, as teachers, and as learners.

We use the terms *personal filters* or *lenses* to describe some of the factors that may impact how we teach and how we learn. These lenses overlay one another and bring to the forefront the complexity of the teaching-learning situation. We will explore the factors that influence how we experience a learning situation, which include but are in no way limited to our perceptions, our culture, our gender, our past experiences, our generational experiences, our level of expertise, and our current social roles (ie, family, work, community). Though each of these filters has an influence on us as teachers and as learners, we cannot always know to what extent they impact any given learning situation. Therefore, we discuss how critical it is to recognize and respect the potential influences of each of these filters. The goal of this chapter is for us to recognize that designing effective instruction requires an appreciation of the dynamic interaction of all of these filters.

Stop and Reflect

Look at Figure 1-1 on page 4. What do you see?
- How old is the person that you see?
- What type of job, if any, do you think this person has?
- Would you describe the person as young or old?
- How would you describe the person? Is she attractive or unattractive?

Plack M, Driscoll M. *Teaching and Learning in Physical Therapy: From Classroom to Clinic* (pp 3-24).

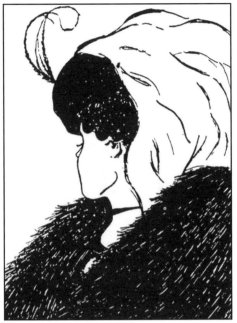

Figure 1-1. Ambiguous woman.

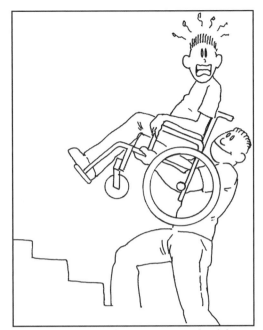

Figure 1-2. Picture of a person in a wheelchair. (© PAX Press, a division of Beneficial Designs, Inc.)

Perception

When you looked at the picture, did you see more than 1 figure? If you look closely, you will see 2 different figures. Generally, people will immediately see one of the figures in the picture and at times struggle to see the other. Depending on how you view the picture of the young woman or the older woman, you will respond to the questions posed very differently. Two people can look at the very same picture and see 2 very different things, which will influence how they respond and react.

Stop and Reflect

What is your reaction to the picture in Figure 1-2? What do you think is going on? What do you think each person is thinking and feeling?

Unlike a simple optical illusion, the cartoon presented in Figure 1-2 can elicit an emotional response that is guided by our own perceptions. These perceptions are influenced by our own personal experiences and cultural beliefs. Based on our perceptions, we make assumptions and judgments about the world around us. For example, depending on your past experiences, you may make different assumptions about what is happening in the cartoon. One person might view this as a positive experience, seeing the man as being very helpful to the young boy in the wheelchair. Another person might view this quite negatively, viewing the man as being overbearing and patronizing without stopping to consider the young boy's feelings.

Steven Covey,[3] in his book titled *The 7 Habits of Highly Effective People*, discusses the concept of internal maps. These internal maps are how we view the world, and they are based on our own value system and beliefs. He describes people as having 2 sets of internal maps: (1) our realities or how things are and (2) our values or how we think things should be. We accept these maps without question because they grow out of our own personal experiences in life. This is how we perceive the world. As a result of our own perceptions of the world, we make assumptions, and we assume that the way we view the world is reality. These assumptions also influence the judgments we make and how we act in certain situations.

As humans, we make assumptions about people all the time. As physical therapists, it is also a significant part of what we do. The minute a patient walks into the room, we begin to collect data on that person and, based on that data, we begin to make assumptions about that person. For example, if a patient walks into the room limping and grimacing, we immediately begin to assume that the patient is in pain. We often use hypotheses to guide our clinical decision-making process. We make hypotheses, test those hypotheses, then, based on the outcome, we begin to revise those hypotheses. Assumptions are like hypotheses, except that people are not always aware of their assumptions and therefore do not always test their assumptions. Very often, our assumptions are accurate, just like our hypotheses; however, there are times when they are not. Making assumptions is not really a problem until we begin to act on our assumptions without first checking the accuracy of them.

Critical Thinking Clinical Scenario

A second-year physical therapy student has just completed her first 4-week full-time clinical rotation. In meeting with the director of clinical education, she described her clinical instructor, who had many years of experience, as awful. When asked why, the student responded that the clinical instructor had poor evaluation skills. She noted that she rarely completed a full examination and often made decisions simply based on a few quick tests.

Reflective Questions

1. What do you think is going on in this scenario?
2. How might the student's limited experience influence her perception of the clinical instructor's skills?
3. How might the physical therapist's expertise influence her approach to the examination?
4. How might the perceptions of each differ?
5. What other explanations might there be for what may have happened in this scenario?

There are always at least 2 people in any teaching-learning situation, each with his or her own perceptions. Whenever you are interacting with one or more person, there are always 2 things going on simultaneously:

1. The intended behavior of the person saying or doing something (ie, the intention)
2. The impact of that behavior or comment on the person on the receiving end (ie, the impact)

The intent and the impact do not always match. Our personal perceptions are often very strong and often color the way we view the entire world; they are very much a part of what we bring to the teaching and learning situation. Our personal perceptions influence both intention and impact. For example, if the student in the previous clinical scenario perceived that the clinical instructor lacked expertise, it may color or influence how that student reacted to the examination and to any feedback the instructor may have offered.

Another example might be the experience of trying to help someone and having that person react negatively to your actions. In the illustration presented in Figure 1-2, the intent of the man may very well have been to offer assistance, whereas the young boy, wanting to be independent, may have experienced his help as unwanted and unnecessary. Intention and impact are essential components of any communication and may influence how learners react to the teaching-learning situation. Examples of how intention and impact may be easily mismatched are provided in Table 1-1.

Stop and Reflect

Have your intentions ever been misunderstood? What were your intentions? What was the impact on the other person? How might this influence your assumptions and actions in the future?

It is important to recognize that a mismatch can easily occur. Also recognize that in any given situation, there are 2 experts:

1. The person behaving is the expert on the *intention* of the action
2. The person on the receiving end is the expert on the *impact* of the action

To minimize the likelihood of these mismatches becoming problematic, clear communication between teacher and learner is essential. If there is any chance that a mismatch between teacher and learner has occurred, it is important to clarify the intent and describe the impact in order to maintain an effective teacher-learner relationship.

One final example might be when a therapist provides a patient with 7 home exercises to complete on a daily basis over a week. The intention of the therapist is to provide a number of options knowing that the patient will likely complete only a few of the exercises. The therapist may have assumed that giving the patient a choice would result in enhanced adherence, with the patient completing at least a few daily exercises. The impact on the patient could very well be that he or she felt overwhelmed with the excessive number of exercises provided. Unless the therapist both checked her assumptions and clarified her intentions with the patient, a mismatch may have occurred. This mismatch may have had a negative impact on adherence and on the development of an effective therapeutic relationship.

Table 1-1. Examples of Mismatched Intention and Impact

Your Intention	The Potential Impact
To be humorous…	Sarcasm, flip, glib, silly, making fun of
To be fair…	Rigid, unyielding, inflexible, unfair
To be flexible…	Wishy-washy, unfair, favoritism, weak, indecisive
To understand someone's thinking (ie, asking "why?")…	Insubordinate, rude, challenging, confrontational

As noted, in clinical practice it is critical to recognize the potential for mismatched communication, particularly when engaging with a number of learners simultaneously. Clarifying the intent and checking the impact of the communication is essential to developing and maintaining an effective teacher-learner relationship. The teacher must continually clarify intentions, and it is important that the learner is made to feel comfortable enough to provide feedback in the event that communication has a negative impact.

Key Points to Remember

- There are 2 experts in every communicative interaction:
  - The provider is the expert on the *intent* of the communication.
  - The receiver is the expert on the *impact* of the communication.
- Clarifying the intent and checking the impact of the communication is essential to developing and maintaining an effective teacher-learner relationship.

Cultural Differences

The US population is becoming increasingly diverse. People from different cultures often bring different values, beliefs, and experiences with them. If we do not appreciate these differences, they may become barriers to effective teaching and quality health care. Different cultures have different beliefs about illness, intervention, prevention, and health promotion. We each tend to think our own beliefs are right and make the most sense; however, to provide effective instruction or health care, we must suspend our own beliefs as we strive to understand our patients' beliefs. This underscores the need to consider culture as another personal filter in any teaching-learning situation.

Stop and Reflect

- Do you believe that if you treat everyone as you want to be treated, then you will be meeting their needs and providing effective care?
- Can you think of a time when this might not be true?

Bennett[4] wrote:

The Golden Rule is typically used as a kind of template for behavior. If I am unsure of how to treat you, I simply imagine how I myself would like to be treated, and then act in accordance. The positive value of this form

of the Rule is virtually axiomatic in US American culture, and so its underlying assumption frequently goes unstated: other people *want* to be treated as I do. And under this assumption lies another more pernicious belief: all people are basically the same, and thus they really *should* want the same treatment (whether they admit it or not) as I would.

Simply stated, the Golden Rule in this form does not work because people are actually different from one another. Not only are they individually different, but they are systematically different in terms of national culture, ethnic group, socioeconomic status, age, gender, sexual orientation, political allegiance, educational background, and profession, to name a few possibilities.

Stop and Reflect

- What does the quote from Bennett mean to you?
- In what ways, if any, does this quote change your perspective on culture as a filter in the teaching-learning situation?

Though it may seem obvious that knowledge of different cultures is critical in teaching and in health care, the process of understanding different cultures cannot be oversimplified. The danger in teaching others about different cultures is the possibility of reinforcing stereotypes. Stereotypes are generalizations that individuals make about people of other cultures. Learning about cultures may at times foster a simplistic view, whereby learners attempt to fit people into categories learned. However, generalizations can be a helpful entry point in understanding more about our learners and our patients. For example, understanding that an Orthodox Jewish male patient may prefer a male therapist may facilitate patient assignments in a busy clinic. On the other hand, if a female therapist in the clinic had a particular strength in managing this patient's dysfunction, it would be important to have a conversation with the patient to ascertain his individual perspective before simply assigning a male therapist. Generalizations are like hypotheses and assumptions; they must be checked. It is critical to check your assumptions with each patient.

Culture is a complex concept with no standard terminology. The Office of Minority Health (OMH) of the US Department of Health and Human Services Institute of Medicine defines culture as the "integrated patterns of human behavior that include the language, thoughts, communications, actions, customs, beliefs, values, and institutions of racial, ethnic, religious, or social groups."[8]

Critical Thinking Clinical Scenario

You have been reviewing the literature on cross-cultural differences. In the literature, it indicates that in dealing with pain, individuals from Italian and Jewish descent tend to complain about their pain, whereas Americans are often more stoic, and those from Irish descent tend to ignore pain.[5-7] You are a health care provider of Irish descent. You were born and raised in New England and your family has lived there for 7 generations. You have 3 patients: 1 patient of Jewish decent, 1 patient of Irish decent, and 1 patient of Italian decent.

Reflective Questions

1. How might your cultural background influence the type of pain questions you ask each of these patients?

2. How might your cultural characteristics possibly impact your reaction to their report of pain?

3. Knowing the influence of culture on one's pain experience, how might you alter the questions you ask to better assess each patient's pain?

It is important to remember that there is often as much variability within cultures as there is across cultures. Purnell[6] and Purnell and Paulanka[7] suggested that subcultures exist within a culture where 2 individuals may have had very different personal experiences and therefore view the world differently. Subcultures are a result of such things as age, generation, nationality, race, color, gender, socioeconomic status, marital status, occupation, physical characteristics, religious affiliation, sexual orientation, and reason for migration. For example, a 62-year-old Asian male business owner who emigrated from China at the age of 4 may have a very different view of Western health care practices than a 62-year-old Asian man who is a new immigrant from China.

Key Point to Remember

It is important to remember that there is often as much variability within cultures as there is across cultures!

There are 2 components to understanding cultures: (1) learning the basic facts and characteristics of different cultures and (2) learning how to effectively engage in cross-cultural encounters. Presenting the specifics about different cultures is beyond the scope of this book; however, there are numerous resources available, including textbooks, research articles, and the like.[5,6,9-14] In addition, Web sites, health care provider brochures, and videos can easily be found to help you learn more about different cultures, especially those most represented in your practice.

Learning about different cultures is not enough, though. It is important to go beyond simply learning facts about different cultures to developing competence in working effectively with individuals from different cultures.[15-17] Cultural competence is the "ability to work effectively in a cross cultural situation." The OMH defines cultural competence as "a set of congruent behaviors, attitudes, and policies that come together in a system, agency, or among professionals that enables effective work in cross-cultural situations."[8] This implies that you have the ability to function effectively as an individual and an organization within the context of the cultural beliefs, behaviors, and needs presented by consumers and their communities.[8]

Purnell[6] suggested that we need to have certain types of knowledge and skills to be culturally competent. Adapted to the teaching and learning situation, to be effective instructors, it is important for us to develop the following knowledge and skills:

- Awareness of our own cultural beliefs and their potential impact on the teaching-learning situation

- Awareness of, and respect for, the needs and beliefs of others

- Adapting our teaching to meet the needs of the learner

As Purnell[6] described, it is insufficient to simply be aware of and respect differences; we must actively seek knowledge about different cultures with the goal of providing care that is congruent with the values, needs, and beliefs of people from different cultures. The Campinha-Bacotes[12,18] indicated that it is equally important to actively engage in cross-cultural encounters that enable us to practice culturally appropriate interactions.

Several stages or processes for developing cultural competence have been presented in the literature. Table 1-2 presents 3 such models.

Inherent in each of these processes is a self-exploration; consciously taking time to reflect upon our own characteristics and how they impact our world view and the teaching-learning situation. Cultural competence is a process, not an endpoint; even if you reach the point of cultural proficiency as described by Leavitt[10] and others, care must be taken to continually check your assumptions with each new patient.

Table 1-2. Processes of Developing Cultural Competence

Leavitt	Mederos and Woldeguiorguis	Purnell
1. Cultural destructiveness— Treating people in a dehumanized manner	1. Exploring one's own culture	1. Unconscious incompetence— Lacking self-awareness of what one does not know about other cultures
2. Cultural incapacity— Bias is present and cross-cultural encounters are ineffective	2. Gaining knowledge of other cultural groups	2. Conscious incompetence— Aware of personal limitations of cultural knowledge
3. Cultural blindness— Treat all people the same with no regard for cultural differences	3. Engaging in cross-cultural encounters	3. Conscious competence— Learning about and validating one's cultural knowledge and providing culturally specific interventions
4. Cultural precompetence— Commitment to appropriate cross-cultural interactions and any inadequacies are acknowledged		4. Unconscious competence— Automatically provides competent cross-cultural care
5. Cultural competence— Respect for any cultural differences; continuous self-assessment and adaptation is present		
6. Cultural proficiency— High regard for any cultural differences and seeks research and advancement of effective approaches to cross-cultural practices		

Adapted from Leavitt RL. Developing cultural competence in a multicultural world—part II. *PT Magazine.* 2003;11:56-68; Mederos F, Woldeguiorguis I. Beyond cultural competence: what child protection managers need to know and do. *Child Welfare.* 2003;82:125-142; Purnell L. The Purnell model for cultural competence. *J Multicult Nurs Health.* 2005;11:7-15.

Critical Thinking Clinical Scenario

You are starting a new position as a physical therapist in an urban hospital serving a large Caribbean population. Patient education will be a significant aspect of your role.

Reflective Questions

Consider the 3 different processes for the development of cultural competence:
1. Where along each of the processes do you currently see yourself?
2. What do you think might be important to know about the Caribbean culture as it relates to health care and physical therapy more specifically?
3. How might you better prepare for your position by moving yourself through these processes?

- Heritage, including country of origin
- Communication, including primary language, verbal and nonverbal cues, touch, and awareness of space and time
- Family roles and practices, such as childrearing, status of the elderly, and views of alternative lifestyles
- Workforce issues, including autonomy and acculturation
- Biocultural ecology, such as physical and metabolic characteristics
- High-risk behaviors, such as use of drugs, alcohol, and tobacco; sedentary lifestyle; and safety practices
- Nutrition, including food rituals and taboos
- Pregnancy and childbearing practices, including birth control and perinatal taboos and practices
- Death rituals, including end-of-life care and burial practices
- Spirituality, including religious practices
- Health care practices, such as health beliefs and explanatory models
- Health care practitioners, including status, use, and perceptions of different types of providers

Purnell[6] and Purnell and Paulanka[7] also provided a model of cultural competence that can be used both as a framework to help us with our own self-exploration and as a means to help us learn more about our learners' or patients' cultures and subcultures. In this model, they presented 12 domains to be explored when attempting to better understand different cultures. Some aspects of these domains include the following:

Purnell[6] suggested that the practitioner can use these 12 domains to formulate questions in obtaining a patient's history. This can be a helpful framework for teachers attempting to better understand their learners.

In practice, the first step to becoming comfortable in cross-cultural encounters is to understand what we bring to the interaction. Self-awareness of our cultural values, beliefs, and practices provides the underpinnings of our knowledge about cultures. As you begin to recognize the different aspects of your own culture, you can begin to explore how other cultures differ. In doing so, it is important to recognize the potential impact of unconscious biases. Engaging with others of diverse backgrounds provides us with opportunities to further enhance our knowledge and skills with cross-cultural interactions. It is through this knowledge and these experiences that we can begin to provide culturally congruent interventions, both in teaching and in patient care.

Stop and Reflect

Reflect on the 12 domains in relation to you and your culture:

- What are your beliefs and/or experiences relative to each of these domains?
- How might your beliefs differ from the beliefs of some of your peers?
- How might your beliefs influence your role as a health care provider?
- What types of questions might you pose to learn more about your patients' or students' cultures?

As you move toward becoming culturally competent on an unconscious level, it is critical to maintain a reflective stance, continually checking your assumptions and validating your actions. Even at the stage where you feel comfortable with multiple cross-cultural encounters, reflection will help prevent you from over-generalizing and stereotyping.

Key Points to Remember

- Cultural competence requires culture-specific knowledge as well as developing skills in engaging in cross-cultural encounters.
- Cultural competence begins with developing self-awareness through reflection on your own cultural experiences and practices.
- Because there is as much variability within cultures as there is across cultures, checking your assumptions is critical.
- Purnell's[6] 12 domains of culture provide an entry point for both self-exploration as well as a means to learn more about your patients and learners.

Generational Differences

As noted earlier, our past experiences influence how we view life and interact with others. As health care providers, you will encounter individuals from across the lifespan. These individuals are influenced by their own family and cultural experiences as well as by their social, political, and historical experiences (ie, generational diversity). In the classroom and in the clinic, we encounter individuals from many generations. It has been proposed that individuals from each generation have their own set of values, ideas, and beliefs. Individuals from the same generation share defining moments in history and common music, television shows, heroes, and passions. Generational commonalities often cut across issues of race, ethnicity, and economics and may shape how individuals from a given generation think and how they view the world around them.[20-26]

For the first time in history, you may find individuals from 4 generations working and learning in the clinic and classroom together:

- The Silent Generation (born 1925-1942)
- The Baby Boomer Generation (born 1943-1960)
- Generation X (born 1961-1981)
- The Millennials (born 1982-2002)[24]

Individuals from each of these cohorts may very well share similar world views because of their shared sociopolitical and historic experiences. It is important to remember, though, that just as there may be as much diversity within cultures as there is across cultures, there may be as much difference within generations as there is across generations.

As a health care provider and as an educator, it is important to understand how generational values and beliefs might impact the teaching-learning situation. It is important that we recognize and acknowledge our own biases as well as the biases that may exist between individuals from different generations. Table 1-3 provides some characteristics common to individuals from different generations. There are times when a certain characteristic may be considered both a strength and a challenge, depending on the context. For example, Gen Xers are generally noted for their desire for work-life balance, which can be viewed as a great personal strength. However, this same characteristic may present a challenge at work, particularly if this individual is being supervised by someone from the Baby Boomer generation who places a high priority on work in his or her life.

Table 1-3. Characteristics Common to Individuals From Different Generations

Generation	Major World Events	Influential Factors	Strengths	Challenges	Learning Preferences
Silent Generation, veterans, GIs (born 1925-1942)	The Great Depression, World War II, Korean War, Cold War, The GI Bill	Values: Conformity, hard work, delayed gratification, duty, honor, authority, order, logic, discipline, job security, loyalty, work before pleasure, thriftiness, focus on children and family, and patriotism	Prioritizes their work life, conforms, adapts, loyal, detail-oriented, thorough, self-reliant, disciplined, hardworking, consistent	Prioritizes their work life, seeks to maintain status quo—change is a challenge, cautious, dislikes conflict, is technologically challenged	Detail oriented, formal presentation style, sequential, teacher as an expert, organized, needs expectations/instructions to be written out, first present theory and then practice
Baby boomer Generation (born 1943-1960)	Lunar landing, Civil Rights Movement, Women's Rights, Political assassinations, Vietnam War, economic prosperity	Values: Work, youth, health/wellness, civil rights, fairness, team oriented, optimism, change, diversity, empowerment, the decline of patriotism, needs immediate gratification	Prioritizes their work life, strong work ethic (ie, equate self-worth with work), driven and hardworking, wants to please, dedicated, good at maintaining relationships, values consensus building, idealistic, challenges the status quo, values relationships, enjoys learning, cooperative/team oriented	Prioritizes their work life, needs significant dialogue and rapport building, egocentric, highly competitive, reluctant to disagree, grade conscious, can be overly sensitive to feedback, may be uncomfortable with conflict, judgmental, egocentric	Organized lectures, detailed handouts, team work, likes to share what they know, small group discussions, likes decision-making and consensus-building activities, debates, needs clearly written expectations, teacher-directed methods
Generation X (born 1961-1981)	Watergate; fall of the Berlin Wall; Gulf War; Emergence of AIDS; personal computers, the Web, and Nintendo; corporate layoffs; Chernobyl	Values: Hard work, maintains work-life balance, job security, deferred gratification, pragmatism, change, cynicism, change in traditional family unit, divorce was common, 2 working parents, flexibility, latchkey kids, independence	Seeks work-life balance, prioritizes leisure activities, highly independent, has high expectations, challenges authority, challenges the status quo, resourceful and adaptable, pragmatic, good at multitasking, outcomes oriented not process oriented, values learning and skill building	Seeks work-life balance, prioritizes leisure activities, has limited tolerance for wasting time, prefers to get to the point, limited tolerance for any information that does not appear to be relevant, focused on the outcomes and may skip steps in the process, limited tolerance for group activities/discussions, direct communication style, cynical, expects instantaneous feedback	Independent/self-directed activities, clear expectations with bullet points, a more informal presentation style, games-guided practice which leads to independence, self-directed modules, flexible learning opportunities (eg, self-paced modules or CD-ROMs), practical application, detailed study guides and exam reviews, teacher must demonstrate expertise
Millennials, Gen Y, Echo Boomers, Nexters, or the Net Generation (born 1982-2002)	Oklahoma City bombing, Columbine shootings, genocides, 9/11 attacks, fall of the Iron Curtain	Values: Optimism, family values, group loyalty, morality, choice, confidence, achievement, civic and social action, racially and ethnically diverse, diversity, revival of patriotism and heroism, grew up with structured and busy schedules, globalism, parents very involved and overprotective (ie, "helicopter parents")	Seeks work-life balance, prioritizes leisure activities, strong work ethic, inclusive/team oriented, expects customer service, high expectations, is technologically savvy, compliant, accepts authority, respectful, confident, assertive and self-reliant, optimistic and enthusiastic, goal-oriented, civic minded and altruistic, embraces change, good at multitasking and non-linear thinking, excels at blending information from many sources	Seeks work-life balance, prioritizes leisure activities, may be overconfident, little tolerance for delays; short attention span, respect must be earned, impatient, may not take criticism well, has a lower tolerance for reading, needs supervision and structure, expects 24/7 service	Visual media is expected, electronic communication, trial and error ("Nintendo logic"), group activities, games/simulations with immediate feedback, external structure (clear expectations and standards), teaching others, practice first then theory, active/experiential learning, case studies, assignments with options, problem-solving scenarios, performance contracts (ie, they set their own goals)

Adapted from Mangold K. Educating a new generation teaching baby boomer faculty about millenial students. *Nurs Educ.* 2007;32:21-23; Henry PR. Making groups work in the classroom. *Nurs Educ.* 2006;31:26-30; Johnson SA, Romanello ML. Generational diversity: teaching and learning approaches. *Nurs Educ.* 2005;30:212-216; Billings D, Kowalski K. Teaching learners from varied generations. *J Cont Educ Nurs.* 2004;35:104-105; Zemke R, Raines C, Filipczak B. *Genererations at Work: Managing the Class of Veterans, Boomers, Xers, and Nexters in Your Workplace.* New York, NY: AMACOM American Management Association; 2000; Gleeson PB. Understanding generational competence related to professionalism: misunderstandings that lead to a perception of unprofessional behavior. *J Phys Ther Educ.* 2007;21:21-28.

Stop and Reflect

How might the following events influence the values, attitudes, beliefs, and behaviors of the people experiencing them? How might it influence an individual's learning preferences?

- The Great Depression
- The Women's Movement
- The assassination of Martin Luther King
- The Vietnam War
- The rise in the divorce rate
- The sale of the first personal computer
- The advent of the Internet
- The attacks on 9/11

Can you think of other events that have shaped your environment across your life span? How have these events influenced your perception of yourself and of those around you?

Critical Thinking Clinical Scenario

You work at a pro bono physical therapy clinic and are trying to raise funds to support the efforts of the clinic. A local community group has agreed to give you some time at their next meeting to give a presentation and to provide them with information about physical therapy and about the clinic. The group is an intergenerational group, and you expect representation from all 4 generations in the audience.

Reflective Question

1. What strategies would you use both in the presentation and in providing information to optimize learning for all members of this group?

Given that multiple generations coexist, misperceptions can occur. For example, in the work environment, members of the Silent Generation typically value loyalty; they place work as a high priority in their lives and often work for the same company for many years. Gen Xers and Millennials, on the other hand, value work-life balance and embrace change. These individuals expect to change jobs multiple times in their lives and may not easily change their social schedules to accommodate the needs of the work environment. This could easily be misperceived as a lack of commitment by members of the Silent Generation. Similar misperceptions can occur in the classroom. Millennials may prefer team work and group performance over the highly individualized and competitive nature of the Boomers. Boomers may perceive this as a lack of ambition, whereas Millennials may perceive the competitiveness of the Boomers as a lack of cooperation.

In planning any teaching-learning activity, generational differences should be considered. Incorporating learning preferences based on generational characteristics will optimally engage the learner. In addition, as with learning styles, using techniques that require learners to move out of their comfort zones (eg, requiring Baby Boomers to use new technologies) may enhance learning. Teaching the same material using a variety of strategies may optimize learning for all participants. For example, if you are teaching a multigenerational community group about health and fitness, you might consider the following:

- Incorporate lectures, handouts, and time for discussion and questions to engage members of the Baby Boomer generation
- Provide a bulleted overview of the major concepts with access to videos and self-paced CD-ROMs to engage members of Gen X on their own time
- Use an interactive game with an experiential component that requires the learners to incorporate all of the components of health and wellness in their daily lives to engage members of the Millennial generation

When planning patient education in the clinical setting for an individual learner, caution should be used in incorporating unfamiliar strategies (eg, CD-ROMs for individuals from the Silent Generation). Patients are already challenged by their own medical issues. Requiring your patients to use unfamiliar strategies may at times add to their stress and may result in a less effective teaching-learning situation.

Critical Thinking Clinical Scenario

In reviewing your patient's chart, you note that her birth date is March 9, 1990. She underwent a recent reconstruction of her anterior cruciate ligament, and you will be seeing her for the first time tomorrow.

Reflective Questions

Considering the typical characteristics of her generation:

1. How much information might you expect your patient to have about her injury and course of treatment before she comes for therapy? What is the likely source of that information?
2. How involved will your patient likely want to be in the decision-making process?
3. How involved will her parents likely be in her course of rehabilitation?
4. What mode(s) of instruction will you consider using?
5. How might you consider communicating with your patient between sessions?

Key Points to Remember

In understanding ourselves and others, it is important to:

- Appreciate generational differences in core values, strengths, and challenges
- Develop clear expectations, which include tolerance and respect for generational differences
- Utilize the typical strengths and qualities of each generation to design effective instructional activities
- Recognize that there is likely as much diversity within generational cohorts as there is across generational cohorts

Andragogy and the Characteristics of the Adult Learner

Our first filter had to do with how we view life, how we perceive the world. Our perceptions are in part a result of our cultural experiences as well, which was our second filter. Another filter or lens that must be considered in any teaching-learning situation, particularly in health care, is the influence of the characteristics of the adult learner. As discussed earlier, many, if not most, of our learners are adults—patients, caregivers, students, colleagues, and other professionals. Even pediatric physical therapists must work closely with parents and caregivers in any teaching-learning situation.

Stop and Reflect

What is the difference between how and why children learn versus how and why adults learn? Consider the following list. What is different? What is the same?

- Their motivation to learn
- Their readiness to learn
- What they bring to the learning situation

Adults bring a great deal of background and experience to any learning situation, which must be both considered and respected. In 1973, Malcolm Knowles, often referred to as the "father of adult learning," coauthored a book entitled *The Adult Learner: The Definitive Classic in Adult Education and Human Resource Development.*[27] This work has been published and updated several times and has become the primary source of information for teachers of adult learners. It is the work of Malcolm Knowles et al[27] along with that of Eduard Lindeman[28] that spawned the field of adult education. It was here that the notion that perhaps children and adults learn differently and that the goal of educating adults may differ from that of educating children was born.

The term *pedagogy* generally refers to the study of teaching; however, in educational theory, the term *pedagogy* more specifically refers to the study of how children learn. Pedagogy traditionally had at its core the transmittal of knowledge as the goal of education. Central to this concept is the teacher as expert. The teacher has full responsibility for the learning situation, including making determinations about what is to be learned, how it will be learned, when it will be learned, and even whether it has been learned. The learner in this situation assumes a rather dependent role. The content of the learning is primarily subject directed and determined by external factors (eg, grade-school curriculum). There is generally a standardized curriculum, and students progress as a unit. The goal of learning is often subject mastery for its own sake, and progression is dependent upon success defined by grades on exams. Children bring limited experience to the situation. In transmitting knowledge, instructors, using a pedagogical approach, tend to rely on lectures, drills, readings, quizzes, and rote memorization.

Andragogy, a term coined by Malcolm Knowles, is defined as the "art and science of helping adults learn."[27] In the early part of the 20th century, educators began to recognize that education was more than simply preparing for a life career or profession. Learning does not end when your formal schooling is finished. Rather, the goal of education, particularly for adults, is a lifelong process of learning and problem solving based on life situations, rather than a process driven by the need to learn a particular subject. Educators began experimenting with assumptions about the characteristics of adult learners and how they learn. These assumptions have formed the basis of the andragogical approach to learning.

Stop and Reflect

When are you most motivated to learn? What motivates you?

Assumptions underlying the andragogical approach to learning include the following:

- *Adults bring a need to know to the learning situation*—Adult learners want to know how learning will occur, what learning is expected, why they are learning what they are learning, and who is teaching them (ie, teacher qualifications).
- *Adults bring an independent self-concept to the learning situation*—Adult learners identify themselves as being in charge of their lives. They are self-directed, want to have some ownership over the learning situation, prefer to be more independent and struggle when they need help or feel dependent on the instructor. They also have an internal

locus of control and have a sense of responsibility for their own learning. They want a choice in how and what they learn and want to be engaged in the decision-making process.

- *Adults bring experience to the learning situation*—Adults bring many different backgrounds, needs, interests, goals, and motivations. Adults learn from each other's experiences and also may have habits and biases that can impact the situation either positively or negatively.

- *Adults bring a readiness to learn, that is life centered, to the learning situation*—Adults are most ready to learn when they perceive a need. They are most interested in learning that is relevant to their current life situation and in solving problems, so learning should be problem centered, not subject centered, as well as goal oriented and value oriented.

- *Adults bring a motivation to learn to the learning situation*—Adults are most responsive to internal motivations (eg, self-esteem, quality of life), although external motivation can be a factor as well. Adults want to be successful and are motivated to learn something that they believe will help them better perform tasks or manage current life situations.

Critical Thinking Clinical Scenario

You are a third-year doctor of physical therapy (DPT) student in the clinic, and you are asked to instruct a patient on a home exercise program (HEP). Your patient is a 42-year-old who has returned to therapy for a recurrent shoulder problem. He is anxious to return to playing tennis. He had a previous HEP but, given that it is a recurrent problem, he does not believe it was effective. This is the first time you have ever instructed a patient on an HEP independently. To save time, you decide to develop the HEP before the patient comes in for his session. When your patient arrives, you introduce yourself and immediately begin to tell him what you want him to do. The patient reacts negatively and seems to question everything you are suggesting. For each exercise you give him, he suggests doing something different.

You describe what happened to your clinical instructor. She suggests that you review the principles of adult learning.

Reflective Questions

1. What characteristics of an adult learner does this patient display?

2. Why might the patient be questioning the exercises you are suggesting?

3. Considering the assumptions underlying the andragogical approach to learning, how might this student have approached this teaching-learning situation differently?

Because adults have a need to know, an important starting point in designing effective adult learning activities in the classroom or clinic is to provide the learner with answers to the following questions:

1. What learning is expected?
2. How will the learning occur?
3. Why are they learning what they are learning?
4. Who is teaching (ie, what are the qualifications of the instructor)?

For example, in working with an adult learner in the clinic, it is not sufficient to simply describe an exercise program you want him or her to follow. You want to be sure to make your expectations explicit, describe how you expect the learner to accomplish the task, and provide solid rationale for why you are asking the learner to do certain activities. In doing so, it is also important that the therapist displays both professionalism and confidence and demonstrates expertise not only in the physical therapy interventions but in the process of teaching.

Remember that adults have a certain readiness to learn when they realize they have a problem or need to know something. Adults may not recognize what it is they need to know, however. They may not realize that something is a problem or that something is important. For example, a patient with diabetes may be focusing on following the diet and exercise program but may not recognize the importance of daily skin checks to prevent potential skin breakdown. It is our role as physical therapists to help our adult learners recognize what they need to know—in this case, the potential consequences of not attending to skin care to increase adherence to performing daily skin checks.

Because adults come to the learning situation with a great deal of experience, this experience must be both considered and respected. The more the teacher can link new learning to something with which the learner is familiar, the more likely the learner will both learn and retain that information. In designing an exercise program, you can ask about the types of movement activities a patient has learned previously. You can then draw analogies between what is currently being learned and what was learned before. For example, you may ask the patient to think about what strategies he has used previously in perfecting his golf game and then have him consider using similar strategies in refining his movement patterns after surgery.

In addition, remember that not all past experiences have been positive ones. It is important for you to recognize potential negative past experiences that may be influencing the learning situation. For example, you may have a patient that you are trying to motivate to engage in a more active lifestyle, but he has never participated in sports or exercise because of a negative experience he had in gym class. Similarly, in the classroom, you may have a learner who has been criticized for asking questions in a previous class so he or she never raises his or her hand in your class. Because of the potential influence of negative past experiences, it is critical that you create a safe learning environment. A safe learning environment is one in which learners feel comfortable making mistakes, asking questions, and bringing their own experiences to bear without fear of embarrassment.

Finally, adults come to the learning situation with their own interests, goals, and motivations and are accustomed to being responsible for their own lives. This should be incorporated into the decision-making process in developing educational activities. To enhance their feeling of ownership and control in the situation, it is important to give adult learners choices. Decisions that are made collaboratively are more likely to be followed. For example, in working with a group of patients or even an individual patient, it is helpful to provide options from which they can choose so that each individual can determine a home exercise program that best meets his or her own personal goals and interests. Linking exercises to activities valued by the individual by collaboratively developing goals moves the learner from a passive recipient to an active participant in the rehabilitation process. It also fosters ownership and an internal motivation to achieve. Inherent in working collaboratively in the teaching-learning situation is the development of functional goals that meet the most urgent personal needs of the learner. Meeting these needs makes it immediately relevant and practical to adult learners, which will enhance their likelihood of participation.

Key Points to Remember

In working with the adult learner, consider the following:

- Choice—Be sure to provide options.

- Voice—Be sure to listen to the learners' needs, interests, goals, and respect their past experiences.

- Relevance—Connect the learning activities to the valued activities of your learners.

- Ownership—Work collaboratively to develop goals that meet the most urgent needs of your learners.

Though there are some distinctions between the way adults learn and the way children learn, it is critical to remember that this is a continuum and not a dichotomy. In fact, both children and adults may learn best when their needs, interests, and experiences are taken into consideration. Though adults have a strong desire to be self-directed, they can be quite dependent in a new learning situation. Andragogy and pedagogy are essentially 2 sets of assumptions, and it is the role of the educator to determine whether to use these assumptions, either in whole or in part, based on the characteristics of the learner and the context of the learning situation.

As educators we must make decisions about which teaching strategies to use based on who our learners are, what they need to know, and what past knowledge and experiences they bring to the situation. At times, a pedagogical approach to teaching and learning may be effective with adults. Certainly in working with students who need to acquire certain knowledge (eg, origins and insertions of muscles), a pedagogical approach such as rote memorization with its concomitant use of exams for assessment purposes may be most effective. Regardless, helping your learners see the relevance of this information to their future practice may enhance their readiness to learn. A pedagogical approach may be an effective strategy in working with patients at times as well. For example, if you are working with a patient who recently had a total hip replacement, use of rote memorization and quizzing may be an effective strategy for teaching total hip replacement precautions. Simultaneously engaging your patient in the collaborative process of designing a home exercise program may be an effective strategy to enhance patient adherence. In either case, however, helping your learner understand what is to be learned, why it is important, how it is relevant, and actively engaging your learner in the process will enhance your learner's motivation and potential success.

Similarly, in working with students in the clinical or classroom setting, the concepts of *choice, voice, ownership,* and *relevance* are equally important. Given the demands of professional curricula, you may not be able to give your students a choice about what they will learn; however, giving them choices in assignments or activities, listening to their own personal goals and interests, linking new knowledge to their prior experiences, and collaboratively developing goals may enhance motivation and self-directed learning.

In part, the decision to use one approach over the other depends on the learner's experience and the context of the learning situation. For example, if the teacher is presenting totally new content with which the learner has no prior experience, the teacher should expect the learner to be more dependent in his or her learning, and a pedagogical approach may be warranted (eg, learning to perform special tests in orthopedics). If the learner needs to accumulate a certain amount of baseline knowledge to perform a task, again, a pedagogical approach may be appropriate (eg, teaching a patient partial weight-bearing gait). If the learner has had a fair amount of experience with the content and needs to master it, however, giving the learner increasing amounts of responsibility and control over his or her own learning may be most effective (eg, working collaboratively with a patient to advance a learned exercise program).

A number of distinctions have been made between how children learn versus how adults learn. One aspect of the learning environment that is the same across the continuum is that all learners like to have fun. Children and adults alike want to feel that the learning environment is both enjoyable and safe. They need to feel that they can make errors and ask questions knowing that they will be respected both for what they know and what they do not know.

Key Points to Remember

- Pedagogy and andragogy are not dichotomous; they are a set of assumptions that run along a continuum.
- Assumptions are to be adopted in whole or in part depending on the needs of the learner; flexibility is critical.
- The challenge for any instructor is to recognize where along the continuum your learner is and then plan your teaching strategies accordingly.
- Regardless of the assumptions used or where along the continuum your learners lie, all teaching situations should be learner centered.
- Choice is essential because in any group of learners you will find individuals along the continuum from
  - Dependent to independent
  - Needing a great deal of direction to little direction
  - Needing a great deal of support to little support
  - Having much experience to little or no experience
  - Having much content knowledge to little or no content knowledge
- The concepts of voice and respect must always be maintained to ensure a safe environment that optimizes learning has been established.
- All learners like to have FUN!

Critical Thinking Clinical Scenario

You are a clinician and an instructor in a physical therapy program. Today, you are presenting on the topic of diagnosis and management of stroke in the young female population. Consider 3 different audiences:

1. A class of first-year physical therapy students
2. A novice clinician who was referred an adolescent female patient who recently had a stroke
3. The mother of the adolescent female who recently had a stroke

Reflective Questions

1. Compare and contrast the characteristics of the learners.
2. How will the assumptions underlying both andragogy and pedagogy guide your approach(es) to these teaching-learning situations?
3. How might you incorporate the concepts of choice, voice, relevance, and ownership in designing the learning experiences?
4. Consider the filters discussed previously and how they may influence how and what you teach.

Learning Styles

Stop and Reflect

- What comes to mind when you think about learning styles?
- If you wanted to learn a new skill, how would you start? What resources would you be most likely to use?

Learning styles are another filter or lens that must be considered in any teaching-learning situation. Very often, when we ask a group of individuals what comes to mind when asked about learning styles, we hear, "I am an auditory learner"; "I am a kinesthetic learner"; "I need to see the details to really understand the big picture"; "I have to understand the big picture before the details make sense." People learn differently. Each one of us, teacher and learner, has a preference for how we learn that is based on our own past experiences. As a result of our experiences, we develop a certain preference for how we take in information from the environment and how we process that information to make it meaningful and useful. Although your preference or style may change and may vary from situation to situation, it remains fairly stable over time.[29]

A variety of learning style inventories are available. Each assessing how the learner takes in information and processes it best from different perspectives. Authors have considered cognitive styles,[30] field dependence versus field independence,[31] environmental preferences,[32] personality styles,[33] and multiple intelligences,[34] to name a few. Each of these researchers focuses on different aspects of the learner and the learning environment. Together, they provide additional information about the potential characteristics of our learners. We will briefly highlight each of these styles and then focus on the Kolb[29] learning style because this is commonly seen in the physical therapy and health care literature.

Messick[30] suggested that individuals have a particular cognitive style with preferences for how individuals acquire information and how they process that information.

1. *Information acquisition:* Learners have a preference for acquiring information through their senses, preferring one mode of sensory acquisition over another (ie, visual, aural, haptic, kinesthetic, smell).
2. *Information processing:* Once information is acquired, the learner takes that sensory information and must process it to make sense of it.
3. Messick[30] suggested that the learner approaches information processing in 1 of 2 ways:

a. A *global* or *holistic approach* in which the learner focuses first on the whole picture and then works to make connections and linkages to the details.

b. An *analytical* or *serial approach* in which the learner focuses on the details first and then works to make linkages and to build a larger, more meaningful picture.

Witkin and Goodenough[35] and later Jonassen and Grabowski[31] focused more on how learners are influenced by their surrounding environment. They described learners as having preferences for being either field dependent or field independent.

1. *Field-dependent* learners prefer collaborative learning and external structure, feedback, and guidance and tend to analyze the big picture more than the details.

2. *Field-independent* learners, on the other hand, prefer independent discovery learning and problem solving, applying knowledge to new situations, are more task oriented, and focus on the details of a situation.

Dunn[32] considered the environmental and cognitive factors as critical to the learning situation. The Dunns focused on 4 major categories:

1. *Environmental factors* (ie, sound, light, temperature, and design)

2. *Emotional factors* (ie, intrinsic versus extrinsic motivation, persistence, conformity versus nonconformity, external versus internal structure, and single versus multitasking)

3. *Sociological factors* (ie, independent versus group work, leader versus follower, routine versus diversity)

4. *Physiological factors* (ie, sensory, time of day, activity versus passivity)

A learner's personality also influences the teaching-learning situation. Myers and Myers[33] developed a personality inventory that is designed to assess both personality type and interpersonal functioning. These authors discussed 4 major personality dimensions that result in 16 different personality types. Each of the 16 personality types has a different approach to problem solving, which is why we include it in this section on learning styles. The 4 major dimensions of the Myers-Briggs Inventory[33] are the following:

1. *Introversion versus extroversion* (ie, internal focus versus external focus)

2. *Sensing versus intuition* (ie, focusing on facts versus feeling)

3. *Thinking versus feeling* (ie, logical and objective versus person-centered and subjective)

4. *Judging versus perceiving* (ie, planned and organized versus organic and spontaneous)

Finally, Howard Gardner[34] presented the concept of multiple intelligences. He suggested that individual learners have particular strengths in 1 or more of 7 categories that the teacher can capitalize on to optimize the teaching-learning situation. Howard Gardner's multiple intelligences include the following categories:

1. *Logical-mathematical*

2. *Verbal-linguistic*

3. *Visual-spatial*

4. *Bodily-kinesthetic*

5. *Musical*

6. *Interpersonal*

7. *Intrapersonal*

As evidenced by the sampling of learning style theories just presented, the learner is influenced by a number of factors both internal and external. Each of the theorists presented has a different focus in assessing learner preferences. What is most important is recognition that each learner brings his or her own preferences to the teaching-learning situation. Teachers, too, bring their preferences, which may or may not be in sync with the learner's.

Stop and Reflect

Think back to a time when, as an adult, you had to learn something new that was quite challenging.

- How did you approach your learning?

- Based on the learning styles just presented, how would you characterize your learning preferences?

- Can you think of a time when you were challenged to learn in a manner that you did not prefer? What did you learn from that experience?

Critical Thinking Clinical Scenario

You are working with a new patient, and you want to be sure your patient education is designed in a way that best meets your patient's needs.

Reflective Questions

1. Considering Howard Gardner's[34] multiple intelligences, what questions might you ask to determine your patient's strengths/preferred mode of learning?

2. Select 1 therapeutic exercise and determine what teaching strategies you would use to meet the needs of each of the 7 types of learners presented by Gardner.

Though the literature presents a number of different learning style preferences, as noted earlier, the Kolb[29] Learning Style Inventory is commonly cited in the health care literature. Kolb's inventory is grounded in the work of a number of experiential learning theorists and psychologists including John Dewey, Jean Piaget, and Kurt Lewin.

Critical Thinking Clinical Scenario

You are working with a patient with a right hemiparesis. You have treated many patients with similar impairments in the past, so you rely on what has worked for your patients over time. When you begin to implement your plan of care, however, the interventions you selected do not seem to be as effective with this particular patient as you had expected.

Reflective Question

1. Describe the problem-solving steps you would take in trying to determine why your interventions are not working and how you might change your plan.

David Kolb[29] described learning as an active "cyclic process in which concepts are derived from and continuously modified by experience." As shown in Figure 1-3, this learning cycle is consistent with Dewey's[1,2] concept of experiential learning and problem solving. Dewey believed that all learning begins with experience. Experiences, especially those that do not fit our expectations, often cause us to observe, step back, reflect, and question. As we ponder the questions raised by these experiences, we begin to pose potential hypotheses or solutions based on some theoretical rationale. Once posed, we begin to test our own hypotheses. After much testing, we find a solution that can be applied to solve the current problem and possibly future problems. This describes the cycle of inquiry, the cycle of problem solving, and the cycle of learning proposed by Kolb.[29]

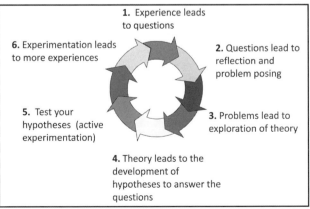

1. Experience leads to questions

2. Questions lead to reflection and problem posing

3. Problems lead to exploration of theory

4. Theory leads to the development of hypotheses to answer the questions

5. Test your hypotheses (active experimentation)

6. Experimentation leads to more experiences

Figure 1-3. The cycle of scientific inquiry.

Stop and Reflect

Consider the steps you identified in resolving the previous clinical scenario. Compare them to the steps described in the cycle of scientific inquiry. How are they similar? How are they different?

Kolb's[29] learning styles grew out of this cyclic process of learning and problem solving. Kolb described learning as having 2 distinct processes:

1. *Prehension* is how we take in or gather information and gain insight from the environment.

2. *Transformation* is what we do with that information to make sense of it and to be able to apply it to solve problems.

Kolb[29] suggested that learners prefer to take in or gather information in 1 of 2 ways. Some learners rely heavily on their senses and experiences and learn best when given concrete examples. Other learners rely more heavily on their powers of thinking and abstraction and learn best when they can link their experiences to theory through analysis and conceptualization. He describes *information gathering* as a continuum, with the 2 ends of the continuum as follows:

- Concrete experience
- Abstract conceptualization

Kolb also suggested that learners generally use 1 of 2 major approaches to making sense of and applying the information they have gathered. Some learners need time to sit back, watch, and reflect upon the information they have gathered, whereas others much prefer to manipulate and experiment with new knowledge. He describes *information processing* as a continuum, with the 2 ends of the continuum as follows:

- Reflective observation
- Abstract experimentation

Stop and Reflect

Are you the type of learner who learns best when you are:

- Given examples?
- Given information that is linked to theory?
- Asked to develop a concept map or drawing to synthesize information?
- Encouraged to use trial and error?
- Given time to practice activities?
- Encouraged to problem solve on your own?
- Encouraged to come up with creative solutions?
- Allowed to take risks and try new things?
- Given time to watch and think before being expected to respond?

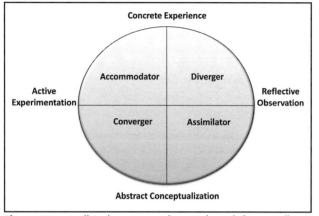

Figure 1-4. Kolb's learning styles. (Adapted from Kolb D. *Experiential Learning: Experience as the Source of Learning and Development.* Englewood Cliffs, NJ: Prentice-Hall; 1984.)

The 2 processes described by Kolb[29] result in the development of 4 major learning styles: diverger, assimilator, converger, and accommodator, which are depicted graphically in Figure 1-4.

- *Divergers* prefer to take in information through their senses, relying on concrete experiences and examples. They make sense of this information through observation and taking time to reflect.
- *Assimilators* tend to take in information by linking their experiences to theory (ie, abstract conceptualization) and similarly make sense of the information through observation and reflection.
- *Convergers*, like assimilators, take information in by linking their experiences to theory but make sense of the information by actively applying the information.
- *Accommodators*, like divergers, prefer to take in information through their senses, relying on concrete experiences and examples, and, like the convergers, need to actively apply the information for it to make sense.

Stop and Reflect

Based on how you think you learn best:
- Identify 2 or 3 characteristics that make you an effective learner. Are they consistent with the characteristics noted in Table 1-4?
- Identify 2 to 3 characteristics that might get in your way or be a barrier to your learning. Are they consistent with the characteristics noted in Table 1-4?

Learners have preferences for how they take in and make sense of information, which leads to their learning styles. Each of the 4 learning styles also has distinct characteristics, unique strengths, and potential challenges to learning. Table 1-4 summarizes key distinctions of each of the 4 learning styles.

Critical Thinking Clinical Scenario

You are a physical therapy student on your second clinical internship. At the midterm evaluation, your clinical instructor noted that you lack initiative and are reluctant to try new approaches. You believe that your clinical instructor moves at a fast pace and expects you to keep up. You explain to her that you prefer to take time to review your texts and make sure that you have solid rationale before trying a different approach with your patients.

Reflective Questions

1. What do you think is influencing this situation?
2. What learning styles are represented in this scenario?
3. What might you suggest to improve the situation?

When individuals with different learning styles, particularly opposing learning styles, are engaged in a teaching-learning situation, conflict may arise. Recognition of the characteristics, strengths, and challenges of each person's learning style may facilitate communication and lead to compromises that can resolve the different perspectives.

Learning styles are a filter that has significant implications for the teaching-learning situation both in the classroom and in the clinical setting. Teacher and learner may have dissimilar styles, which must be recognized and considered in planning any teaching or learning activity, whether one-on-one or in a group.

Though we all have preferred styles, it should be remembered that the most effective learners use all 4 different styles. Therefore, your role as the instructor is to facilitate the use of all 4 styles. Learning styles can be used to either support or challenge your learner. At times, we encourage our learners to use their preferred styles, particularly if the task they are learning is complex. On the other hand, there are times when we challenge our learners by encouraging them to use the opposite learning style. For example, you may be working in the clinic with a student who is an assimilator. Assimilators are typically most comfortable when they have time to organize themselves and think through their session before getting started. When you have a new and complex patient to see, you may want to support the student by giving him or her the time to think and plan before starting. On the other hand, if you have a new patient with a diagnosis that the student has seen several times before, you may want to challenge the student by asking him or her to go in and start the examination without giving him or her time to reflect and plan. By both supporting and challenging your learner appropriately, you will facilitate the development of all 4 learning styles and essentially make your learner a more effective learner.

Table 1-4. Characteristics, Strengths, and Challenges of Kolb's 4 Learning Styles

Learning Style	Personal Goals	Characteristics	Strengths	Challenges	Preferred Learning Strategies
Diverger	Seeks personal relevance Favorite questions: Why? Or why not?	Needs to be personally involved, relationships are important, has an active imagination, sensitive to feelings and can be emotional, learns by listening and sharing ideas, interested in people and culture, believes strongly in his or her own experience, models his- or herself on those he or she respects, excels in viewing situations from many perspectives	Interactive learner, likes to brainstorm, innovative idea people, ambiguity is not a problem, loves to observe and take in a lot of info, sees situations from many perspectives, good listener, conflict negotiators, open minded, are "people people"	Do not ask him or her to act or respond quickly, he or she is too busy chatting and/or brainstorming different ways to approach the problem	Discussions, socratic dialogue, demonstrations, interview activities, storytelling, social networking opportunities, autobiographies, chat rooms, scripted role play, negotiation, consensus development, group activities, brainstorming
Assimilator	Seek facts Favorite question: What?	Needs to know what the experts think and will adapt to what the experts say, learns by thinking through their ideas, collectors of information, less interested in people than ideas and concepts, thorough and industrious, sound theory may be more important than practical use, will continually reexamine facts until it makes sense, schools are designed for these learners!	Analytic learner, theory oriented, looks for how things fit together, adds structure and focus, approaches things in a logical sequence, analyzes, views issues from many perspectives, good organizer, views issues from many perspectives, conceptualizes and creates models	Do not ask him or her to act quickly, he or she needs to gather all the facts, figure out all the angles, analyze and completely think through the situation before acting	Lectures, concept maps, reference guides, theory development, research, creating, decision algorithms, independent work, evidence-based practice, reflection papers, rubrics and checklists, synthesis papers, models, providing structure and sequence creating action plans, visuals, creating drawings
Converger	Seeks usability Favorite question: How does it work?	Learns by testing theories in ways that are practical, uses factual data to build/design concepts, needs hands-on experiences, factual information is more important than interpersonal issues, enjoys problem solving, resents being given answers, restricts judgment to concrete things and has limited tolerance for "fuzzy" ideas, needs to know how it will help in "real life," is a pragmatist	Practical learner, action-oriented, theory-oriented, acts to solve problems once the problem is conceptualized, self-directed, likes practical application and problem solving, experiments, gathers information to solve problems, finds practical use for theoretical ideas	Do not ask him or her to stop and think about all of the angles before diving into the experiment with a solution, unless he or she sees the usability of information he or she may be quick to reject it outright, may be too quick to make some decisions and may spend time solving the wrong problem	Role play, case studies, active learning strategies, games, simulations, fieldwork, applying theory to practice, problem-solving activities, guided practice, logic puzzles/problems, hands-on projects, lab activities, assignments that require the learner to apply theory to practice
Accomodator	Seeks hidden possibilities Favorite question: So what now?	Trusts his or her gut and may reach accurate conclusions even in the absence of any logical justification, adaptable, likes variety, challenges and trial and error, likes to dig in and get things done, risk-takers, most creative, excels in situations that require flexibility, needs to know "what else can we do with this?"	Experimental learner, action oriented and people oriented, likes to test out different approaches, likes challenges and to taking risks, likes to create, set goals, and get the job done	Do not ask him or her to stop and think before acting, these learners like problem solving by trial and error rather than rely on a logical analysis of the situation, these learners like to take risks and prefer to do rather than read	Hands-on activities, films, open-ended activities, practice, creative problem solving, debate, fieldwork, interviews, unscripted role-play, open-ended assignments, innovative, risky activities, creative assignments, storytelling, independent, creative problem solving

Adapted from Kolb D. *Experiential Learning: Experience as the Source of Learning and Development.* Englewood Cliffs, NJ: Prentice-Hall; 1984; McCarthy B. *The 4MAT System: Teaching to Learning Styles With Right/Left Mode Techniques.* Rev. ed. Barrington, IL: Excel; 1987.

Our motto is:

TEACH and LEARN AROUND THE WHEEL

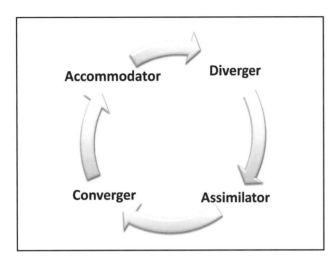

If your learner is a patient in the clinical setting, it is important to remember that your patient may already be challenged by his or her own medical issues and impairments. This may not be a time to challenge your learner/patient further. On the other hand, as he or she nears discharge, you may want your patient/learner to be more proficient at solving problems on-the-spot independently regardless of his or her preferred mode of learning. Clinicians must recognize the preferred style of their patients so they can support them and optimize their learning. On the other hand, clinicians functioning as clinical instructors may choose to incorporate activities that both support and challenge their students to optimize their learning and problem-solving abilities.

Critical Thinking Clinical Scenario

As a new clinical instructor, you are planning learning activities for your student. This is your student's first internship. As part of the welcome packet, you asked her to complete a learning styles inventory so you know that her preference is that of an accommodator. You are an assimilator. You are planning to take your student into the intensive care unit for the first time tomorrow.

Reflective Questions

1. Based on her learning style, what do you see as your student's potential strengths? In what ways might she be challenged?

2. What activities might you plan that would support your student by allowing her to rely on her learning style? How might you challenge her by requiring her to rely on the learning style that is opposite to her own?

3. Given your learning style, where do you see the potential for conflict or misunderstanding?

Key Points to Remember

- To support your learners, select activities that require them to use preferred styles.
- To challenge your learners, select activities that require them to use nonpreferred styles.
- The best learning situations include both challenges and supports.
- Patients are challenged enough by their impairments and functional limitations; use their preferred learning style whenever possible.
- *Teach Around the Wheel!*

If you are teaching a group of individuals, you can assume that you will have learners with all 4 learning styles in the audience; therefore, it is best to incorporate activities that engage all 4 types of learners in the learning process.

Stop and Reflect

Based on how you think you learn best:

- Identify 3 or 4 learning activities/strategies that you find most enjoyable and effective.
- Identify 3 or 4 learning activities/strategies that you dislike or find least effective.

If you take time to speak with your peers about their most and least enjoyable types of learning activities, you may very well find significant differences that may surprise you. Some of your least favorite activities may very well be someone else's favorite learning activities. For example, you may enjoy brainstorming types of activities and dislike too much theory and lecture, whereas your peer may thrive on lectures and note-taking types of activities and dislike small group discussions and brainstorming. When working with others, either in an individual or group teaching-learning situation, it is important to consider a variety of teaching strategies to engage all of your learners. Table 1-4 provides sample activities that build on the strengths of each type of learner.

Key Points to Remember

- Assume all 4 types of learners are in every audience.
- Teach Around the Wheel by including the following:
  - Concrete examples
  - Rationale and theory
  - Time for observation and reflection
  - Time for active experimentation and application

Certainly, the likelihood of administering any one of these inventories to our patients is quite slim. However, Gary Conti and Rita Kolodny[37] developed an easy and nonthreatening instrument called Assessing The Learning Strategies of AdultS, or ATLAS, which can be completed in 1 to 3 minutes depending on your patient's reading level. This valid and reliable instrument enables you to quickly and easily assess your patients' preferred strategies for learning.

The instrument consists of 5 questions organized in a flowchart. Each question has 2 answers from which to select, and, by answering 2 to 3 questions, the learner is identified as belonging to 1 of 3 groups of learners: navigators, problem solvers, or engagers. As with the learning styles inventories, each group of learners has distinct preferences for how they approach learning and problem solving.

•   *Navigators* prefer a structured, organized, logical approach; seek external resources to enhance their learning; tend to be perfectionists; and like clear objectives, deadlines, and feedback.

•   *Problem solvers* prefer a less structured approach with a lot of options; prefer trial-and-error learning, learn best by sharing and hearing stories and concrete examples; and tend to procrastinate and have difficulty starting and stopping when learning a task.

•   *Engagers* prefer to be actively engaged in something they enjoy; learning needs to be fun and meaningful; they enjoy working in groups; and they are emotionally invested in learning and take pride in their accomplishments.

A review of the learning styles, preferences, and strategies presented suggests similarities, differences, overlap, and even some apparent contradictions. As with culture, characteristics of the adult learner, generational differences, and the like, learning styles is simply another filter to be considered in learning more about our learners and about who we are as learners.

Summary

In this chapter, we presented an overview of the individual characteristics that may influence the teaching-learning situation in the classroom or clinic, including perceptual differences, cultural differences, generational differences, differences of the adult learner, and learning style differences. We described these different characteristics as filters or lenses, which must be considered in designing any teaching-learning experience (Figure 1-5).

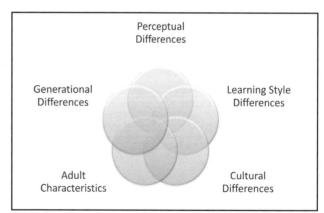

Figure 1-5. Filters that help up to understand our learners and ourselves.

Having examined each of these filters, you can begin to recognize how they can potentially interact to influence our abilities to teach and to learn effectively. However, we cautioned that there is an inherent danger whenever one tries to categorize differences. For example, in considering someone of a different culture or a different generation, it is important to remember that there is as much intracultural and intragenerational diversity as there is intercultural or intergenerational diversity. Singular categories cannot capture the complexity of any individual, which is why we consider each a lens or filter. Each filter or lens adds to the complexity of your learner and your learning situation.

Key Points to Remember

- Clarifying the intent and checking the impact of your communication is essential to developing and maintaining effective teacher-learner relationships.

- To be an effective teacher, it is important to understand how you learn and how that may be similar to, and different from, how your learners learn.

- To be an effective teacher, it is important to provide your learners with the following:
  o Choice
  o Voice
  o Relevance
  o Ownership

- To be an effective teacher, it is important to consider your learner from a number of lenses or filters:
  o Cultural differences
  o Generational differences
  o Characteristics of the adult learner
  o Learning style preferences

- There is as much diversity within cultures and generations as there is across cultures and generations.

- You can use learning style preferences to both support and challenge your learner.

- You can assume that each audience consists of individuals with different learning style preferences; therefore, to be effective, you will want to teach around the wheel.

- To teach and learn around the wheel, you want to incorporate the following:
  o Concrete examples
  o Theory and evidence
  o Time for reflection
  o Time for active experimentation

References

1. Dewey J. *Experience and Education*. New York, NY: Simon & Schuster; 1938.
2. Dewey J. *How We Think*. Amherst, NY: Prometheus Books; 1991.
3. Covey S. *The 7 Habits of Highly Effective People*. New York, NY: Simon and Schuster; 1989.
4. Bennett MJ. Overcoming the golden rule: sympathy and empathy. In: Bennet MJ, ed. *Basic Concepts of Intercultural Communication: Selected Readings*. Yarmouth, MA: Intercultural Press; 1998:191-214.
5. Lattanzi JB, Purnell LD, eds. *Developing Cultural Competence in Physical Therapy Practice*. Philadelphia, PA: F.A. Davis; 2006.
6. Purnell L. The Purnell model for cultural competence. *J Multicult Nurs Health*. 2005;11:7-15.
7. Purnell LD, Paulanka BJ. *Transcultural Health Care: A Culturally Competent Approach*. Philadelphia, PA: F.A. Davis; 2008.
8. Office of Minority Health. What is cultural competency? Available at http://www.omhrc.gov/templates/browse. aspx?lvl=2&lvlID=11. Accessed April 26, 2008.
9. Leavitt RL. Developing cultural competence in a multicultural world—part I. *PT Magazine*. 2002;10:36-48.
10. Leavitt RL. Developing cultural competence in a multicultural world—part II. *PT Magazine*. 2003;11:56-68.
11. Romanello ML. Integration of cultural competence in physical therapist education. *J Phys Ther Educ*. 2007;21:33-39.
12. Campinha-Bacote J, Campinha-Bacote D. A framework for providing culturally competent health care services in managed care organisations. *J Transcult Nurs*. 1999;10:290-291.
13. Campinha-Bacote J. The process of cultural competence in the delivery of healthcare services: a model of care. *J Transcult Nurs*. 2002;13:181-184.
14. American Physical Therapy Organization. Tips to increase cultural competence. Available at http://www.apta.org/AM/Template.cfm?Section=Cultural_Competence1&Template=/TaggedPage/TaggedPageDisplay.cfm&TPLID=48&ContentID=20219. Accessed May 21, 2009.
15. Shore S. A curricular model of cross-cultural sensitivity. *J Phys Ther Educ*. 2007;21:53-59.
16. Hayward L, Canali A, Hill A. Interdisciplinary peer mentoring: a model for developing cultural competent health care professionals. *J Phys Ther Educ*. 2005;19:28-35.
17. Gordon SP. Making meaning of whiteness: a pedagogical approach for multicultural education. *J Phys Ther Educ*. 2005;19:21-27.
18. Campinha-Bacote J. Cultural desire: the key to unlocking cultural competence. *J Nurs Educ*. 2003;42:239-240.
19. Mederos F, Woldeguiorguis I. Beyond cultural competence: what child protection managers need to know and do. *Child Welfare*. 2003;82:125-142.
20. Mangold K. Educating a new generation teaching baby boomer faculty about millenial students. *Nurs Educ*. 2007;32:21-23.
21. Henry PR. Making groups work in the classroom. *Nurs Educ*. 2006;31:26-30.
22. Johnson SA, Romanello ML. Generational diversity: teaching and learning approaches. *Nurs Educ*. 2005;30:212-216.
23. Billings D, Kowalski K. Teaching learners from varied generations. *J Cont Educ Nurs*. 2004;35:104-105.
24. Zemke R, Raines C, Filipczak B. *Genererations at Work: Managing the Class of Veterans, Boomers, Xers, and Nexters in Your Workplace*. New York, NY: AMACOM American Management Association; 2000.

25. Gleeson PB. Understanding generational competence related to professionalism: misunderstandings that lead to a perception of unprofessional behavior. *J Phys Ther Educ.* 2007;21: 21-28.

26. Stumbo T, Thiele A, York AM. Generic abilities as rank ordered by baby boomer and generation X physical therapists. *J Phys Ther Educ.* 2007;21:49-52.

27. Knowles M, Holton E, Swanson R. *The Adult Learner: The Definitive Classic in Adult Education and Human Resource Development.* Woburn, MA: Butterworth-Heinemann; 1998.

28. Lindeman EC. *The Meaning of Adult Education.* 4th ed. Orono, Ontario: Harvest House Ltd; 1989.

29. Kolb D. *Experiential Learning: Experience as the Source of Learning and Development.* Englewood Cliffs, NJ: Prentice-Hall; 1984.

30. Messick S. The matter of style: manifestations of personality in cognition, learning, and teaching. *Educ Psychol.* 1994;29: 121-136.

31. Jonassen DH, Grabowski BL. *Handbook of Individuals Differences, Learning, and Instruction.* Hillsdale, NJ: Lawrence Erlbaum; 1993.

32. Dunn R. Learning style: state of the science. *Theor Pract.* 1984;23:10-19.

33. Myers IB, Myers PB. *Gifts Differing: Understanding Personality Type.* Palo Alto, CA: Davis-Black; 1995.

34. Gardner H. *Frames of Mind: The Theory of Multiple Intelligences.* New York, NY: Basic Books; 1993.

35. Witkin HA, Goodenough DR. Field dependence and interpersonal behavior. *Psychol Bull.* 1977;84:661-689.

36. McCarthy B. *The 4MAT System: Teaching to Learning Styles With Right/Left Mode Techniques.* Rev. ed. Barrington, IL: Excel; 1987.

37. Conti G, Kolodny R. Identifying learning strategy preferences of adults: Assessing The Learning Strategies of AdultS (ATLAS). Available at http://www.conti-creations.com/atlas. htm. Accessed May 4, 2008.

Reflection and Action Learning
Keys to Self-Awareness, Problem Solving, and Continuous Improvement in Practice

Chapter Objectives

After reading this chapter, you will be prepared to:
- Recognize the value of reflection in clinical practice and professional development.
- Describe reflective practice including the elements underlying the reflective process.
- Link reflective practice to critical thinking and clinical decision making.
- Apply the elements of reflection to enhance critical thinking in practice.
- Develop effective questions to facilitate critical thinking and reflective practice.
- Utilize the questioning process as a basis for creative problem solving.

"Having experiences does not necessarily mean that you have learned from them." -Dewey[1]

"Without an ability to reflect ... practitioners are forced into haphazard, reactive patterns of behavior when faced with professional dilemmas." -Brown and Gillis[2]

Stop and Reflect

Have you ever known someone who does not seem to learn from his or her experiences? Someone who seems to make the same mistake over and over again? Why do you think that might be?

As we learned in the previous chapter, John Dewey[3] believed that our experiences are the basis for learning. Dewey believed that experience is not enough, however; it is what we do with our experiences that allows us to learn from them. In this chapter, we explore the concept of reflection as a means of making sense of and learning from our experiences.

The reflective process enables us to search for connections to prior learning and past experiences so that we can make sense of our current experiences in the context of what we do and do not know. The reflective process helps us continually build new neuronal connections by linking new knowledge to prior learning. The more we can link new knowledge or new experiences to what we already know, the more sense it makes and the easier it is to learn.

Conscious reflection also facilitates deeper learning (ie, learning beyond simple rote memorization). Through reflection, we can begin to look at our own situation from multiple perspectives. The reflective process provides us the opportunity to reframe problems, question our own assumptions, and analyze our own experiences.[1,4–10] It is also through this process that we can connect our personal experiences, preferences, and beliefs to the experiences of others, including our patients, in the clinical decision-making process.[11]

Reflection has been widely used in higher education to facilitate deeper learning. Recently, researchers have begun to study the reflective process and its importance in educating physicians, nurses, physical therapists, and other health care providers.[12–22] In physical therapy specifically, it has been considered the hallmark of professional practice.[23] It is considered the key to critical thinking[9,24,25] as well as the link to the development of clinical expertise.[26,27] Reflection provides an

Plack M, Driscoll M. *Teaching and Learning in Physical Therapy: From Classroom to Clinic* (pp 25-42).

Table 2-1. Abstract Concepts Essential to Professional Development in Physical Therapy

Core Values	Essential Affective Behaviors of Physical Therapist
• Accountability • Altruism • Care and compassion • Excellence • Integrity • Professional duty • Social responsibility	• Cultural competence • Professional ethics • Communication • Interpersonal skills • Leadership • Self-assessment • Clinical judgment • Lifelong learning

opportunity to actively manipulate information, encode it further, and transform it into learning that lasts (ie, enhances memory pathways).[9,11,24,25]

Reflection is particularly important in physical therapy, where becoming a professional requires much more than simply gaining knowledge and skills. Reflection helps us make sense of what it means to be a professional and enables us to recognize and assimilate the attitudes and behaviors essential to quality care.[28,29] In physical therapy, for example, it enables us to make sense of abstract concepts such as the Core Values of Professionalism from the American Physical Therapy Association (Table 2-1).[30,31]

In this chapter, we explore the reflective process, what it is, why it is important, and how to facilitate it. We describe how reflection is the basis for critical thinking, self-assessment, and lifelong learning, which are all critical to the development of expertise in practice. Finally, we provide you with some strategies to facilitate the process in yourself, in your learners, and in others.

Stop, Do, and Reflect

In Table 2-1, select 2 of the core values on the left-hand side of the table, and think about how they might link to some of the essential affective behaviors noted on the right-hand side of the table. For example:
- In what ways do the core values of care and compassion influence how you interact on an interpersonal level with your patients?
- In what ways might the core values of excellence and integrity influence how you self-assess?

Compare and Contrast
- How does your response to the questions above differ from the responses you provide to basic factual questions?
- How was your approach to answering the questions above different from your approach to completing multiple-choice exam questions?

Reflection is critical in physical therapy because evidence-based practice and client-centered care require us to analyze best evidence while considering our own values and assumptions as well as the values, beliefs, and goals of each patient. The reflective process requires us to take time to consider the situation from the view of our patient and his or her family as well as from the view of other stakeholders such as the doctor or insurance provider. It facilitates critical thinking by engaging each of us in recognizing our own assumptions and how those assumptions might impact our therapeutic relationships and the clinical decisions we make. As learners and clinicians, reflection also helps us develop a questioning attitude and the skills needed to continually assess our own knowledge and recognize the gaps in our own knowledge and understanding, which is essential to quality care—particularly given our rapidly changing global health care environment.[20]

Key Points to Remember
- Reflection:
  - Facilitates deeper learning
  - Provides us the opportunity to view our own experiences from multiple perspectives
  - Enables us to reframe problems, question our own assumptions, and analyze our own experiences
- Reflection is the hallmark of expert practice.

Reflection: Defined

So what is *reflection*? Reflection is a generic term with many definitions. Boyd and Fales[32] defined it as the process of examining an experience that raises an issue of concern. They described it as an internal process we use to help refine our understanding of an experience, which may lead to changes in our perspectives. It is both the cognitive and affective behaviors we engage in to gain new insights into, and a deeper understanding of, our own experiences.[5]

Donald Schön's[7] work is often cited in the reflective practice literature. He describes 2 types of reflection: *reflection-in-action* and *reflection-on-action*. We, as learners, teachers, and therapists, are often faced with unique and ambiguous problems in the clinical setting during which we are forced to stop, think, and problem solve in the midst of what we are doing. For example, you may walk into a patient's room in an acute-care setting with a plan to work on ambulation. As you begin to transfer the patient from sit to stand, he complains that he is faint. Immediately, you change your plan to accommodate a very different situation than you had anticipated. At the very moment when you recognized that something was not right, you began to reflect and question what was going on in that situation and how you would need to quickly adapt. Schön[7] calls this reflection-in-action.

In clinical practice, reflection-in-action requires us to function on 2 levels simultaneously:

1. Attending to the task of interacting with the patient
2. Continually questioning, observing, assessing, and adjusting our thoughts and actions throughout the session[20]

Based on the previous example, throughout the session, you want to be sure that you are continually interacting with your patient and want to ensure that trust, confidence, care, and compassion are maintained. Simultaneously, you are continually assessing outcomes and making decisions about any changes you might need to make given the dynamic situation in play. Though some of this is done on a relatively unconscious level, the more we can focus on the decisions we make and how we make them, the more we can learn from our everyday experiences.

Literature suggests that expert clinicians routinely use the reflective process.[27] In addition to reflecting in the moment, after each patient interaction, expert clinicians stop to reflect on what they did and ask themselves what worked, what did not work, and why? Again, in the example above, once you have quickly adapted, modified, and completed your session, as a reflective practitioner, you would take a moment to think about what happened and what signs you may have missed in bringing the patient to standing too quickly. Schön[7] refers to this as reflection-on-action. Conscious use of the reflective process is essential to developing expertise.[27]

There is 1 more component of this reflective process that is very important and often missed. Once you have taken the time to think about what happened, the logical next step would be to think about how you might do things differently next time and perhaps anticipate potential problems before they even arise. Building on the work of Schön,[9] Killion and Todnem[6] described this process as *reflection-for-action*. It is by consciously

taking this next step that we enhance our future practice and patient care.

In a study of expert clinicians, Jensen et al[27] noted that the use of the reflective process was a key factor that set expert clinicians apart from their peers. Expert clinicians routinely engage in reflection and continually search for new strategies to improve their approaches to patient care. Reflection is integral to competent practice, and it is a skill that can and must be learned and practiced by novice clinicians in both the academic and clinical settings.[10,20,33-37] Though we may frequently stop to think about how a particular session has gone, we do not always consciously analyze the situation sufficiently to enhance our own practice, nor do we routinely take it to the next step to determine how what we learned from the experience might improve how we practice next time. Understanding the complexity of the process and practicing the components and elements of reflective thinking will increase the likelihood that you will become a reflective practitioner and skillful clinician.

Key Points to Remember

- There are 3 types of reflection:
  - Reflection-in-action
  - Reflection-on-action
  - Reflection-for-action
- All 3 types of reflection are essential to quality clinical practice.

We have completed a number of research studies, written a number of articles, and conducted numerous workshops on reflection with physical therapy students and clinicians as well as educators, medical students, residents, physicians, and other health care providers.[12,13,22,38-40] Through this process, we have developed a number of frameworks to help new learners begin to recognize and apply the different elements of the reflective process. Recognizing each of the elements of reflection can prompt us to more fully analyze our experiences and become more conscious of the decisions we make and the factors that have influenced those decisions. By engaging in this process, we can begin to move toward more expert practice.

The frameworks we have developed are based on the works of numerous reflective theorists, the most commonly cited of which are Donald Schön[7] and Jack Mezirow.[25] Table 2-2 provides a definition of the reflective elements described by Schön[7] as well as Killion and Todnem.[6] To help you put these elements into context, we have provided some quotes from student reflections that illustrate each of these elements in Table 2-2.[6,7,9,22,38]

Table 2-2. Schön's Reflective Elements

Reflective Element	Sample Quotes
Reflection-in-action Occurs while the novice is in the midst of an activity	"These unexpected conditions made me start to think about our initial plan for G… Time constraints and his delayed responses forced the group to eliminate some of the tests we wished to perform… I felt rushed to think of which tests… were the most important …Interventions that we planned for G. The day before had to be modified on the spot."
Reflection-on-action Occurs after the novice has completed the action/encounter	"This week helped me to get over the difficulty… when someone challenged an idea I had I'd back down and lose confidence. I['d] feel angry… that they are trying to get me. But this week I realized that… people challenging my thoughts allowed me to look at things from all angles. I learned so much by standing my ground and pursuing a difference in opinion. The challenge… helped me… see things from different perspectives… [I] realized that I can be misunderstood at times. … I want to improve this because… I must be able to communicate properly. It is vital to the patients' safety."
Reflection-for-action The novice begins to anticipate situations before being faced with them and/or begins to plan for the future to improve the present situation/outcome	"I realize now that my frustration made me raise my voice and made other people feel something against me… I don't think I acted like a professional. Next time, I would talk to my professors about how I felt… and how I thought… we needed more time to reflect on our own… [I learned that] taking things to a professional level with my teachers at this point and asking my classmates instead of interrupting them could have helped me to overcome this challenge."

Critical Thinking Clinical Scenario

The following is a quote from a reflective essay written by a student after having worked with his first patients as a student physical therapist. He was initially uncomfortable with the emotions that his patient displayed:

"When he [our patient] remembered his friends in the war and he became teary-eyed, my first reaction was, "Oh my gosh what do we do now?" in my head but at the same time I put my hand on his shoulder to let him know it was ok. He had his arms in the air, and when I put my hand on his shoulder, they dropped to the side and he sighed a deep breath out. It was like a double nonverbal communication. It was beautiful."

The following is a quote from a reflective essay written by a student after working on a project with a group of students from his class:

"From this challenge, I learned that I am not always going to have everything my way and … maybe if I listened closer and asked questions [of] my classmates … [perhaps] I will get that interest in them and that enthusiasm that I need. I think the only way that we all can grow is if we work together. I know now that if I listen, I will learn from my classmates, as well as my teachers, and be more challenged than I am now."

Reflective Questions

1. Which of Schön's reflective elements do you recognize in each of the quotes?

2. What do you think each of the students learned from this experience?

3. What do you think each student will do differently next time he or she is faced with a similar situation?

People often suggest that reflection is just something that we do naturally. We have started a number of workshops by asking people if they believe that they reflect. Most people say, "Of course I do, I think all the time, doesn't everyone?" Sure, people stop to think about what they are doing and to solve whatever problems they face. However, Mezirow[25] believes that being a reflective practitioner requires much more than just stopping to think, solving problems based on what we already know, or daydreaming about the future. Reflection is much more than just exploring our thoughts or feelings. According to Mezirow,[25] to be a reflective practitioner, it is important that we continually question our experiences, what we know, and how we know it. Stopping to question what just happened can help us further analyze and make sense of our experiences and learn from them.

Key Points to Remember

Reflection:

- Is much more than just stopping to think and solving problems based on what we already know

- Is much more than just exploring our thoughts or feelings

- Requires us to continually question our experiences, what we know, and how we know it

Mezirow's[25] work provides a different perspective, adds another dimension to the reflective process, and offers us another framework from which to explore the reflective process.

Critical Thinking Clinical Scenario

Students were working together in groups on a particular case study. At the end of the day, 1 student went home and reflected. She wrote in her journal: "There was an instance when a group member's frustration was hindering the progress of the entire group. Some people felt hurt or left out, even though they did not verbalize it. After going home, I was disappointed that I did not even attempt to offer a solution or acknowledge the problem. I did not stand up for what I thought was right. In the end, I realized it's much easier to believe in an idea than to do something about that idea."

Reflective Questions

1. What do you think was going on in this scenario?
2. Whose perspectives did the student take into consideration?
3. How might you have approached this situation differently?
4. What assumptions did this student make regarding the situation?
5. Why do you think she did not say anything at the time?

The questions raised in the Critical Thinking Clinical Scenario are reflective questions, yet they go beyond the concepts of reflection-in-action, on-action, and for-action. They require us to analyze the situation from different perspectives. Mezirow[25] contends that reflection is a higher-order, conscious-thought process. He offered 3 additional elements to the reflective process: content reflection, process reflection, and premise reflection. He suggested that taking time to analyze a situation using these 3 elements of reflection may help clarify our understanding of, and assumptions about, our current situation. Behaviors may result that reflect changes in underlying values, attitudes, and beliefs, which is critical to becoming professionals. The questions posed in the scenario above are based on Mezirow's reflective framework.

Content reflection involves the analysis of the problem or situation from the perspectives of all those involved.[25] This is common in quality patient-centered practice where we are required to routinely consider the perspectives of the patients, the caregivers, the families, the nurses, third-party payers, and all those involved in patient care. By exploring the perspectives of all of the individuals involved in the patient's care, we can begin to determine what factors may be influencing the situation and from there be better prepared to develop the most appropriate and effective plan of care for that patient. Content reflection can help us better understand the personal, environmental, social, and contextual factors that might influence a patient's beliefs and abilities to engage in therapy and in following through on an established home program.

Only after we have analyzed the situation from all of these perspectives can we effectively begin to determine how we might approach the situation or what strategies we might choose in addressing the problem. The more we know about our patient situation, the more equipped we are to help our patients develop effective strategies. Mezirow[25] termed this *process reflection*. As practitioners, we use process reflection when analyzing a situation to determine the problem-solving strategies we will choose, determine the efficacy of the strategies chosen, and perhaps explore what other strategies might be available.

Finally, *premise reflection* is the most difficult of Mezirow's[25] reflective constructs because it requires us to question and analyze our own assumptions or the assumptions underlying the problems with which we are faced. Assumptions are taken-for-granted beliefs—often accepted without thinking—and as a result they are difficult to recognize, especially personal assumptions. How often have you made assumptions about individuals based on their disability, their culture, their race, their size, or their socioeconomic status? We all make assumptions; premise reflection enables us to recognize those assumptions and to question them before we make judgments or decisions based on our own engrained, taken-for-granted, unconscious, and unquestioned notions.

Premise reflection also occurs when we question why a particular problem exists. For example, when we stop to question why a particular patient is not entitled to certain medical treatment, why certain disparities exist in health care, or why we are required to treat 4 to 6 patients in 1 hour, we are using premise reflection. To recognize our own assumptions and biases and how they might impact our clinical decision-making process, as well as our role as patient advocate, requires significant skill in premise reflection. Descriptions of Mezirow's reflective elements and illustrative quotes from student reflections are presented in Table 2-3.[22,25,38,41,42]

Table 2-3. Mezirow's Reflective Elements

Reflective Elements	Sample Quotes
Content reflection The novice attempts to explore the problem to better understand it	"I learned that … the sit to stand transfer has many domains. We discussed … strength, biomechanics, flexibility, endurance, and the affective domain. … Initially, I viewed Mrs. E's sit to stand transfer basically as a strength issue. As my group analyzed Mrs. E's sit to stand technique, I revised my opinion of Mrs. E's problem and realized that her problem may lie in all of the domains."
Process reflection The novice begins to explore the strategies and/or processes involved in an experience or problem-solving situation. The novice might begin to explore other possible strategies.	"I spent time meeting [with] my group prior to meeting the [patient], and there we shared our ideas. … I had a flow chart that I wrote out the night before, which we could have followed. When it was time to meet … the [patient], none of us used the flow chart … we adapted to diff[erent] situations."
Premise reflection The novice recognizes and begins to explore or critique his or her own assumptions, values, beliefs, and biases. The novice may begin to seek multiple perspectives and/or alternative explanations.	"In the beginning, I felt like I was getting the easier patient. What a silly assumption! … The lesson gained was far more valuable. I realized that the reason I felt this … was because I don't feel confident in my skills. … I realize … patients can be equally challenging and yet equally rewarding. There is no such thing as an easy or difficult patient. … How I choose to perceive [sic] the situation is what ultimately counts."

Critical Thinking Clinical Scenario

The following are quotes from reflective essays written by students after having worked with their first patients as student physical therapists:

"Working with a real patient is very different from working and practicing on my fellow classmates. … Many times in class we were not only given a problem … but a solution to go with it. It prevented me from going through the valuable thought process of "What intervention should I choose?" "Why am I choosing this intervention?" etc. Instead, I allowed the thinking to be done for me and then understand, afterwards, why, what, etc?"

"What I found most helpful in this course is that you should never judge a book by its cover. You should approach each patient with an open mind. Before I met Mr. B, my judgment [was] that he was going to be a difficult [patient] because of what I read in his past medical history (PMH). After a few moments, I realized there was a great deal of life, history, and joy in him. I saw that personality and thought how could I have missed that. I feel it was from reading his PMH and judging him by it without ever meeting him, I was close minded."

Reflective Questions

1. Which of Mezirow's reflective elements do you recognize in each of the quotes?
2. What assumptions might each of these students have held before working with these patients?
3. What do you think each of the students learned from this experience?
4. What do you think the instructor reading these quotes might have learned?
5. What do you think each of the students will do differently next time they are faced with a similar situation?

Atkins and Murphy[43] did a meta-analysis of the many definitions of reflection present in the literature, and, as a result, they described 3 elements essential to the reflective process (Figure 2-1). First is a trigger event. A *trigger event* is typically a personal awareness of an uncomfortable feeling and/or thought (ie, positive or negative). As a result of this trigger event, we pause and begin to critically analyze our own feelings and thoughts, why they exist, and how they relate to the experience itself or to some prior learning. This analytic process (ie, the reflective process) generally results either in the development of a new perspective or confirmation of the practitioner's original perspective.

For example, a therapist is working with a young child and has provided the caregiver with a list of activities that she should be doing with the child throughout the day to improve the child's motor abilities. When the caregiver and child return for a follow-up session, the therapist inquires about the home activities she suggested. The caregiver tells the therapist that she has not had time to work with the young child. The therapist's initial reaction may be one of annoyance and frustration with the caregiver because she knows how important the activities are for this child. However, if she takes the time to step back, ask questions, and analyze the situation, she might find that the caregiver is responsible for several other young children (content). Although the caregiver is anxious to work with the child, she has no additional support at home (process). The therapist might also realize that she assumed that the caregiver did not value the therapeutic activities she had developed (premise). Taking time to analyze the situation from multiple perspectives may help the therapist reframe her approach, enabling her to work with the caregiver to problem solve different strategies to meet the needs of the child

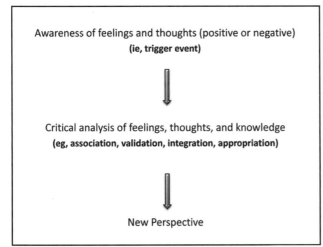

Awareness of feelings and thoughts (positive or negative)
(ie, trigger event)

Critical analysis of feelings, thoughts, and knowledge
(eg, association, validation, integration, appropriation)

New Perspective

Figure 2-1. Reflective process. (Adapted from Atkins S, Murphy K. Reflection: a review of the literature. *J Adv Nurs.* 1993;18:1188–1192.)

within the constraints of her current situation. Rather than annoyance and frustration, reflection may have resulted in a shift in perspective for the therapist, which may make her interactions much more productive. This analytic process will enable you to make more informed clinical decisions.

Reflection as the Basis for Critical Thinking

We noted in Chapter 1 that Kolb[4] described reflection as 1 element of the learning cycle; he viewed it as the link between our concrete experiences and what sense we make of them. Brookfield[24] viewed reflection as a link to critical thinking and defined critical thinking as a direct outcome of the reflective elements of both Mezirow[25,41] and Schön.[7,9] He believed that we become critical thinkers by taking time to revisit our experiences and process them from a number of different perspectives before drawing conclusions.

Critical thinking is what allows us to recognize the assumptions, beliefs, and values that underlie our decision-making processes. Critical thinking enables us, as clinicians, to solve problems, justify our own actions, and even anticipate potential outcomes. As critical thinkers, we use the analytical process of reflection to extract deeper meaning from our experiences, apply it to new situations, and ultimately enhance our abilities as expert clinicians.

Critical Thinking Clinical Scenario

A student returns from clinic and is debriefing with her director of clinical education (DCE). The student shares her frustration by saying that she had a terrible clinical instructor (CI). When the DCE asked her to elaborate, the student said that her CI's exams were always very fast and she neglected to perform a number of special tests. When probed, the student indicated that the treatment sessions seemed to go okay and that the patients were generally satisfied.

Reflective Questions

1. In describing this scenario, what type of reflection was the DCE facilitating in the student?
2. What other factors might the student consider in judging the performance of her CI? (content reflection)
3. What assumptions might the student have made about her CI? (premise reflection)
4. What strategies might the student consider in checking her assumptions about the CI? (process reflection)
5. How might the student approach this situation differently in the future? (reflection-for-action)
6. We know that expert therapists make many rapid unspoken decisions when working with patients. How might the student better understand the decisions made? (process reflection) What might the CI do to make her thinking process more transparent for the student?

Key Points to Remember

According to Brookfield,[24] being a critical thinker requires us to:
- Use the reflective elements described by Schön[7,9], Killion and Todnem[6], and Mezirow[25] as we process and make sense of what we do and do not know:
  - Reflection-in-action
  - Reflection-on-action
  - Reflection-for-action
  - Content reflection
  - Process reflection
  - Premise reflection
- Identify and challenge the assumptions underlying ideas, values, beliefs, and actions.
- Recognize and challenge the context within which a problem exists that can influence how we think and act.
- Explore alternative explanations and solutions.
- Become a reflective skeptic (ie, question everything; do not accept theory or evidence for fact but rather challenge everything in context).

Reflection: Why Is It Important in Clinical Practice?

Initially, Schön[9] analyzed the curricula in a number of professional programs and stated that many programs favored what he called *technical rationalism* over problem solving and professional development. That is, the focus was on attainment of knowledge and skills, almost to the exclusion of the development of professionalism and critical thinking. This has significant implications for physical therapists. In physical therapy, expert practitioners use their own intuition and personal thoughts and feelings to inform the gathering, analysis, and interpretation of clinical data. Through the reflective process, they continually elicit multiple perspectives and seek alternative solutions as they question their own personal assumptions, which ultimately better informs their clinical decision-making efforts.[27,41,44] Reflection is integral to the development of expertise, and, as such, it is important that students and novice clinicians be given opportunities to both develop and practice the skills of reflective practice, along with the technical knowledge and skills needed to develop clinical expertise.

In addition to enhancing our clinical decision-making skills, reflection is key to self-assessment, which is critical to professional development and lifelong learning. It is through the reflective process that we begin to hone our self-assessment skills.[20,31] Self-critique is what allows us to recognize the limits of our own knowledge, and it is only once we recognize our own limitations that we begin to seek new knowledge and skills. It is this ongoing critique that leads to continuous improvement in practice and encourages lifelong learning.

Finally, through the reflective and critical thinking processes described by Schön,[7,9] Mezirow,[25] and Brookfield,[24] we can begin to recognize our own values, beliefs, attitudes, and assumptions and how they might differ from those of our colleagues, patients, and families. Integrating both the perspective of the practitioner and the patient in the clinical decision-making process ultimately enhances patient adherence and outcomes.

Key Points to Remember

Reflection:

- Facilitates self-assessment, which facilitates lifelong learning
- Facilitates critical thinking
- Informs the clinical decision-making process
- Is integral to the development of expertise

Facilitating Reflection Through the Use of Questions

We have explored the definitions and elements of reflection, but why is it so important to know the elements of reflection? Reflection, like any other skill, needs to be practiced and perfected. Unless we develop skill in all aspects of the reflective process, we cannot truly become critical thinkers. By taking time to think about how you analyze your experiences, you will know what elements of reflection you typically use and which ones you do not.

Often, new learners and new clinicians find it relatively easy to reflect back on their experiences and analyze them from many perspectives (ie, reflection-on-action, content reflection); they are able to figure out what strategies to use and even what they might do differently next time (ie, process reflection and reflection-for-action). What is most difficult for new learners and new clinicians is being able to think on their feet and to recognize the assumptions they bring to different situations (ie, reflection-in-action and premise reflection). Reflection, particularly reflection-for-action and premise reflection, are critical to the development of expert clinicians.

What can you do if you find that you consistently use some elements of reflection but not others? Questions are at the heart of the reflective process. We can use questions to begin to elicit different types of reflection and facilitate deeper learning. Continually stopping to question what we know, how we know it, and why we know it can help us develop higher-order critical thinking skills. Questions help us facilitate the reflective process in ourselves and in others, both in the classroom and in the clinic. Developing the skill of asking good questions is critical not only to your own professional development but to providing quality care. Asking your patients probing and reflective questions will provide you not only with a rich, detailed history but a better understanding of your patients' health beliefs, as well as the personal, social, environmental, and contextual factors that may influence their participation.

Questions encourage self-assessment and critical thinking. They help you recognize and consider different perspectives and different solutions and uncover your own ingrained, taken-for-granted assumptions. Good questions not only facilitate a more in-depth analysis of the situation from multiple perspectives but they encourage synthesis of these different viewpoints. Questions enable you not only to evaluate what is really happening in a given situation, but also your role in that situation.

Being able to ask yourself and others good reflective questions is an art and needs to be practiced. When asked to reflect, either verbally or in writing, very often, new learners simply revert to telling a story.[45-47] They simply describe their experiences and do not take the critical step toward analysis proposed by Atkins and Murphy.[43]

By pausing to question and think about the elements of reflection, either personally or with others, you can begin to move beyond recall and storytelling to higher cognitive thinking (ie, analysis, synthesis, evaluation). Good questions encourage you to use the breadth of reflective elements and fully explore the situation. It is through this higher-order reflective process that critical thinking skills are developed.

Key Points to Remember

Questions:

- Help you recognize and consider different perspectives and different solutions
- Encourage you to use the breadth of reflective elements and fully explore the situation
- Help you uncover your own ingrained and taken-for-granted assumptions
- Facilitate a more in-depth analysis of the situation from multiple perspectives
- Encourage the synthesis of these different viewpoints

The keys to good questioning are:

1. Establish a comfortable, nonthreatening learning climate
2. Recognize that questioning is an art and needs to be practiced
3. Stimulate higher cognitive thinking (ie, synthesis and evaluation) rather than just recall

Using questions to facilitate the different elements of Schön's[7,9] work enables us to think on our feet (eg, reflection-in-action), review our performance (eg, reflection-on-action), and develop plans for improving our performance in the future (eg, reflection-for-action). This will result in a more comprehensive analysis of any given situation and in more fully informed clinical decisions. Table 2-4 provides examples of questions that can be used to prompt the reflective process.[9,22,38,40] These types of questions can be used to facilitate personal reflection as well as to elicit reflection on the part of learners, peers, and even patients.

Using questions to facilitate the different elements of reflection described by Mezirow[25] can help us explore situations from multiple perspectives (eg, content reflection), develop strategies to manage different situations (eg, process reflection), and begin to recognize the assumptions we hold in a given situation (eg, premise reflection). Table 2-5 provides examples of questions we can use to facilitate the process.[22,25,38,40,41] As above, these questions can be used to facilitate personal reflection as well as to elicit reflection on the part of learners, peers, and even patients.

The questions provided are simply exemplars that you can use for entry into the reflective process. The purpose of considering a variety of questions that elicit each of the different reflective elements is to give you multiple opportunities to broaden your view and sharpen your thinking on any situation. Reflective thinking is not a linear process; rather, questions lead to new understandings, and new understandings often trigger more questions. Just as Kolb[4] described learning as a cyclic process, so, too, is the reflective process that leads to deeper learning.

Table 2-4. Sample Reflective Questions That Facilitate Schön's Elements of Reflection

Schön's Elements	Sample Questions
Reflection-in-action	- Am I getting the results I want? - What could I change right now to improve my results? - What am I missing? - That didn't work. Now what?
Reflection-on-action	- What happened? - Why did it happen? - Could it have been different? - What else might be playing into the situation? - What might the other person have been thinking? - How did my actions impact the outcome? - What was I feeling at the time?
Reflection-for-action	- What might I do differently next time? - What would I do if...? - What plan can I put in place so that it does not happen again? - How could I do it even better next time? - What would happen if...? - What will I do next time I see a patient like this?

Table 2-5. Sample Reflective Questions That Facilitate Mezirow's Elements of Reflection

Mezirow's Elements	Sample Questions
Content reflection	Content reflection typically answers *what* questions: • What else might be going on? • What is causing this problem? • What else do I need to know? • What might the patient be thinking/feeling? • What am I missing? • What else do I need to ask the patient about her history?
Process reflection	Process reflection typically answers the spirit of the *how* questions: • How else could I approach this problem? • How else can I get the information I need? • How did I come to this conclusion? • What strategies might you use to improve your teaching?
Premise reflection	Premise reflection typically answers the spirit of the *why* questions: • Why do you think you need to know this? • Why did you make that decision? • Why should I question a doctor's orders? • How did you expect the patient to react? • What assumptions do you hold in this situation?

Critical Thinking Clinical Scenario

You are a clinical instructor, and your student shares the following experience with you. "This happened in a physical therapy clinic where I was volunteering. It was the first time I ever observed physical therapy. There were 2 physical therapists. One therapist was cheerful, always listened to her patients' problems, chatted with them a great deal, and spent a lot of time with each patient. The other would see his patients as quickly as possible, he never seemed to smile and really did not chat much with his patients. Some of his patients would come to me and tell me that they did not think therapy was very helpful. Even though I knew that was not true, I usually just listened. I did not know what to do. I just knew in the future I wanted to be like the first therapist—taking as much time as possible with each patient and making sure that I am always pleasant and smiling."

Reflective Question

1. You realize that the intern may be making some assumptions in this scenario, and you want the intern to more fully analyze what was happening before just drawing her conclusions. What questions would you pose to elicit each of the following reflective elements?

    o Reflection-in-action?
    o Reflection-on-action?
    o Reflection-for-action?
    o Content reflection?
    o Process reflection?
    o Premise reflection?

Critical Thinking Clinical Scenario

You are working with a patient who recently had a right total knee replacement (TKR). She had a TKR on her left knee 5 years ago. You do your evaluation, develop a plan of care, provide a brief treatment, and send her home with a home exercise program. She returns the next visit frustrated stating, "This is a waste of time; I know I'll never be able to walk without a cane so I'm not coming back."

Reflective Questions

1. What does this have to do with the reflective process?
2. Considering the different reflective elements we have discussed, what questions might you ask your patient to better understand her thinking?
3. Considering the different reflective elements discussed, what questions might you ask yourself to determine what happened and what you should do next?

Reflection as the Basis for Higher-Order Processing

Another framework we have used in facilitating the reflective process is Bloom's taxonomy. More than 50 years ago, Benjamin Bloom[48] designed a method of classifying learning objectives along a hierarchy from simple to complex. To this day, Bloom's taxonomy is taught in almost any course related to teaching and learning, and it will be discussed in detail later in this text. This hierarchy can be used as a framework to facilitate higher-order thinking through the reflective process. This hierarchy in the cognitive domain moves from the most basic knowledge and comprehension, through application and analysis, to the highest levels of synthesis and evaluation.

The process of facilitation can start at any point along the hierarchy. For example, you may be working with a student who is evaluating a patient with a frozen shoulder and things do not go well. As a clinical instructor, you will need to determine where along the taxonomy your student's skills are lacking: Is it that he or she does not have sufficient knowledge of the shoulder anatomy? Is he or she having difficulty analyzing the movement dysfunction? Is he or she having difficulty synthesizing all of the information he or she gathered from the tests and measures that were used? Using the questioning process will help you and your learners more clearly delineate problems and develop the best strategies to help you perform better next time.

For ease of application in the reflective process, the 6 levels of the cognitive domain have been collapsed to 3 levels.[39,48] Table 2-6 describes each of these 3 levels and provides sample reflective prompts.

Critical Thinking Clinical Scenario

You are a new clinical instructor and are currently supervising a student in the clinic. You ask the student to develop a plan of care for your patient with cystic fibrosis. The student returns with an inadequate plan. You want to help your student, but you need to first figure out where she is struggling.

Reflective Questions

1. Considering each level of Bloom's taxonomy, what types of questions would you ask the student to be able to identify where her knowledge is lacking?

2. How would your strategies for helping this student differ if you found that she was lacking knowledge compared to having difficulty synthesizing all of the information that was gathered?

Reflection: Activities That Engage Learners in the Reflective Process

Many strategies are available to help you perfect the reflective process. Some educators have used journal writing as a means of helping learners describe their

---

Table 2-6. Sample Reflective Questions That Facilitate Higher-Order Thinking Using Bloom's Taxonomy

Level	Sample Questions
Level I—Knowledge and Comprehension The learner may describe the experience for the purpose of understanding or making meaning; explain what happened; describe his or her thoughts, feelings, and actions; and state the results of his or her actions. The more skillful reflector would begin to articulate gaps in knowledge (ie, surprise, confusion).	• What steps would you take in managing a patient with encephalitis? (Knowledge) • What do you know about patients with juvenile diabetes? (Comprehension) • What are the indications and contraindications for ultrasound? (Knowledge) • What is your approach to interviewing patients? (Comprehension) • What is the typical presentation of an individual with this disorder? (Knowledge)
Level II—Analysis and Application The learner may attempt to deconstruct the experience; analyze what happened; differentiate between perceptions, feelings, thoughts, facts, etc; examine alternative explanations; explore something about the experience that stands out as interesting, different, confusing, or unique; raise questions; and explore why this particular experience stands out for him or her. The more skillful reflector analyzes the experience from multiple perspectives beyond the self.	• What do you know about the pathophysiology of juvenile diabetes that will help you determine what exercises to prescribe for this patient with cystic fibrosis? (Application) • How will your treatment for the 2 patients we just saw with right hemiparesis differ? (Analysis) • What can you tell me about the gait on this child with cerebral palsy that is abnormal? (Analysis)
Level III—Synthesis and Evaluation The learner may begin to draw conclusions based on an analysis of the experience; hypothesize different strategies for the future; recognize learning beyond the description of the experience; and articulate personal learning from the experience. The more skillful reflector would base conclusions on synthesis of multiple perspectives.	• Based on your analysis of what just took place, how would you approach the situation differently next time? (Synthesis) • What is your plan of care for this patient with spastic diplegia? (Synthesis) • Has your patient's physiological response to the exercise regimen you prescribed improved at all? (Evaluation) • Having worked with this patient in the hospital, what recommendations do you have for his discharge? (Evaluation) • What is the prognosis for this patient? (Evaluation)

experiences and begin to use the reflective and analytic or critical thinking processes.[19,21,38,45,49-53] Some have encouraged students to write about critical incidents while in the clinical setting.[12,54,55] A critical incident is anything that surprises or confuses you; something that seems to go against what you know or understand; something that you react to in an unexpected manner.[24] Journal writing can help you process critical incidents after they have occurred. This is what Atkins and Murphy[43] were referring to when they discussed trigger events. For example, after seeing a very preterm infant in the neonatal intensive care unit, one medical student wrote in her reflections about how she was concerned with the significant resources being used for these babies because they would likely have a compromised outcome. She was clearly upset and having the opportunity to share her personal reflections prompted an important discussion about the cost of medical care, treatment outcomes for preterm infants, and how our assumptions can impact the clinical decisions we make. Without time to write and share reflections, this important discussion might not otherwise have taken place during that clerkship.

Learners often have mixed opinions about journal writing. Some find the process effective in helping them delve into their experiences, whereas others consider it time consuming and tedious and feel that it has no relevance. There are definite benefits to maintaining a reflective journal, however.[50,52] It is a record over time that allows us to revisit not only the experience but our reflections on that experience. It becomes a recursive process allowing for deeper learning each time we revisit and explore our writing. Nonetheless, it can be time consuming. Other less time-consuming forms of written reflection, including reflective essays, critical incidents, and structured questions, can be used.[10,12,22,24,40,55,56] These, too, serve the purpose of making you stop to think, analyze, and learn from your experiences.

Written journals and essays are most often done in isolation, which can be problematic because we tend to process our experiences strictly from our own lenses. More experienced reflectors and questioners will be able to consider multiple perspectives in the analytic process; however, it is often difficult to question our own thought processes, recognize our own assumptions, or pose alternative solutions without prompting. This is the real benefit of interactive journals, electronic discussion boards, or blogs (ie, that is, if those engaged in blogging stop to reflect, analyze, and question that which is written). Blogs are examples of a type of public journal commonly used by Generation Xers and Nexters that can facilitate just this type of interactive reflection.[28,29,57-59] Even posting a thought-provoking question on Twitter can elicit interesting responses—responses that may make you change your perspective and think differently.

> ## Stop, Do, and Reflect
>
> Have you ever read or participated in a blog? If so, what was the level of discussion like? Were people simply sharing opinions and facts? Did they justify their thoughts with substantiated facts or simply opinion? Did you note any level of analysis? Did they attempt to evaluate what was being written before drawing any conclusions? Did they discuss strategies for change? Were there any assumptions being made? Did anyone question the assumptions?
>
> Next time you read or participate in a blog, consider the reflective frameworks discussed earlier. Think about the reflective elements as you read. Consider the types of questions you might ask to reveal assumptions or to broaden and deepen the discussion on the blog.

To facilitate the reflective process and deepen the discussion, using an interactive process, we can pose questions to the writer or act as a "critical other" or "devil's advocate."[24] The writer can then reflect on the questions posed, which will enable the writer to think more deeply about his or her writing. To truly facilitate the reflective process, as the reader, you would not simply give advice; rather, you would pose questions to extend the writer's thought processes, encouraging higher-order critical thinking. By posing questions, using the theories of Mezirow,[25] Schön,[7,9] and Bloom,[48] you can facilitate the depth and breadth of reflection noted above.

Verbal reflective techniques can be used as an alternative to written reflections, such as reflective questions, reflective dialogue, after-action reviews, and action learning sets.[12,60-64] Each of these techniques uses dialogue to facilitate the reflective process. Again, the dialogue can be prompted by critical incidents or even by videos, patient stories, or particular literary works. The reflective component encourages us to share thoughts, feelings, reactions, as well as an analysis of our experiences. Again, we can pose questions to encourage each other to think critically, uncover taken-for-granted assumptions, consider multiple perspectives, and explore multiple strategies before coming to a conclusion.

As noted earlier, however, without guidance, journals can become diaries simply containing facts and opinions rather than analytic tools for learning. It is important to remember that it is this analytic process that is closely linked to the development of the critical thinking skills essential to effective clinical decision making. Because reflection and journal writing do not come naturally for many, facilitation is essential. Posing reflective questions can further facilitate this process. For example, you can ask students to submit written clinical incidents and then respond to them by posing questions for them to ponder—this may facilitate further analysis. Choosing questions that incorporate more than one element of reflection can also further facilitate both the depth and breadth of critical thinking. In the final section of this chapter, we offer a strategy that uses questions to facilitate reflection in solving complex problems.

Key Points to Remember

Writing can be effective in facilitating reflection and higher-order thinking. Consider using written journals and logs based on critical incidents.

An interactive process may be a more effective means of facilitating the breadth and depth of reflection. Consider using the following:

- Interactive journals
- Electronic discussion boards
- Blogs and other social networking tools (eg, Twitter)

Verbal reflective techniques can be used as an alternative to written reflections. Consider using the following:

- Reflective questions
- Reflective dialogue
- After-action reviews
- Action learning sets

In all instances, asking questions rather than giving advice can enhance reflective thinking and processing.

Action Learning: Using Reflection and Action to Solve Real World Problems

Stop and Reflect

Have you ever had a child ask you a question that made you stop in your tracks to really ponder your response? Did that question cause you to think about some of the things you just take for granted? Did it make you question what you know or how you know it? (eg, Why is the sky blue? How does a big, heavy plane fly?)

Consider this

Michael Marquardt, in his text entitled *Action Learning in Action: Transforming Problems and People for World-Class Organizational Learning,*[63] tells the story of a pizza man. In this story, a group of individuals was tasked with identifying innovative strategies to provide support services for a government laboratory. The group was a homogeneous mix of individuals who had worked in the organization for some time, and they kept coming up with the same ineffective solutions. Working late one evening, they decided to call for a pizza delivery. The pizza delivery man arrived and on a whim they asked him to join in the discussion. Of course, he knew little to nothing about providing support services for government laboratories. Like a young child, he made comments and asked a lot of naïve questions, which made the group stop and really think about some of the things they had just been taking for granted. For the first time, the group began to question some long-held assumptions. The end result was an innovative solution that had the potential to save the company $35 million dollars!

Action learning (AL) is a powerful method of learning in groups that ties reflection to action as the group strives to solve real world problems. The groups are typically small, diverse groups of individuals (ie, 4 to 8 individuals) committed to solving problems and helping each other learn from their experiences. Ideally, action learning groups consist of individuals who are familiar with the problem as well as those naïve to the issues. AL typically consists of cycles of reflection facilitated by questions that are followed by the development of an action plan based on what was learned from the group. These cycles lead to learning, growth, and continuous improvement in practice for all participants. Furthermore, this process generally leads to more creative and innovative problem solving as the learning of the whole is greater than the sum of its parts.[63–65]

AL is ideal for solving problems that are:

- Important to the individual or organization
- Complex, with no easy solution
- Ambiguous, with no black or white answer

Ideally, the individuals involved have some authority to influence change, and the more complex and important the problem is, the more powerful and valuable is the learning. Table 2-7 provides the steps to AL.[63,65–67]

Action learning facilitates questioning of yourself and others and draws on the group so that you can learn from one another. Action learning uses the reflective process to enhance and capture what was learned through experience. It encourages continuous improvement by implementing the action plans that emerge from the learning process. Finally, as Marquardt[63] wrote, "What makes action learning so powerful in solving problems is its inherent ability to employ a systemic, holistic, and comprehensive approach. Asking layers of questions and reflecting on possible responses to those questions forces group members to think beyond symptoms to root causes." Just as in physical therapy where treating

Table 2-7. Steps to Action Learning

1. Present the problem/issue.
2. Raise questions.
3. Reframe the problem (find the root cause).
4. Explore potential solutions.
5. Explore alternative solutions.
6. Reflect on what was learned.
7. Develop an action plan (ie, what would I do differently next time, or what should I do now?).
8. Implement the action plan.
9. Observe and evaluate the outcomes of that plan.
10. Return to the group to reflect on the plan, the action, and its outcome.
11. Revise the plan—which is the start of a new cycle of action learning.

the symptom without finding the root cause is ineffective, solving problems without first finding the root cause is ineffective as well.

Key Points to Remember

How AL differs from a typical problem-solving session:

- Learning and team development are just as important as solving the problem.

- Group members are as diverse as possible (ie, not just the experts).

- Questions are used to facilitate reflection and problem reframing and always precede the development of strategies for action.

- Dialogue, not debate, and questions, not advice, are encouraged, with the goal of getting all ideas on the table rather than attempting to convince anyone of any given solution.

Key Points to Remember

Questions enable us to "diverge and examine from a systems perspective before we converge towards solution."[68]

Questions help us consider:

- Different perspectives
- Different contributing factors
- Different solutions
- Different strategies
- Personal assumptions

Questions help us:

- Clarify situations
- Provide context to a situation
- Open up new possibilities and new ways of thinking
- Unpack complex ideas
- Offer new insights

As discussed previously, questions can help us consider different perspectives, different contributing factors, different solutions, different strategies, and personal assumptions. Questions can help us clarify our thinking, provide context to the situation, open up new ways of thinking, and offer new insights. Most importantly, good questions enable the group to broaden their thinking and examine the situation from a systems perspective before attempting to converge on any one solution. The frameworks of Schön,[7,9] Mezirow,[25] and Bloom[48] previously presented can be used to frame questions that facilitate the process. Particularly good questions are nonjudgmental, elicit exploration and reflection, and make group members think. Krystyna Weinstein[65] also provide some particularly thought-provoking questions you might consider (Table 2-8).

Action learning is commonly used in business[62-64] and has been reported in medicine,[69] nursing,[61,70] and physical therapy.[12] This process may be particularly helpful in the clinical environment because students and clinicians are continually faced with complex problems with no black or white solutions. Because of the fast pace and the typical one-to-one model of the physical therapy clinical environment, this process can be particularly challenging to implement. There are few opportunities available for learners to work in groups to solve problems. Technology can offer unique solutions, however, and may be particularly engaging for Generation Xers and Nexters.

Table 2-8. Sample Thought-Provoking Action Learning Questions

• What is stopping you from… ?	• What would your ideal solution look like?
• What would happen if you… ?	• What else might you do in this situation?
• What strategies have you tried?	• What worries you most about… ?
• What other strategies might you consider?	• Are you being totally honest with yourself?
• What's at the back of your mind?	

Stop and Reflect

Think of a time when you were faced with a challenging situation while on your clinical rotation. Maybe you were having difficulty communicating effectively with your clinical instructor and you could not quite determine the cause of the problem. How might a "virtual action learning set" through the use of an online discussion group have helped you determine the cause of the problem and develop strategies to improve your communication with your clinical instructor?

We and others have been successful in using electronic discussion boards, online journals, and blogs to encourage dialogue, collaboration, reflection, and critical thinking with students in physical therapy, medicine, and nursing in the classroom and in the clinical setting.[12,28,58,59,71–75] Students can engage in virtual action learning groups on the electronic discussion board or by using blogs to solve their own clinical dilemmas and critical incidents as well as to facilitate their own learning in the fast-paced clinical environment. We have found that students value the input of their peers and were able to work through their dilemmas in these virtual environments. Input was primarily in the form of questions, and the students commented that the questions really made them think about their incidents differently and analyze them in a way that they would not have done without prompting from their peers.[12,28] Table 2-9 summarizes the advantages of virtual action learning sets.[63,65–67]

Key Points to Remember

Action learning is:

- A method of solving problems using cycles of reflective questions followed by the implementation of action plans.
- A method of solving problems by working in small groups to ask questions and draw on the knowledge of the group.
- Different than brainstorming because you are using questions to facilitate the thought process rather than offering suggestions and recommendations to simply solve the problem.

Keys to action learning

- Questions precede the development of the strategies for action and are used to facilitate reflection and problem reframing to get at the root cause.
- Dialogue, not debate—the goal is to get all the ideas out on the table, not convince anyone of any given solution.
- Action learn focuses on the learning as much as it does on the problem solving.

Table 2-9. Advantages of Virtual Action Learning

- Virtual action learning (VAL) provides you with a mechanism to gather peer support as you solve your own clinical dilemmas.
- VAL facilitates critical thinking and fosters deeper learning as you think through your peers' dilemmas and develop questions that help them analyze their own situations more deeply.
- VAL facilitates independent thinking and self-directed problem solving in the clinic setting where you might otherwise tend to rely more heavily on your clinical instructor to help you solve your dilemmas.
- You are free to engage in the discussion when it is most convenient for you, when you have had time to review the comments and questions posed and reflect on your own thoughts without the pressure of having to provide an immediate response.
- The discussion board becomes a permanent record of all of the discussions related to your dilemma as well as the dilemmas your peers faced, which you can revisit throughout your clinical experiences and use as a resource for other dilemmas or incidents you might face.
- VAL can also provide a degree of anonymity, allowing learners to post critical incidents and raise thought-provoking questions in a safe learning environment.

Summary

Experience is at the core of learning, and reflection is what enables us to learn from our experiences. Reflection is more than just stopping to think and act based on what we already know. It requires us to consider all of the factors that may be influencing a given situation and to explore the multiple possibilities available for solving dilemmas, which may prevent us from coming to decisions prematurely. Reflection requires us to question what we already know and what we often take for granted. We can engage in the reflective process by ourselves or with others, in writing or verbally, face-to-face or electronically. Being able to view situations from many perspectives is the basis for critical thinking. Skillful reflectors are critical thinkers, and critical thinking is the basis for effective clinical decision making, which is at the heart of quality practice.

Because of the fast-paced nature of the clinical environment, there is an ever-increasing need for creative thinking and excellent clinical decision making. New ideas can come from thinking "outside-the-box." Posing appropriate questions can result in creative thinking and making new connections rather than a simple regurgitation of basic factual knowledge. The skill of reflection is not innate; it must be learned over time and requires practice. Focusing on the elements of reflection and use of reflective questions in the classroom and the clinic may help us facilitate higher levels of critical thinking and problem solving in ourselves and others.

Key Points to Remember

- Reflection is a critical element to learning from experience.
- Reflection is more than just stopping to think and act based on what we already know.
- Reflection requires us to view situations or problems from many perspectives.
- To facilitate deeper and broader thinking, consider the following reflective processes:
  o Reflection-in-action
  o Reflection-on-action
  o Reflection-for-action
  o Content reflection
  o Process reflection
  o Premise reflection
- The learner is encouraged to move through the cognitive hierarchy from lower-level thinking to higher-level thinking.
- Questions are paramount to the development of reflective practitioners and critical thinkers.
- Questions help us consider:
  o Different perspectives
  o Different contributing factors
  o Different solutions
  o Different strategies
  o Personal assumptions
- Questions help us:
  o Clarify situations
  o Provide context to a situation
  o Open up new possibilities and new ways of thinking
  o Unpack complex ideas
  o Offer new insights
  o Encourage systems thinking
- Skillful reflectors are both skillful questioners and critical thinkers.
- Action learning can facilitate learning in groups as they use questions and the reflective process to solve real-world problems.
- Action learning can facilitate learning in groups as they use questions and the reflective process to solve real-world problems.

References

1. Dewey J. *Experience and Education.* New York, NY: Simon & Schuster; 1938.

2. Brown SC, Gillis MA. Using reflective thinking to develop personal professional philosophies. *J Nurs Educ.* 1999;38:171–175.

3. Dewey J. *How We Think.* Amherst, NY: Prometheus Books; 1991.

4. Kolb D. *Experiential Learning: Experience as the Source of Learning and Development.* Englewood Cliffs, NJ: Prentice-Hall; 1984.

5. Boud D, Keogh R, Walker D. *Reflection: Turning Experience Into Learning.* New York, NY: Kogan Page/Nichols Publishing; 1985.

6. Killion J, Todnem G. A process for personal theory building. *Educ Leadersh.* 1991;48:14–16.

7. Schön DA. *Educating the Reflective Practitioner.* San Francisco, CA: Jossey-Bass Publishers; 1987.

8. Sugerman DA, Doherty KL, Garvey DE, Gass MA. *Reflective Learning: Theory and Practice.* Dubuque, IA: Kendall/Hunt Publishing Company; 2000.

9. Schön DA. *The Reflective Practitioner: How Professionals Think in Action.* New York, NY: Basic Books; 1983.

10. Johns C. *Becoming a Reflective Practitioner.* 2nd ed. Oxford, UK: Blackwell Publishing; 2004.

11. Zull J. *The Art of Changing the Brain: Enriching the Practice of Teaching by Exploring the Biology of Learning.* Sterling, VA: Stylus Publishing; 2002.

12. Plack MM, Dunfee H, Driscoll M, Rindflesch A, Hollman J. Virtual action learning sets: a model for facilitating reflection in the clinical setting. *J Phys Ther Educ.* 2008;22:33–41.

13. Blatt B, Plack MM, Mintz M, Simmons S. Acting on reflection: does student performance on a standardized patient examination improve with reflection and revisiting the "patient"? *J Gen Intern Med.* 2007;22:49–54.

14. Crofts L. Learning from experience: Constructing critical case reviews for a leadership programme. *Intensive Crit Care Nurs.* 2006;22:294–300.

15. Larin H, Wessel J, Al-Shamlan A. Reflections of physiotherapy students in the United Arab Emirates during their clinical placements: a qualitative study. *BMC Med Educ.* 2005;5:3.

16. Kidd J, Nestel D. Facilitating reflection in an undergraduate medical curriculum. *Med Teach.* 2004;26:481–486.

17. Brady DW, Corbie-Smith G, Branch WT. "What's important to you?": the use of narratives to promote self-reflection and to understand the experiences of medical residents. *Ann Intern Med.* 2002;137:220–223.

18. Branch WT Jr, Paranjape A. Feedback and reflection: teaching methods for clinical settings. *Acad Med.* 2002;77:1185–1188.

19. Williams RM, Wessel J, Gemus M, Foster-Seargeant E. Journal writing to promote reflection by physical therapy students during clinical placements. *Physiother Theory Pract.* 2002;18:5–15.

20. Westberg J, Jason H. *Fostering Reflection and Providing Feedback: Helping Others Learn From Experience.* New York, NY: Springer Publishing Company; 2001.

21. Kalliath T, Coghlan D. Developing reflective skills through journal writing in an OD course. *Organ Devel J.* 2001;19:61–70.

22. Plack MM, Santasier A. Reflective practice: a model for facilitating critical thinking skills within an integrative case studies classroom experience. *J Phys Ther Educ.* 2004;18:4–12.

23. Shepard KF, Jensen GM, eds. *Handbook of Teaching for Physical Therapists.* Boston, MA: Butterworth-Heinemann; 1997.

24. Brookfield SD. *Developing Critical Thinkers: Challenging Adults to Explore Alternative Ways of Thinking and Acting.* San Francisco, Calif: Jossey-Bass; 1987.

25. Mezirow J. *Fostering Critical Reflection in Adulthood: A Guide to Transformative and Emancipatory Learning.* San Francisco, CA: Jossey-Bass Publishers; 1990.

26. Benner P. From novice to expert. *Am J Nurs.* 1982;82:402–407.

27. Jensen GM, Gwyer J, Hack LM, Shepard KF. *Expertise in Physical Therapy Practices.* Boston, MA: Butterworth-Heinemann; 1999.

28. Chretien K, Goldman E, Faselis C. The reflective writing class blog: using technology to promote reflection and professional development. *J Gen Intern Med.* 2008;32:2066–2070.

29. Kalet AL, Sanger J, Chase J, et al. Promoting professionalism through an online professional development portfolio: successes, joys, and frustrations. *Acad Med.* 2007;82:1065–1072.

30. American Physical Therapy Association (APTA). *Professionalism in Physical Therapy: Core Values.* Alexandria, VA: American Physical Therapy Association; 2004.

31. May W, Stroker G. Critical thinking and self-assessment: the key to developing professional behavior. Paper presented at: National Clinical Education Conference; March 23, 2001; San Francisco, CA.

32. Boyd E, Fales A. Reflective learning: key to learning from experience. *J Hum Psychol.* 1983;23:99–117.

33. Shields E. Reflection and learning in student nurses. *Nurs Educ Today.* 1995;15:452–458.

34. Jensen G, Denton B. Teaching physical therapy students to reflect: a suggestion for clinical education. *J Phys Ther Educ.* 1991;5:33–38.

35. Kern DE, Branch WT Jr, Jackson JL, et al. Teaching the psychosocial aspects of care in the clinical setting: practical recommendations. *Acad Med.* 2005;80:8–20.

36. Shapiro J, Rucker L, Robitshek D. Teaching the art of doctoring: an innovative medical student elective. *Med Teach.* 2006;28:30–35.

37. Plack MM, Greenberg L. The reflective practitioner: reaching for excellence in practice. *Pediatrics.* 2005;116:1546–1552.

38. Plack MM, Driscoll M, Blissett S, Plack T, McKenna R. A method for assessing reflective journal writing. *J Allied Health.* 2005;34:199–208.

39. Plack MM, Driscoll M, Cuppernull L, Marquez M, Maring J, Greenberg L. Inter-rater reliability of assessing reflective journals from a pediatric clerkship using Bloom's taxonomy. *Ambul Pediatr.* 2007;7:285–291.

40. Dunfee H, Plack MM, Driscoll M, Rindflesch A, Hollman J. Assessing reflection and higher order thinking in electronic discussion threads in the clinical setting. *J Phys Ther Educ.* 2008;22:60–66.

41. Mezirow J. *Transformative Dimensions of Adult Learning.* San Francisco, CA: Jossey-Bass; 1991.

42. Cranton P. *Understanding and Promoting Transformative Learning: A Guide for Educators of Adults.* San Francisco, CA: Jossey-Bass; 1994.

43. Atkins S, Murphy K. Reflection: a review of the literature. *J Adv Nurs.* 1993;18:1188–1192.

44. Borrell-Carrio F, Epstein RM. Preventing errors in clinical practice: a call for self awareness. *Ann Fam Med.* 2004;2:310–316.

45. Kerka S. Journal writing as an adult. *ERIC: Learning Tool Practice Application Brief.* 2002;22:84–89.

46. Kerka S. Journal writing and adult learning. *ERIC Dig.* 1996;174:1–4.

47. Woodward H. Reflective journals and portfolios: learning through assessment. *Assessment and Evaluation in Higher Education.* 1998;23:415–423.

48. Bloom BS, ed. *Taxonomy of Educational Objectives: Book 1 Cognitive Domain.* New York, NY: Longman; 1956.

49. Williams RM, Wessel J. Reflective journal writing to obtain student feedback about their learning during the study of chronic musculoskeletal conditions. *J Allied Health*. 2004;33:17–23.

50. Boud D. Using journal writing to enhance reflective practice. *New Dir Adult Contin Educ*. 2001;90:9–18.

51. Edwards R, White M, Gray J, Fischbacher C. Use of a journal club and letter-writing exercise to teach critical appraisal to medical undergraduates. *Med Educ*. 2001;35:691–694.

52. Jarvis P. Journal writing in higher education. *New Dir Adult Contin Educ*. 2001;90:79–86.

53. Kessler PD, Lund CH. Reflective journaling: developing an online journal for distance education. *Nurs Educ*. 2004;29:20–24.

54. Branch W, Pels RJ, Lawrence RS, Arky R. Becoming a doctor: critical incident reports from third year medical students. *New Engl J Med*. 1993;329:1130–1132.

55. Gould B, Masters H. Learning to make sense: the use of critical incident analysis in facilitated reflective groups of mental health student nurses. *Learn Health Soc Care*. 2004;3:53–63.

56. Pee B, Woodman T, Fry H, Davenport E. Practice-based learning: views on the development of a reflective learning tool. *Med Educ*. 2003;34:754–761.

57. Lagu T, Kaufman EJ, Asch DA, Armstrong K. Content of weblogs written by health professionals. *J Gen Intern Med*. 2008;23.

58. Leppa CJ. Assessing student critical thinking through online discussions. *Nurs Educ*. 2004;29:156–160.

59. Low S. Supporting student learning during physical therapist student internships using online technology. *J Phys Ther Educ*. 2008;22:75–82.

60. Bressmann T, Martino R, Rochon E, Bradley K. An action learning experience for speech-language pathology students: on the experience of having dysphagia for a day. *Can Lang Pathol Audiol*. 2007;31:127–133.

61. McGrath D, Higgins A. Implementing and evaluating reflective practice group sessions. *Nurs Educ Pract*. 2006;6:175–181.

62. Marsick VJ, Watkins KE. *Facilitating Learning Organizations: Making Learning Count*. Brookfield, VT: Gower; 1999.

63. Marquardt M. *Action Learning in Action: Transforming Problems and People for World-Class Organizational Learning*. Palo Alto, Calif: Davies-Black Publishing; 1999.

64. Yorks L, O'Neil J, Marsick VJ, eds. *Advances in Developing Human Resources: Action Learning: Successful Strategies for Individual, Team and Organizational Development*. The Academy of Human Resource Development; 1999.

65. Weinstein K. *Action Learning: A Practical Guide for Managers*. 2nd ed. Burlington, VT: Gower Publishing Company; 1998.

66. Yorks L, O'Neil J, Marsick VJ. Action learning: successful strategies for individual, team, and organizational development. San Francisco, CA: Berrett-Koehler; 1999.

67. McGill I, Beaty L. *Action Learning: A Guide for Professional, Management, and Educational Development*. 2nd ed. Philadelphia, PA: Kogan Page; 1995.

68. Marquardt M. *Leading with Questions*. San Francisco, CA: Jossey-Bass; 2005:33.

69. Balslev T. Action learning in the paediatric neurology clinic. *Med Educ*. 2004;38:564–565.

70. Douglas S, Machin T. A model for setting up interdisciplinary collaborative working in groups: lessons from an experience of action learning. *J Psychiatr Ment Health Nurs*. 2004;11:189–193.

71. Kamin CS, O'Sullivan P, Deterding RR, Younger M, Wade T. A case study of teaching presence in virtual problem-based learning groups. *Med Teach*. 2006;28:425–428.

72. Cook DA, Dupras DM, Thompson WG, Pankratz VS. Web-based learning in residents' continuity clinics: a randomized, controlled trial. *Acad Med*. 2005;80:90–97.

73. Oliver M, Shaw GP. Asynchronous discussion in support of medical education. *JALN*. 2003;7:56–67.

74. Sandars J, Langlois M, Waterman H. Online collaborative learning for healthcare continuing professional development: a cross-case analysis of three case studies. *Med Teach*. 2007;29:e9–e17.

75. Drevdahl D, Dorcy KS. Using journals for community health students engaged in group work. *Nurs Educ*. 2002;27:255–259.

The Brain
How Current Concepts in Brain Function May Inform Teaching and Learning

Chapter Objectives

After reading this chapter, you will be prepared to:

- Describe some of the key structures and systems in the brain involved in learning, memory formation, and memory retrieval.

- Differentiate between declarative and nondeclarative memory.

- Discuss memory formation and retrieval and the various brain structures and systems implicated in each.

- Discuss current research on the impact of emotion on attention and memory formation.

- Recognize the potential impact of stress and emotion on the learning environment.

- Recognize the role of emotion and meaning on gaining our learners' attention.

- Recognize the role of establishing context for learning by connecting new information to prior knowledge and personal experiences.

- Evaluate current research related to brain function and its potential implications on teaching and learning.

- Recognize the need for future research that may enable educators to link current concepts in brain research to educational strategies.

Stop, Do, and Reflect

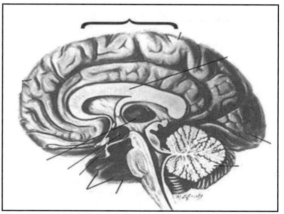

Figure 3-1. Structures of the brain. (Reprinted with permission from the National Institute on Alcohol Abuse and Alcoholism.)

- In the diagram in Figure 3-1, how many of the structures in the brain can you name?

- What are their functions?

- Which structures are most involved in learning, memory formation, and memory retrieval?

You may be wondering why you need information about the brain's structure in a book on teaching and learning. You are not likely to do neurosurgery! You are an educator in the health care environment, someone who wants to be an effective instructor. That is the main reason for including a section on the brain and how it functions. To teach as effectively and efficiently

Plack M, Driscoll M. *Teaching and Learning in Physical Therapy: From Classroom to Clinic* (pp 43-64).

as possible, it is important for us to work in concert with brain organization and function, not at cross-purposes with it.

In any teaching-learning situation, we want to engage learners as fully and as quickly as possible; we want to make complex information meaningful and accessible; and we want our learners to gain and retain the information we are providing. Whether in the clinic or the classroom, we will have patients and students with different life experiences and different levels of background knowledge. Learning more about how the brain works, how neurons communicate with one another to form and reactivate connections, and how to enhance retrieval of prior knowledge may help optimize the educational experience. In this chapter, we will examine some of the cortical, subcortical, and deep cortical structures and mechanisms critical to the learning process.

Advances in technology have enabled researchers to better visualize what is happening in the brain during learning activities more than ever before. It is important to remember, however, that information from neuroimaging studies cannot be applied directly to the classroom or clinic, nor should it be.[1] What we can do as educators, however, is analyze research findings to help us support or refute our observations about effective instruction in the classroom or clinic.

This chapter is intended to provide a broad and basic overview of neuroanatomy as it relates to teaching and learning. We describe some of the major structures of the brain related to learning, memory formation, and memory retrieval. We do not intend for this to be an in-depth study of neuroanatomy. Current literature on brain function as it relates to memory and learning is vast, and we acknowledge that what is to follow may be considered an oversimplification of the complex workings of the brain and its myriad interconnecting systems. Recognizing the complexity of the human brain and that brain research is truly in its infancy, we discuss some of the potential implications for effective teaching and learning, with the caveat that further research is needed to make any direct links to the classroom or clinic. In particular, we explore the implications of stress in the learning environment, as well as the impact of emotion, attention, and prior knowledge on learning. Much of the information has been available to educators through the work of educational theorists and cognitive psychologists, and brain research has provided potential links to neuroanatomical function. Though we note that direct links from current brain research to the classroom cannot be made (yet!), the goal of this chapter is to pique your interest in the ongoing pursuit of information related to the potential application of brain research to teaching and learning.

Neuroimaging

Current technology enables us to visualize what is happening in the brain during various activities in ways that were impossible before the advent of techniques such as positron emission topography (PET), magnetic resonance imaging (MRI), and functional magnetic resonance imaging (fMRI).[2] Before these techniques became available, researchers relied on the study of pathology, autopsied brains, and more static studies. These new technologies allow researchers to observe the activity level in various parts of the brain while the individual is engaged in different tasks. Using PET scans, fMRIs, and even more recently diffusion tensor imaging (DTI) and magnetoencephalography (MEG), scientists can observe the level of activity in the brain during various tasks, enabling them to begin to map the function of the brain.[2]

Ongoing research with neuroimaging tools continues to add to our knowledge of topics such as how adolescents and adults respond differently to cognitive and decision-making tasks[3-5]; how the reward circuitry is engaged during various learning tasks[6]; and how practicing various motor and cognitive skills can impact the size and activity level in different parts of the brain.[7,8] Through brain research and neuroimaging, we know that learning results in physical changes in the brain; networks are developed among neurons, and these connections can be reactivated. The term *neuroplasticity* has been used to describe this ability of the brain to change in terms of structure and function based on learning.[7,9-12]

Learning how the brain functions may have implications for how we plan instruction. For example, brain research tells us that adolescents may have more difficulty inhibiting impulses when in social situations, and they tend to assess risk at a lower level (ie, minimize the danger of a given activity) than adults.[13-15] Recognizing this, as a physical therapist, we may want to take extra steps in working with our adolescent patients to develop strategies to remind them of their weight-bearing restrictions particularly when they are in school and around peers.

Brain Structure and Function

Brain Function and Learning on a Macrolevel

There has been a proliferation of popular writing about the brain and decision making in business and marketing,[16] the brain and physical exercise,[17] and the application of principles of brain research to everyday life.[18] These texts have piqued the interest of many professionals and laypeople in basic brain anatomy and function. In the following pages, we provide an overview of some key terms and concepts related to major brain structures and their function (see Figure 3-1).

One of the first authors to apply what we know about the brain to the teaching-learning experience in the university setting was James Zull. In his book, *The Art of Changing the Brain*,[11] Zull described 3 major functions of the cerebral cortex as *sensation, integration,* and *motion* and noted how these functions not only form the foundation of all nervous systems but provide the underpinnings of experiential learning. Incoming data from the external world (eg, sights, smells, and sounds) are routed to areas of the brain that can interpret them appropriately. The brain continues to extract meaning from these data and integrates that meaning with prior knowledge to develop new meaning. Developing new meaning often results in new thoughts, plans, or actions.

Zull[11] noted that concrete experience, the first phase of Kolb's[19] learning cycle, corresponds with the reception of sensory data in the sensory cortex and is the first step in the learning process. The second phase of Kolb's learning cycle requires us to integrate the incoming information to make meaning of the incoming data using varying degrees of observation and reflection. In the third phase of the cycle, we begin to connect our observations to what we know (ie, prior knowledge) and formulate hypotheses about our experiences, which depend on activity in the frontal cortex as well as other cortical and subcortical areas. Finally, in the fourth phase of Kolb's learning cycle, we begin to actively test those hypotheses and/or implement the various "plans" we developed, which requires activity in the motor cortex.[11] As we implement our plans and ideas, we are faced with new experiences. As a result, each experience shapes and reshapes how we learn and how we view the world.

Critical Thinking Clinical Scenario

You are a clinical instructor working with a first-year student physical therapist during her first exposure to clinical education. She is in clinic 1 day per week for 10 weeks, and she wants to observe a surgical repair of the anterior cruciate ligament (ACL). In the current hospital setting, this is possible, but you would need to rearrange a number of things for this to happen, and the student would miss time observing direct physical therapy interventions. You are just not sure whether the possible benefits of this observation are worth the efforts required to set it up, particularly because it is so early in your student's education.

Reflective Questions

1. Given the description of Kolb's learning cycle, how might this observation enhance your student's learning?

2. How might this experience enhance her understanding of clinical practice?

3. How might this experience help prepare her for when she takes her course in the management of patients with musculoskeletal dysfunction?

4. What new information and/or shift in perspective might the student develop as a result of the observation?

5. Which learning preference might best appreciate this opportunity?

6. What could the clinical instructor do to maximize this learning experience for students with different learning preferences?

The Neuron: The Basis for Brain Function and Learning

Any review of the learning process must begin with a description of a *neuron*, which serves as the basis for all learning. What distinguishes neurons from other cells that make up the human body is their ability to "communicate" with each other and form increasingly complex networks based on sending and receiving physical, electrical, and chemical signals.

Figure 3-2 depicts a neuron with its cell body, axon, and dendrites. Learning occurs when neuronal connections are developed; retrieval of prior learning occurs when these connections are reactivated or the elements of the memory are reconstructed.[9,20] *Dendrites* receive incoming chemical signals generated by the electrical impulses from the axons of other neurons. Electrical impulses travel down the *axon* to the axon terminal where one or more chemicals, called *neurotransmitters*, are released. Examples of these chemical neurotransmitters include dopamine, serotonin, epinephrine (adrenaline), norepinephrine, and acetylcholine.[21] These neurotransmitters spread

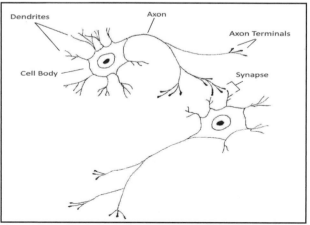

Figure 3-2. Depiction of a neuron, cell body, axon, and dendrites. (Reprinted with permission from Lisa Mogilanski.)

across the tiny space or *synaptic cleft* between the end of the axon and the dendrite of another neuron.[20,22] On the surface of the neighboring dendrite are receptors specifically shaped to receive certain incoming neurotransmitters. These neurotransmitters can be either excitatory or inhibitory. Once the neurotransmitter fits into the receptor, there is a change in the membrane permeability. Because there can be thousands of dendrites on a single neuron, the number of incoming signals is vast. If enough excitatory signals arrive on the dendrite at the same time, the neuron will initiate an electrical impulse down its axon, beginning another potential neuronal connection. The nervous system communicates via these neurotransmitters and electrical impulses. Any increase or decrease in these neurotransmitters will impact this neural transmission and communication. This simple description fails to convey the vast tangle of networks that develop throughout our lives as we continually form new neuronal connections through learning.

A basic adage of neurologists and others involved in applying brain research is, "the more nerves fire, the more nerves wire."[22-25] The task of effective teachers is to tap into and connect new information with whatever prior knowledge or neuronal connections related to that information exist in the learner. Repetition, practice, analogies, multiple modes of presentation, and hands-on activities all related to a single concept will result in multiple neuronal connections being strengthened through the "firing" or transmission of electrical and chemical signals across multiple synapses. Even the act of thinking about a new adaptation of a physical therapy intervention observed in the clinic, for example, can result in neurons being stimulated to form new connections.

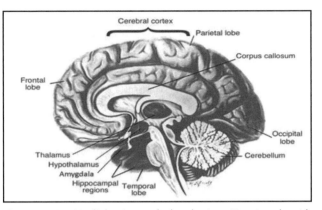

Figure 3-3. Medial view of the brain. (Reprinted with permission from the National Institute on Alcohol Abuse and Alcoholism.)

cerebellum, thalamus, amygdala, and hippocampus, that are involved in human survival. These structures support critical life functions and are also involved in our learners' readiness to learn (eg, arousal, attention, motivation), as well as their ability to learn and form and retrieve memories.

Figure 3-3 depicts a medial view of the brain that shows some of these subcortical and deep cortical structures of the brain. Although we generally refer to brain structures in the singular, it is important to recognize that almost all of the structures are paired, with the exception of those at the midline.

The *brainstem* is located at the base of the brain where it joins the spinal cord and coordinates sensory and motor information between the body and brain. It contains the midbrain, pons, and medulla. It regulates functions related to survival such as respiration, blood pressure, heart rate, and sleep. The brainstem also includes the *reticular formation*, which is a functional system that serves to regulate our level of arousal as well as our sensory input and motor behavior (including posture and locomotion).[26]

The *cerebellum*, a small 2-hemisphere structure, is located just superior to the brainstem and tucked under the occipital lobes. The cerebellum accounts for about 11% of the total brain mass; only the cerebrum is larger.[26,27] Physical therapy clinicians and students alike will recognize the importance of the cerebellum in maintaining posture and balance and in coordinating automatic movements.

Recently, researchers identified functional linkages between the cerebellum and the frontal cortex that suggest there is an important role for the cerebellum in cognitive and executive functioning as well.[9,28,29] It is believed that the cerebellum is involved whenever we are called upon to coordinate thoughts, attention, and feelings; to sequence information; to prioritize plans; or to figure out how long it will take us to do something.[28,30] Not surprisingly, given the importance of these types of functions in interpersonal interactions, the cerebellum is considered to play an important role in our social skills as well.[28,30]

Stop and Reflect

A first-year physical therapy student is learning basic medical terminology along with other content in various courses. The word *extension* has now developed new meaning for this student.

- What possible meanings might the word *extension* have had for a person prior to physical therapy school?

- What other words have new meaning for you now?

- How could the instructor have used the prior connections to teach the meaning of the word in a physical therapy context?

- List as many different study strategies as you can think of to learn medical terminology, to capitalize on the adage, "the more nerves fire, the more nerves wire."

Subcortical and Deep Cortical Structures and Functions

Before addressing the parts of the brain most clearly recognized as being involved with direct instruction, it is important to mention the subcortical and deep cortical structures of the brain, such as the brainstem,

Researchers continue to examine the nonmotor contributions of the cerebellum in studies of neuropsychological disorders,[31] verbal memory,[32] and cognitive development.[33] Recent brain research suggests that the function of the cerebellum is much more complex than anyone initially thought. The cerebellum actually functions to support our cognitive processes by linking information from portions of the brain that perform mental tasks with those that gather sensory information. The cerebellum performs this function on a subconscious level, essentially freeing up the conscious part of the brain for additional cognitive activity.[34]

The *thalamus* is sometimes referred to as a relay station because it projects fibers to and receives fibers from all regions of the cortex. All incoming sensory data, except for olfactory data (ie, smell), first pass through the thalamus, where they are processed and directed to the appropriate parts of the brain for further processing. As with other sensory data, olfactory data are directed to the cortex for interpretation through the thalamus; however, it also bypasses the thalamus and is forwarded directly to the amygdala to be analyzed for danger. Through its myriad connections, the thalamus is thought to be involved in sensory, motor, learning, and memory activities as well as cortical arousal.[26]

The *amygdala* is where sensory information is evaluated on a subconscious level for potential threat. If the amygdala considers incoming sensory data such as a loud noise or violent movement to be dangerous, it alerts the hypothalamus. The amygdala also connects emotional content (positive or negative) to a person's memory of an experience, making it more likely to be remembered in the future.

The *hypothalamus*, among other functions, initiates the physiological responses associated with the fight, flight, or freeze reaction when danger is perceived. When you have been frightened by something and experience a sudden increase in your heart rate and respiration, it is your hypothalamus that helped coordinate these reactions. Your hypothalamus also plays a key role in maintaining your body's homeostasis or balance (eg, sleep-wake cycle, regulation of food and water intake, body temperature, hormone secretion).[22,26]

The *hippocampus*, another structure with connections to the amygdala and hypothalamus, plays an important role in the formation and retrieval of certain types of memories. Though the mechanism remains unclear, some scientists suggest that over time the memory is consolidated (ie, all sensory data related to that particular memory become linked), and at that point, the hippocampus may no longer be needed to retrieve the memory; the memory is likely stored in other cortical regions and is now considered stored in long-term memory.[20,35-38]

The *basal ganglia* are a collection of cells deep within the brain, that consist of the caudate nucleus, putamen, globus pallidus, and subthalamus. The putamen and caudate nucleus are also known as the *striatum*, which receives input from the cortex. Though the function of the basal ganglia is not fully understood, it is known to be involved in the initiation of voluntary movement and in the formation of memories related to skills, habits, and routinized behaviors.[22]

Before leaving the subcortical and deep cortical structures of the brain, we must briefly consider the essential role of various *neurochemicals* (eg, neurotransmitters, neurohormones, neuropeptides) in brain function. During learning and memory formation, not only are there structural changes in the brain, but there is evidence of neurochemical changes as well. These neurochemicals have modulatory effects on learning and memory formation. For example, the neurotransmitter acetylcholine is linked to the processing of sensory information and memory formation and has an influence on an individual's level of arousal and readiness to learn.[21] The neurotransmitter dopamine has been implicated in learning based on rewards and reinforcement, as well as movement and memory consolidation.[39,40] Neuropeptides have also been shown to influence arousal, concentration, motivation, stress response, and memory formation.[21] Finally, varying levels of circulating neurohormones (eg, catecholamines, glucocorticoids) have been shown to either enhance or impair learning and memory formation.[21] A broad range of neurochemicals impact the function of all brain structures and therefore affect our abilities to attend, learn, form, and retrieve memories.

Stop and Reflect

Each of the previously described brain structures is likely to be familiar to you from course work in anatomy or neuroanatomy. Select a couple of the structures, and think about your prior knowledge of them.

- In what ways might knowledge of these structures impact patient care?
- In what ways might knowledge of these structures impact teaching and learning?

What, if any, shift in perspective have you had about these structures and the teaching-learning situation?

Cortical Structures and Function

All the brain structures discussed above often operate on an unconscious level; they detect potential threat, influence what we attend to, and make it possible for us to remember much of what is presented. These structures continuously coordinate physiological responses and allow us to form factual, experiential, emotional, and motor memories. They comprise a relatively small portion of the brain, yet they make it possible for us to learn.

Our ability to reflect on experience, make appropriate decisions, plan ahead, discuss our feelings, and act reasonably depends primarily on our cerebral cortex.[9,25] As noted previously, current research suggests that the cerebral cortex relies on its connections with other structures such as the cerebellum to perform these functions well.[28,30]

Figure 3-3 shows the *cerebral cortex*, whose 3 pound weight belies the fact that it is the "greediest" organ of the body and consumes more than 20% of the body's energy.[9,25] Sylwester[9] described the cerebral cortex as being composed of hundreds of millions of highly specialized mini-columns of neurons that process units of information to allow us to make meaning and use of incoming sensory data. The 6 layers of the cerebral cortex enable us to receive incoming information, process that information, and respond to it appropriately.

The cerebral cortex is typically described in terms of the *right* and *left hemispheres*. Both sides of the brain are involved in all activities and are connected primarily through the corpus callosum. Though there remains much debate, current thought suggests that the right hemisphere is dominant for visual-spatial functions (eg, getting gist or big picture) and attention, whereas the left hemisphere is dominant for language and skilled movement. Although dominance is noted, it is important to remember that the corpus callosum allows for interaction between the hemispheres for many functions, including language and movement.[22,41]

The cerebral cortex consists of the *occipital, temporal, parietal*, and *frontal lobes*. The lobes derive their names from the skull bones above each area.

The *occipital lobes*, in the posterior portion of the cortex, process visual stimuli, which is the most highly evolved special sense. There is great specificity among the visual processing neurons in the occipital lobe, with different areas devoted to different aspects of vision such as distance, depth perception, motion, and color.[9,22]

The *temporal lobes*, located on each side of the brain, above the ears, are primarily responsible for processing auditory stimuli (eg, language, music perception, and comprehension), face and object recognition, and aspects of long-term memory. The temporal lobe is also involved in language comprehension.[9,22]

The *parietal lobes*, located near the top of the brain, contain a strip of cells called the somatosensory cortex that processes information related to sensation such as touch and temperature, as well as the body's sense of position in space.

Remember Zull's[11] conceptualization of Kolb's[19] learning cycle presented earlier? All learning begins with concrete experience, which generates incoming sensory information. Whether you are a student physical therapist, clinical instructor, or patient, the sights and sounds associated with entering a very busy physical therapy gym, for example, will present a great deal of incoming visual, auditory, and somatosensory stimuli that need to be processed for a person to understand what is happening. Clinicians who regularly work with patients in this setting may have forgotten how potentially over stimulating the gym area can be for a patient or student experiencing it for the first time. Allowing time to get one's bearings, look around, and ask questions can help the learner process the many incoming sensory stimuli before focusing on the demands of the treatment itself.

Critical Thinking Clinical Scenario

Think back to the first time you entered a complex environment. For example, think about the first time you entered a hospital room, an intensive care unit, or a busy physical therapy gym. Think about the sounds, the activities, the scents. Did you feel a sense of being overwhelmed by different sensory input? Think about entering the same scenario today; would you be equally overwhelmed, or perhaps have you made sense of the environment and so it feels less overwhelming? Now imagine working with a young patient who requires surgery and will be entering a hospital for the first time.

Reflective Question

1. What strategies might you use to help prepare your patient so that he or she is not so overwhelmed by the sights, sounds, scents, etc, of the environment?

The *frontal lobes*, more than any of the other brain structures, are what make us uniquely human. This area of the brain, comprising 41% of the cerebral cortex, has continued to grow and expand over the past thousands of years because of the increasingly complex and more sophisticated tasks that we as humans have undertaken.[9] The frontal lobes enable us to process, plan for, and respond to potential threats and challenges identified by our more primitive structures. They play a critical role in our ability to properly sequence our thoughts and actions.[10] Researchers suggest that the frontal lobes, with their interconnections to the sensory processing areas of the brain, allow us to temporarily hold information in our working memory needed for us to respond to an environmental demand or retrieve relevant information for problem solving.[20] Not only does this area of the brain contribute to our ability to focus attention, reflect on the past and future, and problem solve, it enables us to be conscious of these abilities.[10,20,25]

In addition, the frontal lobe plays a significant role in the planning, execution, and control of movement. Of course, the frontal cortex, as all brain structures, does not act in isolation. It requires linkages with subcortical and deep cortical structures for many of its functions (eg, prefrontal cortex and cerebellum [executive function]; amygdala [arousal and attention]; hippocampus and striatum [memory]; parietal, temporal, and occipital lobes [sensory input]; basal ganglia [movement initiation]; and cerebellum [movement control]).

The *prefrontal cortex* is the forward-most portion of the frontal lobes. It is often described as the "CEO" of the brain because it coordinates and integrates almost every function of the brain and is responsible for the highest order of processing. Ongoing studies of the adolescent brain indicate that this area of our brain continues to mature, especially in terms of increased mylenization, well into our twenties.[3,9]

Damage to any area of the frontal lobes, particularly the prefrontal cortex, through trauma or cerebral vascular accident can result in problems with "executive function," defined by Squire and Kandel[20] as "the ability to direct one's actions toward future goals" (p. 95). Difficulties with executive function include problems in planning, coordination, and inhibition of impulses, any of which can pose a challenge in the teaching-learning situation. Suggestions for providing patient education to individuals who demonstrate impairments in executive function appear in Chapter 9.

Beneath the cortex (ie, gray matter) is an area described as *white matter*. This description is derived from the *myelin*, or white fatty covering, of many axons. Myelin functions to speed the transmission of electrical impulses along the axons. The white matter within the cortex facilitates communication throughout the central nervous system. The axons within the white matter form 3 major bundles or large tracts:

1. *Commissural fibers* make connections between the 2 cerebral hemispheres. A good example of commissural fibers is the corpus callosum.

2. *Association fibers* make connections within a single hemisphere. Short association fibers connect within the same lobe; long association fibers connect different lobes.

3. *Projection fibers* make connections between the cortex and the rest of the nervous system. A good example of a bundle of projection fibers is the internal capsule, which connects the basal ganglia and thalamus, among other structures.[26]

These fibers serve to integrate information from multiple regions of the nervous system. For example, it serves to link sensory and motor information, speech and language information, and auditory information with visual information. It is the complexity of these interconnections that allows us to process, integrate, coordinate, and act upon the multiple types of sensory information we receive.

For example, as you are sitting at your desk, you may begin to feel a sensation of being cold. This subconscious sensory information is brought to the conscious level in the cortex where a decision needs to be made. Your brain begins to connect this sensation with other incoming sensory input (eg, you feel a cool breeze, you see an open window, and you hear trees rustling outside), and you then make a conscious decision as to whether you should close the window, turn up the thermostat, or find a sweater.

Movement: A Sample of the Complexity and Interconnectedness of Brain Function

Before leaving this section on brain structure and function, it is worth reinforcing that these structures do not work in isolation. Rather, it is the interconnectedness of these structures that enables us to learn and function effectively. Performing a goal-directed movement is an excellent example of the complexity of this process and provides a basis for you to understand how we both teach and learn movement, which will be explored in future chapters. Bear et al[22] described a goal-directed movement as requiring 3 levels of activity:

1. *Strategy*—Before initiating a movement, we must first obtain sufficient sensory information to determine where we are in space and what surrounds us. From there, we must determine the goal of our movement as well as the best approach to use in achieving that goal. This planning may require input from multiple areas of the cortex, including the parietal lobe (sensory input), the prefrontal lobe (planning, abstract thinking, decision making, and anticipating potential consequences), motor cortex of the frontal lobe (movement activity), the temporal lobe (auditory input), the occipital lobe (visual input), and some of the deep and subcortical structures such as the basal ganglia and thalamus. We need to link information from each of these structures to strategize in planning a motor act.

2. *Tactics*—Once we have decided on the goal of the movement, we must determine the appropriate sequence, timing, direction, etc, needed to achieve a smooth movement. This requires activity in the motor cortex of the frontal lobe as well as activity from the cerebellum. The cerebellum is intimately involved in ensuring that movement occurs smoothly, timely, and with precision. Through various feedback loops, the cerebellum functions to continually adjust the movement to ensure successful achievement of the goal.

3. *Execution*—Implementing the movement requires activation of the appropriate muscles to perform the movement. This requires activity in structures in the brainstem, spinal cord, peripheral nervous system, and muscles or effectors. Once movement is initiated, ongoing neuronal feedback among cortical cells and neurons in the basal ganglia, thalamus, and cerebellum is required to again continually adjust our movement and posture.

This is a relatively simplistic description of how goal-directed movement occurs; however, it demonstrates the complexity of movement and the vast number of brain structures required in the control of movement. This clearly complicates our task of helping our patients learn effective movement strategies.

Key Points to Remember

- It is the interconnectedness of brain structures and systems that enables us to learn and function effectively.
- Learning requires a coordinated effort among the following:
  - Cortical
  - Subcortical
  - Deep cortical structures
  - Functional neurochemical systems
- Function requires neuronal communication:
  - Between hemispheres
  - Within hemispheres
  - Between the cortical and subcortical structures throughout the nervous system
- The frontal lobes, in particular the prefrontal cortex, are the areas of the brain that make us uniquely human. Damage in this area has major implications for all aspects of the teaching-learning process.
- The brain sculpts itself (changes physically) based on interaction with the environment (neuroplasticity).
- We are all wired differently based on our previous experiences.
- Theories and information about how the brain functions are being continually updated based upon advances in neuroscientific techniques.

Memory Formation as the Basis for Learning

How do we know we have learned something? As a clinical instructor, how will you know whether or not your student knows enough about gait training to allow him or her to assist patients? How will you know if your patient has learned an exercise sufficiently

enough to perform it correctly at home? The answer to these questions has to do with memory. The only way we can gauge success in teaching is by assessing our learner's ability to retrieve and implement the knowledge and skills we taught. One way a learner can tell if he or she has learned something is if he or she can demonstrate that knowledge. In these examples, the learner must retrieve the knowledge from what is referred to as *long-term memory*. How initial attention to something ultimately results in long-term memory is an integral part of the learning process. Because memory is inextricably intertwined with learning, it is essential for educators to use what we know about the process of memory formation to facilitate learning.

We have explored the function of various cortical and subcortical structures of the brain as the foundation for teaching and learning. Memory formation is the basis upon which we learn. Memory formation, like many other processes throughout the brain and body, requires the use of multiple memory systems, multiple neuroanatomical structures, and multiple neurochemical systems throughout the brain.[36,37,40,42-45] In this section of the chapter, we provide a broad overview of what memory is and how it is formed.

Two Types of Memory

Researchers generally describe 2 major types of memory, although the words they use to label them vary. Squire and Kandel[20] provide a concise history of various approaches to the study of memory in their comprehensive book, *Memory: From Mind to Molecules.* Though they use the terms *declarative* and *nondeclarative* to classify the 2 types of memory, others use the terms *explicit* and *implicit*, respectively, to describe these same processes.[20,22,37,46]

Declarative or explicit memory refers to memories that can be verbalized, declared, or made explicit. Declarative memory is subdivided into semantic memory and episodic memory.

- *Semantic memory* refers to our memory for factual information, general knowledge about which we can speak or write, and information that is available for conscious recall. These are memories of people, places, and things that are not connected to a specific event (time or place). Semantic memory allows us to remember something and describe it.

- *Episodic memory*, the other type of declarative or explicit memory, is more autobiographical and allows us to remember when and under what circumstances we learned that information; it is specific to a certain time and place. It represents a more complex aspect of memory than being able to label or describe something.

Declarative memory enables us to make comparisons with what we already know. Declarative memories are encoded in terms of relationships among multiple events, which enable us to generalize across similar concepts.[20,46] Explicit or declarative memories are also shaped over time and with each new related experience.[22,47] Although the hippocampus is most directly involved with the formation and retrieval of long-term declarative memories, our long-term memories are thought to be stored throughout the cerebral cortex.[20]

Nondeclarative or implicit memory occurs earliest in human development, when the baby has not developed sufficient language to describe the memory. It includes memory for any automatic behaviors and skills, conditioned responses, and unconscious awareness of past experience.[20,37,46] Nondeclarative memory includes several categories of memories: procedural, emotional, and classical conditioning.[22] The 2 types of memory we are most concerned with are procedural and emotional memory:

- *Procedural memory*, is our memory for skills and habits such as piano playing and bicycle riding. This type of memory forms the basis for motor learning and for how we teach movement, which will be discussed in a future chapter. Nondeclarative procedural memories require repetition and practice over a longer period of time and are less likely to be forgotten than declarative memories. For example, you may not remember how you learned to tie your shoe, but you can tie your shoe with ease.

- *Emotional memory*, is our memory that has been associated with positive or negative arousal. Emotional memory formation—fear, in particular—has been the subject of significant ongoing research.[37,38,48-51]

Critical Thinking Clinical Scenario

You are working with a patient who has diabetes. You notice that the patient is wearing new shoes and that there is an area of redness on your patient's foot when the shoe is removed. You had instructed your patient about the importance of foot care and examination of the feet on a regular basis. At that time, your patient expressed little interest in following your recommendations. Now, your patient appears concerned about the redness and comments, "I haven't been checking my feet, and I am afraid I have developed a bad blister; now I know why you want me to check my feet every day. I'm going to use different shoes and pay more attention to my feet."

Reflective Questions

1. Why might this patient be more diligent about foot care and self-examination in the future?

2. What memory process is being engaged in this patient?

3. How might your knowledge of brain function help explain this new desire to be more diligent?

4. How can the physical therapist help this patient remain diligent?

How Memories Form

Once a person attends to incoming sensory information, the potential for learning occurs, and this act of learning is linked to the process of memory formation and memory retrieval. Memory used to be considered in terms of where learned information was stored in the brain, a physical location that was determined after something was learned.[52] Memory was also thought of as a process of recording and storing experiences almost like on videotapes or CDs.[29] There remains much that is still unknown about how memory works, but current researchers concur that there are multiple memory systems involved in memory formation and memory retrieval, each with projections to multiple cortical, subcortical, and deep cortical areas requiring input from various neurochemical systems of the brain.[20,36,37,45]

Current thought suggests that the hippocampus, along with other parahippocampal and cortical regions, is involved in the consolidation and retrieval of most declarative and nondeclarative memories[20,22]; the striatum in the basal ganglia with input from several cortical and subcortical structures is critical for the development and retrieval of procedural memories[22]; and the amygdala is essential in the development and retrieval of emotional memories.[38,53-55] As you will see later, not only do the structures of the brain play a critical role in our memory formation and retrieval, but so do neurotransmitters, neurohormones, and other neurochemicals.

Although multiple structures are involved in the memory formation, it is important to remember that these structures do not work in separate and independent ways. There is fluid interaction among all the neural pathways.[20] Once incoming information is attended to, these stimuli must be scanned for relevance (threat and meaning) and routed to the appropriate areas of the brain for analysis.

As previously described, most incoming sensory information is routed through the thalamus. The thalamus processes this sensory information and directs it to the appropriate sensory-processing areas of the cerebral cortex and other areas (eg, visual data to the visual cortex, which covers the occipital lobe). A small portion of incoming information makes its way to our consciousness, and this information forms the basis of what we consider our thoughts, conscious visual, auditory, and language-based memories.

Often, people use a multistep framework to conceptualize the various aspects of memory formation and retrieval. As long as we do not consider this model as depicting actual places and discrete systems in the brain, this analogy can help us make sense of how we encode, store, retrieve, and integrate new information into existing neuronal networks (Figure 3-4). Typically,

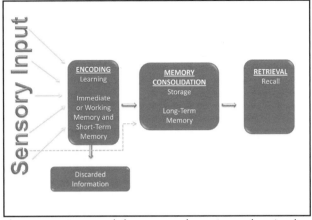

Figure 3-4. Framework for memory formation and retrieval.

information moves from sensory input to immediate or working memory to short-term memory and after some time is consolidated into long-term memory, although it has been noted that some memories can move directly from sensory input to long-term memory.[22]

The neural connections that make up a memory lie in many different areas of the brain, often near the part of the cortex involved in the original processing. For example, memory traces of a student physical therapist's first day in an acute-care setting, with its myriad visual, auditory, and olfactory cues, may be scattered among the occipital lobes, temporal lobes, hippocampus, and prefrontal cortex as well as the amygdala, especially if some of the sights, sounds, and smells from that day were emotionally charged. Whether the student's experience was positive or negative, it was likely emotionally charged, and as a result the amygdala was involved in coordinating memory formation.[37,53] If the student visits a hospital again years later, memories of that first internship may easily be triggered by the various sights, sounds, and smells in the environment. Just as the amygdala was involved in coordinating the actions of the cortical, subcortical, and neurochemical systems in the formation of this emotional memory, it is likely involved in the reformation and retrieval of this emotional memory.[53,56]

The frontal lobes, especially the prefrontal cortex, hold new information for a few seconds in what Squire and Kandel[20] referred to as *immediate memory* and others describe as working memory.[22] Much of the incoming information will be discarded and never make it into our short- or long-term memories. When incoming information is considered important enough for more analysis, it is routed to the hippocampus for further processing and consolidation into our long-term memory.

Whether one refers to this aspect of the memory formation as immediate or working memory, researchers agree that time and capacity are limited in working memory. For declarative memories, often, rehearsal or repetition is what allows us to maintain and begin to encode information in our working memories.[22] Active manipulation (ie, further processing) of the data is necessary to move information from working memory to long-term memory. Examples of active manipulation include focusing on the meaning or relevance of the information to be learned to one's own life, grouping discrete pieces of information into meaningful units, creating a story or song based on the content, or employing other mnemonic devices.[18,20,25] Additional strategies for memory enhancement will be discussed in the next chapter.

Critical Thinking Clinical Scenario

A physical therapist has returned to school to pursue his doctor of physical therapy degree. He is overwhelmed by the amount of new information he is expected to learn in the differential diagnosis course. During class, he feels like he understands exactly what is being presented. Then, he goes home and draws a blank when trying to apply the information to the case assigned for homework. There are several topics, related to symptoms he's seen in his patients, that are really clear for him, but some of the other information being presented is totally new to him.

Reflective Questions

1. What might be going on in this scenario?
2. What might be helping the therapist's learning?
3. What might be interfering with his mastery of the material?
4. Has something like this ever happened to you?
5. How might knowing that past experiences can both help and hinder learning help them in the future as a learner and as a teacher?

Key Points to Remember

- Memory formation is the basis for learning.
- There are 2 types of memory:
  - Declarative or explicit, which consists of semantic and episodic memory.
  - Nondeclarative or implicit, which includes skill or procedural memory as well as emotional memory.
- Multiple regions of the brain are involved in the formation and retrieval of different types of memory.
- Active manipulation, or the processing of sensory data, is essential to the formation of long-term memory and learning.

Potential Implications for Teaching and Learning

As noted earlier in the chapter, we currently cannot make a direct link from brain research to the classroom.[1,57] What we can do as educators, however, is remain abreast of current brain research and become critical consumers of the research (ie, continually question and analyze what science is telling us and reflect on how it may or may not apply to our own practices). Teaching, like physical therapy, is both an art and a science. Our role as evidence-based practitioners is to understand and appropriately apply current research in designing effective teaching-learning situations. As noted earlier, it is important that we work in concert with brain function and not at cross-purposes. What becomes challenging, as in all of health care, is that new and at times conflicting information is being discovered daily and it takes time for consensus to be developed among scientists. What we currently know about the brain is quite limited; as research continues, new knowledge will be developed, and it will be up to us to determine how and when to apply that knowledge not only in the clinical setting but in the classroom setting. In addition, application of all new knowledge requires systematic assessment and evaluation, both in the classroom and in the clinic.

Having discussed brain structure and function, we will now explore some potential implications that current brain research might hold for us as educators. We raise questions about and explore the possibility of some links from brain research to classroom practice and make the recommendation that we continue to explore current research to determine when and how to best apply theory to practice. Only future research will be able to solidify the direct links between brain research and classroom teaching. In the next section of this chapter, we explore the following questions:

- How might emotion and stress impact the learning environments?

- What strategies might we use to gain the attention of our learners?

- How might establishing context for learning by making connections to prior knowledge and personal experiences influence learning?

Learning and Emotion: The Learning Climate

Educators have long recognized the importance of the learning climate in the teaching-learning situation.[58] What does current knowledge of brain function tell us about stress and its impact on learning? Though much of the recent research on the amygdala has been related to fear responses and fear conditioning, some studies have suggested that the amygdala plays a role in both positive and negative experiences, and it has been linked to enhanced learning and the formation of memories, particularly emotional memories.[37,38,53] Emotionally arousing stimuli can increase our level of alertness, and, as a result, emotionally charged experiences, whether negative or positive, are often more readily remembered.[29,53,59,60]

In addition to the nature of the emotion (negative or positive), however, it is important to pay attention to the intensity of emotional arousal as well. Emotions can range from highly negative to highly positive. Some degree of emotional stress may actually help us remember important information and events. Too much stress (ie, high intensity), on the other hand, can actually lead to impaired learning, impaired memory, and maladaptive behaviors (eg, anxiety disorders). This is particularly true of explicit or declarative memory formation.[51,53,60] In addition, in situations perceived as highly emotionally charged, memory for the major details of the situation may be enhanced, whereas memory for the broader details surrounding the situation may actually be impaired.[37]

Consider this classroom example. You are presenting a talk on physical therapy interventions for wound care to a group of first-year physical therapy students who have never been exposed to the subject. You begin your talk by showing a slide of a horrific wound filled with maggots being used for therapeutic purposes. This may well arouse a significantly negative emotional response from some students. They may very well remember the slide that aroused such emotion but forget much of the discussion about the intervention. Similarly, if you are teaching students about motor development and you decide to have some of your students bring in their children or children they know, the students might be so by engaged in having fun with the children (ie, positively emotionally charged) that, again, they fail to remember the details of the children's movement patterns. In each situation, it would be important for the instructor to direct the students' attention to the key points of the lesson and to clarify the connection between the emotionally charged slides or children's performance and the content being taught.

How much stress or emotional arousal is too much? Despite a significant body of literature on the effects of stress on learning and performance, there is no clear answer as to how much is too much. The results of these studies are complex and at times conflicting.[53,61] For example, animal studies have shown that different types of stress may impact male animals and female animals differently. Acute stress may impede learning in female animals while enhancing learning in male animals; uncontrollable stress may enhance performance in female animals while hindering performance in male animals.[61] Even in humans, fMRI studies have demonstrated different patterns of amygdala excitation in men and women when presented with emotionally charged information.[53] Acute stress may enhance learning and memory formation, whereas chronic stress may lead to maladaptive behaviors such as anxiety and depression. This, too, depends on when, how, and what type of stress is applied.[53,60]

Many factors can influence the degree to which stress enhances or impedes memory, including the severity of the stress, individual differences (eg, life experiences), the phase of memory formation during which stress is perceived, gender, age, and context.[62] Even the type of task involved may be a factor in whether stress is a help or a hindrance. For example, in animal studies, a high-stress environment enhanced learning of simple tasks, whereas a low-stress environment enhanced learning of complex tasks.[61]

To understand the impact of stress on learning, the role of the neurochemicals that underlie stress reaction such as cortisol and noradrenaline must be considered as well. Both noradrenaline and cortisol, released under stress, potentially impact the prefrontal cortex, hippocampus, and amygdala. Mildly stressful stimuli result in increased release of noradrenaline, which has been correlated with increased activation of the amygdala and hippocampus and enhanced consolidation of emotional memories. Similarly, increased levels of cortisol have been shown to enhance encoding and consolidation of memory but impede memory retrieval.[53]

The effects of stress on learning and memory have been and continue to be studied using a variety of strategies, from animal studies to human studies, from neurobiological studies to neuroimaging studies, and as noted, seemingly conflicting results have been reported.[53,61] Just as we caution not to make direct links between neuroimaging and classroom teaching strategies, the same caution holds for making direct links between animal studies and human behavior.

It is safe to say that stress in the learning environment is a complex phenomenon. What we do know at this point is that emotionally charged information is better remembered than neutral information. However, individual differences as well as the intensity, frequency, timing, duration, predictability, and controllability of the stress will all influence an individual's response to stressful situations.[21,53] Shors[61] suggested that stress in the learning environment cannot be categorized as either "good" or "bad." Too little stress can lead to boredom and inattention; too much stress can impede attention and learning.

Whether we work in the classroom or the clinic, our environments have the potential to enhance or obstruct learning. It is important for us to remember that stress may be differentially experienced (ie, not everyone reacts to stress in the same way).

Stop and Reflect

The clinical instructor wants to confirm that the student can identify the origins and insertions of various muscles related to the impairment of the patient with whom she is currently working. The clinical instructor feels that the quickest and most efficient way to determine whether she knows the information is to ask her to answer questions throughout the patient's session.

- How might the student react to being questioned in front of the patient?
- How might the patient react in this situation (ie, how stressful might it feel for the patient)?
- How might the level of stress impact the student's ability to answer the questions posed (ie, retrieve information)?
- How else could the clinician have obtained the desired information?

Fostering a sense of safety and comfort or adding an element of humor and enjoyment can emotionally charge a learning environment in a positive way, which may enhance the learning experience. We can encourage the use of positive emotion through clinical examples, social interaction, and appropriate humor. As a clinical instructor, it may be important to consider that periodically engaging your learner in conversations about common interests, hobbies, or favorite subjects in physical therapy school may put your learner at ease. This sense of ease can help minimize your learner's stress level, which may potentially enhance your learner's memory retrieval and enable your learner to more readily respond to questions about previously learned material.

As educators, our goal is to optimize learning and retention in our learners and patients; minimizing the likelihood that our learners feel threatened (ie, excessively stressed) in the learning environment may facilitate that process. Of course, as our learners progress, particularly in the clinical setting, it may be important to increase the level of stress in a controlled manner so they can adapt and develop strategies to manage the increasingly complex demands of clinical environment. It is also important to remember that learners experience stress differently; what may be just enough stress to arouse and engage one learner may feel overly stressful for another learner. To optimize learning, it is our role to monitor the effects of stress (positive or negative) on our learners and modify accordingly.

Critical Thinking Clinical Scenarios

As we noted, learners differentially experience stress; what is stressful for one learner may not be considered stressful for another. Consider the following teaching-learning scenarios:

- A clinical instructor continually asks her student on-the-spot questions to help her learn to think on her feet.
- An instructor mocks a student for asking a "silly" or "stupid" question.
- An instructor routinely uses sarcastic humor in the classroom.

Reflective Questions

1. Have you ever experienced a stressful situation that helped your learning? Hindered your learning?
2. If you were the student in each of these scenarios, how stressful would it be for you?
3. In what ways might your learning be impacted in each of these situations?

Critical Thinking Clinical Scenario

Your patient has recently had a TKR and it is day 1 postsurgery. Your clinical instructor asks you to assist in helping him stand for the first time. The patient says he is not ready to stand. He is afraid it is going to hurt too much, and he doesn't want to work with a student physical therapist.

Reflective Questions

1. What do you think is going on with the patient?
2. How might your knowledge of brain function help you better understand the patient's reactions?
3. How might you change the environment to support your patient and enhance his motivation?

Critical Thinking Clinical Scenario

You are teaching a home exercise program to your 60-year-old patient who recently had back surgery. She is fearful of pain and feels stressed about doing the exercises on her own. Although she is motivated to improve, she just cannot seem to remember the exercises you want her to perform.

Reflective Questions

1. What do you think is interfering with the patient's ability to complete the home exercises appropriately?
2. What else could the clinician do to facilitate the patient's learning and retention?
3. How might knowledge of the structure and function of the brain help you analyze this scenario?

Key Points to Remember

- Emotional arousal, either positive or negative, increases learners' attention.
- Excessive emotional arousal, either positive or negative, may increase retention of major details of the situation to the detriment of the finer details.
- Multiple factors may influence the degree to which stress can enhance or impede memory, including the severity of the stress, the phase of memory formation during which stress is perceived, context, and type of task involved.
- Individual differences, intensity, frequency, duration of stress and its predictability and controllability will all influence an individual's response to stressful situations.
- Learners experience stress differently; what may be just enough stress to arouse and engage one learner may feel overly stressful for another learner.
- To optimize learning, our role as educators is to monitor the effects of stress (positive or negative) on our learners and modify the environment as possible.

Learning and Attention

"To learn, you must pay attention" is the title of a recent article in the *Proceedings of the National Academy of Sciences* related to understanding learning from a molecular level.[63] Again, intuitively as educators, most of us would agree that this makes sense. Researchers tell us that this need for attention is particularly true for explicit or declarative memory formation and retrieval.[47] Again, this makes perfect sense. With so much incoming sensory information available all the time, how do we know what is important and where to direct our attention?

We know from the previous section that it is important to consider the emotional climate of the learning environment. Both positive and negative emotions may increase the likelihood that an experience, event, or stimulus will be attended to and remembered.[38,64] Emotionally threatening input is processed, prioritized, and attended to more readily than other emotionally charged or neutral input. Researchers suggest that the amygdala may actually recognize a fear stimulus and begin to influence other cortical, subcortical, and deep cortical structures and neurochemical systems to act before we are even fully cognizant of the stimulus itself. Further, threatening input may negatively impact certain memory systems.[22,38,51,53]

Recently, researchers have suggested also that selective attention to details will increase the likelihood that those details will be remembered, and this selective attention is mediated by interactions between the cortex and hippocampus.[65] Attention is needed both during the formation and retrieval of explicit memories.[47] Explicit memory formation also requires more than attention to a single detail or sensory modality (ie, sight, sound, smell); rather, all of the sensory input must be integrated into a representative whole. It requires attention to the entire context of the experience, including the internal and external cues that represent the entire experience. Researchers suggest that this attention and integration occurs at the level of the hippocampus and is mediated by dopamine neurotransmitters and other neurochemical systems.[47] Attention is a complex process that does not occur in a single neuroanatomical structure, rather it represents "a family of processes that functions in different behavioural contexts, with different time frames and at different hierarchical levels of the central nervous system".[47]

So what might this mean for us as educators? How can we help our learners attend? What strategies might we use to help focus our learners' attention in the learning environment?

Stop and Reflect

Think back to some of the teaching-learning experiences you had as a learner:

- What was the best experience you had as a learner? What made it so great?
- What did the instructor do to engage your attention?
- How might that relate to what you learned in this chapter about the brain and how it functions?

If you think about some of the great presentations you have attended in which you were fully engaged, did the instructor do something to grab your attention at the beginning of the presentation? Perhaps he used a joke, a story, or a thought-provoking question; perhaps he made you think back to something with which you were already familiar; or perhaps he presented the material in a unique manner. Again, intuitively, good educators know that before you begin teaching you have to gain the attention of your learners; then, of course, you want to maintain it throughout your presentation. We will discuss many strategies to help you do just that in the next chapter.

For now, consider this example of using some type of emotional "hook" to engage the attention of your learners. Imagine that you are presenting to a class of doctor of physical therapy students about the history of, and evidence base for, a new physical therapy intervention. It may not arouse much emotion in a class of doctor of physical therapy students. If you wanted to increase the likelihood that students will attend to and begin processing the information being presented, consider beginning with a clinical example illustrating the successful application of this intervention and include anecdotal information about the instructor's excitement and the patient's feelings of accomplishment. This "story from the clinic" can provide a positive emotional context for the lecture material and increase its priority for processing.

Similarly, when a clinical instructor prefaces a discussion of contraindications for a specific physical therapy intervention with mention of something that had gone seriously wrong with a patient in the past, the student physical therapist is very likely to pay attention. In this example, hearing that someone was hurt represents an emotional hook that will grab the student's attention more effectively than beginning with a list of facts. Could it be in both of these examples that by using emotionally arousing input you move the content from being neutrally charged to potentially positively or negatively emotionally charged, thereby increasing arousal through the amygdala and its projections? Once again, only future research will be able to tell us for sure.

In addition to emotional charge, novelty, change in voice tone, sudden movements, and mention of our names are all salient details in the environment that may signal that something has changed that might be important and perhaps we should attend to it. Imagine that you, as the instructor, become frustrated with several students who appear to be text messaging, whispering to one another, and generally not engaged with the lecture. You might raise your voice and tell the students to pay attention or leave the classroom. Suddenly, your raised voice and words take precedence and gain the attention of the chatting students and perhaps for several students seated nearby. Because this situation may feel threatening to at least some students, their attention immediately shifts to your reprimand and away from the information you were presenting about the new therapeutic intervention. The sudden change in the learning climate, the change in your tone of voice, your movement, the mention of a student's name all served to shift the focus and attention of your learners. Indeed, for effective instruction to continue, you will need to summarize the key points you presented before continuing with new information; however, at that point, you likely have their full attention.

Emotion, novelty, and sudden environmental changes (eg, sights, sounds, smells, or movements) are all factors that typically engage our attention. As humans, we know we are more likely to attend to salient stimuli (eg, novelty, sudden changes, and sudden movements) in the environment. Though there remains some debate, researchers suggest that salient stimuli are perceived by the amygdala and sent to the cortex, and it is this interaction that results in our increased attention.[38] This increased amygdala-cortical activity with its concomitant neurochemical activity can increase our level of arousal and motivation and lead to enhanced learning and memory formation. Is this potentially a neuroanatomical or brain-based reason for incorporating emotion, novelty, movement, sights, smells, sounds, and other salient stimuli in our teaching strategies?

Stop and Reflect

How might you use this information about the power of salient stimuli to help your study group get the most out of a 3-hour session to review course material for a major exam?

Key Points to Remember

- Information related to survival or threat will be processed before information associated with emotions in general.
- Information with any emotional connection will receive higher priority for processing than neutral information.
- Emotion and salient stimuli (eg, novelty and movement) can attract our learners' attention.

Learning and the Role of Prior Experiences and Personal Meaning

We know from an earlier chapter that adults bring a great deal of experience to the teaching-learning situation, and it is important that we as instructors respect and connect with that experience. Why is that, though? Is it possible that it has something to do with memory formation and memory retrieval? If we can link information to memory pathways that have already been established, will that make learning new information easier or more efficient?

In the early 1990s, there was a surge of interest in prior knowledge and its effects on learning and memory. In 1994, Tobias[66] completed a study on interest and prior knowledge. His research suggested that there is a linear relationship between interest and prior knowledge, and when we work on something of interest, we make more personal connections and become more emotionally involved. He found that increased interest stimulated more pleasant emotions, activated more personal connections, and resulted in the use of deeper strategies for learning. Interest and prior knowledge facilitated learning. Scientists use association studies to correlate behavioral measures (ie, task outcomes) with fMRI studies. These studies confirm that learning is both more effective and more efficient in the presence of prior knowledge, and if we associate new learning with prior learning, we can enhance the formation of certain types of memories.[67,68]

The work of Della Libera and Chelazzi[69] in 2009 suggests that our selective attention is influenced by our past experiences and, more specifically, by the outcomes of those experiences. We learn to attend to, or ignore, a stimulus based on the consequences of our previous experiences with that particular stimulus. Muzzio et al[47] described a type of internal "map" that is developed by the hippocampus to represent a given contextual experience and suggested that this map is acquired through learning and is reshaped through experience. Similarly, based on their research findings, Della Libera and Chelazzi[69] postulated that learning is the result of an accumulation of experiences, and each experience influences how we will act in the future when faced with similar circumstances. Pastalkova et al[70] also noted that during learning, neurons fire in the hippocampus of animals in a sequence that suggests that they recall past experiences as they plan future actions. In Chapter 1, we described how Kolb,[19] an educational theorist, proposed a cyclic learning process that is quite consistent with current findings in brain research. He suggested that each new concrete experience potentially reshapes how we view our next experience. Each experience shapes our thinking and it is through this ongoing cycle that we learn.

The filters described in detail in Chapter 1 also may reflect some of the different neuronal connections that form when individuals have had different experiences. For example, the young adults of the Millennial generation have had multiple experiences with technology as a major component of their educational experience. What we might term as comfort with technology most likely derives from extensive neuronal networks that were developed in using computers in multiple ways to support their learning. Medina[18] also noted that culture may impact the degree to which people will find meaning in, and attend to, aspects of a potential learning situation.

In learning, to make sense of our everyday experiences, we link back to our past experiences. Our memory, through vast networks of connections, allows us to analyze whether incoming sensory information is important and whether it is related to something we already know. If, based on our personal experiences, information is of interest or meaningful to us, we are more likely to attend to it. Once again, however, it is important to remember that individuals have different experiences, so not everyone will attend to incoming stimuli to the same degree.

In the scenario that opened this section of the chapter, the clinicians who attended the lecture on computerized prostheses probably had different professional experiences, resulting in the development of different neuronal connections. It may have been helpful if the presenters tried to link to those different experiences by asking questions about the participants' experiences with different types of prostheses or microprocessors and computers or by showing pictures of the more commonly used prostheses. Even the learner with no prior experience with patients with prostheses may have been engaged by a question about microprocessors or computers, with which he or she may have had some experience. In asking a variety of questions to engage the audience, it is possible that the presenters may have been able to reactivate trace memories and various neuronal networks in all members of the audience. Might this have increased the likelihood that the presenters would have gained the attention of more audience participants?

Critical Thinking Clinical Scenario

You are a first-year student physical therapist, and you see on the course schedule the topic "universal precautions" and wonder what information will be covered. The word *precautions* draws your attention, yet you have no idea of the content to be addressed in this class.

Reflective Questions

1. Why might the word *precautions* grab your attention?
2. What connections to past learning might the instructor make?
3. How might the cultural background of the student or instructor influence this learning experience?

Stop and Reflect

Consider some of the different filters presented in Chapter 1. In particular, think about individuals from different generations and/or different cultures. Consider also what you learned in this section on the potential importance of linking learning to prior knowledge and meaning.

- Think of a time when prior knowledge helped your learning or perhaps a lack of prior knowledge may have hindered your learning.

Key Point to Remember

Connecting to prior knowledge and past experiences may help grab your learner's attention and enhance the efficacy and efficiency of learning and memory formation.

Emotion, attention, past experiences, and *personal meaning* are important in all learning situations. For example, you may be in a school building, hear a loud alarm, and observe people stop what they are doing and move toward a door labeled "Exit." Clearly, this loud sound drew everyone's attention away from what they were doing and had meaning for them. Imagine being from a very different cultural background, where you may not have recognized the importance of the sound, nor would the sound necessarily have any meaning for you. You likely would have attended to the sound because it was a novel stimulus, but its meaning would have been lost without prior experience or memory of what to do in that situation. Once you have had the experience of a fire drill—or worse, a real fire—however, it likely would have aroused some emotion in you, and the next time you heard the sound of the alarm you may very well have reacted rather quickly. Having already had the experience of needing to react to a fire alarm, the next time you hear the same sound, you likely would be emotionally aroused, you would attend to the stimulus, you would recognize the potential consequences of the stimulus, you would make meaning of the experience, and it would influence how you would respond.

What does this all mean in the classroom or clinic? To design effective teaching and learning experiences, it is important to consider *emotion, attention, past experiences,* and *personal meaning.* Can using an emotional hook help us focus our learner's attention? Will linking new knowledge to prior knowledge help our learners make sense of their experiences and enable them to more easily learn the material being presented? If we present material to our learners in a way that is personally relevant/meaningful, will they become more emotionally aroused, ready to attend, and therefore learn and remember? From the educational literature as well as the neuroscience and cognitive neuroscience literature, emotion, attention, past experience, and personal meaning all appear to be critical components in memory formation, memory retrieval, and learning. The science of learning continues to progress; our role as educators is to be critical consumers of the research so that we may determine when and how to appropriately apply research findings to enhance the art and science of teaching and learning in the classroom and clinic.

Memory and Aging

Researchers confirm that changes in memory do occur as we age.[12,20,71] People have more difficulty finding the word they want to say or remembering where they put their car keys. Cognitive functions such as attention and memory are differentially affected with age. For example, selective attention appears to be preserved; on the other hand, memory, particularly short-term memory, appears to be more impaired than long-term memory, and declarative memory more impaired than procedural memory. A decline in the rate of processing information and the ability to process information from multiple sources simultaneously are contributing factors.[71]

Why memory deteriorates is less clear. It has been shown that with age there are changes in the frontal cortex, which is critical for working memory and executive functioning (eg, planning, organizing). There is evidence of neuronal, neurochemical, metabolic, and receptor changes in the cerebral cortex and in the hippocampus.[71] Others note changes in subcortical areas, especially the areas involved in the development of neurotransmitters such as dopamine.[72] Still others cite cellular and intercellular changes as a result of oxidative damage and neuro-inflammation within the brain itself as facilitators of age-related decline.[71]

On an optimistic note, there is a great deal of research being conducted on strategies to minimize age-related cognitive decline. Research on neuroplasticity shows that the adult brain is adaptable, and researchers continue to study factors that may slow or prevent cognitive decline in older adults.[12] Among the most promising approaches are physical activity; social involvement in family, friendship, and/or community networks; and cognitive stimulation.[73-75] There is consensus among researchers as well that exercise, especially aerobic exercise as little as walking 20 minutes a day, can improve cognitive and memory function as well as decrease risk for physical and cognitive deterioration.[76,77] In addition, Rebok et al[78] have reported on the benefits of cognitive stimulation in senior citizen volunteers. Volunteering in schools to promote literacy resulted in improved physical, social, and cognitive functioning in the elders.

Rebok et al[78] also described a number of the techniques found to enhance memory in older adults. One strategy that they found effective was the use of mnemonics. The challenge with using mnemonics is that they target memory and do not necessarily take into consideration other forms of age-related cognitive decline (eg, sensory, cognitive processing). Besides a decrease in memory formation, we know that other sensory changes often accompany increasing age such as vision loss, hearing loss, and auditory processing loss. Mahncke et al[12] studied a "brain plasticity-based training" that was adapted from a program previously used successfully with children. They used a computer-based program that provided sensory and cognitive exercises that became increasingly more complex and demanding with use. A variety of tasks were required targeting recognition, discrimination, sequencing, memory, and the like. They used novelty and rewards to facilitate the process as well. Their adult participants demonstrated learning and improved performance after dedicating only 1 hour per day to the activities. These promising results are in part attributable to what we now know about the brain and its ability to adapt to the demands placed upon it.

As health care providers and educators working with the elderly, it is important to consider strategies to help manage age-related cognitive decline. Allowing enough time for your elderly patient to process information is critical. Providing multimodal patient education materials may also enhance retention; however, care must be taken to ensure that the different modes of delivery are complementary and not distracting. Using memory cues such as logbooks or timers may prompt recall. Of course, we cannot overlook perhaps the most commonly used technique to enhance memory: writing down something to be remembered![78] Tapping into activities that are personally relevant by asking questions about other personal experiences related to the topic at hand can recruit episodic memory processes. Connecting the activity to something your patient finds fun (eg, dance, gardening, other hobbies) may pull in the emotional component of learning and retention as well. Finally, remember that gaining full attention to the incoming stimulus is an essential prerequisite to learning; therefore, keeping distractions to a minimum is critical.

Critical Thinking Clinical Scenario

Refer back to the scenarios of the 74-year-old patient with the total knee replacement and the 60-year-old patient with recent back surgery. You are at the point that you want to begin stair climbing with your 74-year-old patient, but he is feeling stressed, is fearful, and is having difficulty using the proper sequence in climbing the stairs. Despite your reminders, he continues to ascend and descend stairs the way he has always done it, which may be unsafe. Similarly, your 60-year-old patient, although apparently motivated, returns each week and tells you that she just could not seem to remember how to perform her home exercises safely.

Reflective Questions

Recognizing that part of the difficulty your patients may be experiencing in remembering the steps and sequencing his stair climbing appropriately or remembering her home exercise program could be in part the result of age-related cognitive and sensory decline:

1. What assumptions might some therapists hold about your patient's nonadherence to proper stair-climbing activities and performance of the prescribed home exercise program?
2. How can understanding age-related cognitive decline help to modify the assumptions that some may hold about an elderly patient's adherence to prescribed activities?
3. What strategies might you use to assist your patient in safely climbing stairs both in the clinic and in his home and in performing his home exercise program?

Key Points to Remember

- A decline in sensory function (eg, vision loss, hearing loss, and auditory processing loss) and the rate of processing information as well as the ability to process information from multiple sources simultaneously contribute to the decline in cognitive function and memory.
- Cognitive functions such as attention and memory are differentially affected with age.
  - Selective attention appears to still be preserved.
  - Short-term memory appears to be more impaired than long-term memory.
  - Declarative memory appears to be more impaired than procedural memory.
- Age-related changes include changes in the following:
  - The frontal cortex, which is critical for working memory and executive function (eg, planning, organizing).
  - Neuronal, neurochemical, metabolic, and receptor changes in the cerebral cortex and in the hippocampus.
  - Subcortical areas, especially the areas involved in the development of neurotransmitters such as dopamine.
  - Cellular and intercellular changes as a result of oxidative damage and neuroinflammation within the brain itself.
- To facilitate learning, memory formation, and memory retention in your aging patients:
  - Allow enough time for your elderly patient to process information.
  - Provide multimodal patient education materials (eg, written materials, videos, audio recordings, pictures).
  - Develop mnemonic strategies for remembering important information.
  - Use memory cues (eg, logbooks, timers).
  - Use personally relevant activities.
  - Use emotion to enhance learning and retention by making activities fun.
  - Optimize attention by minimizing distractions.
  - Provide for aerobic exercise.
  - Provide social contacts.

Summary

This chapter provides a general overview of some key structures of the brain, their functions, and how they may be involved in learning and memory. Perhaps the point most central to the application of brain research to teaching and learning is the incredible degree of complexity and interconnectedness that exists among all of the structures of the brain. From the neurons, at the cellular level, to the larger cortical and subcortical structures, brain structures never work in isolation. As educators, we have known for some time that our effectiveness as teachers and learners depends on us connecting new information to prior learning and using emotion to gain the attention of our learners and potentially enhance retention of the material being presented. We also know the importance of creating an environment, both in the classroom and in the clinic, that is conducive to learning. For us, this means continually monitoring the level of stress involved in learning. Some degree of mild stress may enhance learning; however, it is critical to remember that too much stress may impair learning and retention. Of equal importance is recognizing that stress is perceived differentially by individuals (ie, what may not be perceived as stressful by one person may be perceived as stressful by others). Monitoring the stress in the learning environment is essential to good teaching and learning. Finally, we know that using a variety of strategies to present new material allows us to engage our prior knowledge and recruit multiple memory pathways, which in turn strengthens neuronal connections. Though much is now known about how the brain functions, much still remains to be learned. Given the central role that student and patient education has in health care, it is important for us to stay informed about the latest findings in applied brain research.

Our goal in this chapter was to pique your interest in how much we know and how much we are still learning about brain function. As we said earlier, although we cannot make direct links from animal studies to human conditions or from molecules and neuronal connections to observed behaviors (yet!), pondering the potential links between the findings of cognitive psychologists and neuroscientists and the behavioral observations of educators and clinicians in the classroom and clinic certainly raises a number of interesting questions worthy of further study.[57] The field of neuroscience, along with the related fields of neuropsychiatry and neuropsychology, is developing rapidly. Researchers in education and psychology view learning from a behavioral perspective; neuroscientists view learning from anatomical and molecular perspectives. As these perspectives continue to converge, we will continue to gain greater insight into how we learn and therefore how we teach in the classroom and in the clinic, benefiting our learners and patients alike. As educators, rigorously exploring basic brain research to determine whether the findings apply in the classroom and clinic settings provides excellent opportunities to add to the scholarship of teaching. These are exciting times for scientists, clinicians, and educators alike!

Key Points to Remember

- To teach as effectively and efficiently as possible, it is important for us to work in concert with brain organization and function, not at cross-purposes with it.

- Understanding brain structure and function may enhance our ability to be effective in the teaching-learning situation.

- Memory is the basis for learning and includes the following:
  o Declarative memory (semantic, episodic)
  o Nondeclarative memory (procedural, emotional, and classical conditioning)

- Understanding what memory is, how it is formed, and what strategies can be used to enhance memory formation and retrieval may optimize our teaching and learning.

- Current information on brain structure and function may have implications for us as educators. As educators in the classroom and the clinic, it is important to
  o Recognize the role of stress and emotion in creating optimal learning environments.
  o Gain our learner's attention through the use of emotion and meaning.
  o Establish context for learning by connecting the new information to our learner's prior knowledge and personal experiences.

- The aging brain requires special consideration to enhance memory formation and retrieval.

- There is still much for us to learn about the brain, its structure, its function, and how it relates to teaching and learning.

References

1. Goswami U. Neuroscience and education: from research to practice? *Nat Rev Neurosci.* 2006;7:406-413.
2. Bandettini PA. The year in cognitive neuroscience 2009: what's new in neuroimaging methods? *Ann N Y Acad Sci.* 2009;1156:260-293.
3. Giedd J. The teen brain: insights from neuroimaging. *J Adolesc Health.* 2008;42:335-343.
4. Choudhury S, Blakemore S, Charman T. Social cognitive development during adolescence. *SCAN.* 2006;1:165-174.
5. Stevens M, Kiehl K, Pearlson G, Calhoun V. Functional neural networks underlying response inhibition in adolescents and adults. *Behav Brain Res.* 2007;181:12-22.
6. Galvan A, Hare T, Parra C, Penn J, Voss H. Earlier development of the acumbens relative to the orbitofrontal cortex may underlie risk-taking behavior in adolescents. *J Neurosci.* 2006;26:6885-6892.
7. Draganski B, Gaser C, Busch V, et al. Changes in grey matter induced by training. *Nature.* 2004;427:311-312.
8. Ebert T, Pantev C, Weinbruch C, Rockstroh B, Taub E. Increased cortical representation of the fingers of the left hand in string players. *Science.* 1995;270:305-307.
9. Sylwester R. *How to Explain a Brain.* Thousand Oaks, CA: Corwin Press; 2005.

10. Goldberg E. *The Executive Brain*. New York, NY: Oxford University Press; 2001.

11. Zull J. *The Art of Changing the Brain: Enriching the Practice of Teaching by Exploring the Biology of Learning*. Sterling, VA: Stylus Publishing; 2002.

12. Mahncke HW, Connor BB, Appelman J, et al. Memory enhancement in healthy older adults using a brain plasticity-based training program: a randomized, controlled study. *Proc Natl Acad Sci*. 2006;103:12523-12528.

13. Lamm C, Zelazo P, Lewis M. Neural correlates of cognitive control in childhood and adolescence: disentangling the contributions of age and executive function. *Neuropsychologia*. 2006;44:2139-2148.

14. Leon-Carrion J, Garcia-Orza L, Perez-Santamaria F. Development of the inhibitory components of the executive functions in children and adolescents. *Int J Neurosci*. 2004;114:1291-1311.

15. Gardner M, Steinberg L. Peer influence on risk taking, risk preference, and risky decision making in adolescence and adulthood: an experimental study. *Devel Psychol*. 2005;41: 625-635.

16. Ariely D. *Predictably Irrational*. New York, NY: HarperCollins; 2008.

17. Ratey J. *Spark*. New York, NY: Little, Brown & Co; 2008.

18. Medina J. *Brain Rules*. Seattle, WA: Pear Press; 2008.

19. Kolb D. *Experiential Learning: Experience as the Source of Learning and Development*. Englewood Cliffs, NJ: Prentice-Hall; 1984.

20. Squire L, Kandel E. *Memory: From Mind to Molecules*. 2nd ed. Greenwood Village, CO: Roberts and Company Publishers; 2009.

21. Gulpinar MA, Yegen BC. The physiology of learning and memory: role of peptides and stress. *Curr Protein Pept Sci*. 2004;5:457-473.

22. Bear MF, Connors BW, Paradiso MA. *Neuroscience: Exploring the Brain*. 3rd ed. Baltimore, MD: Lippincott Williams & Wilkins; 2007.

23. Hebbs D. *The Organization of Behavior: A Neuropsychological Theory*. Mahwah, NJ: Laurence Erlbaum Associates; 2002.

24. Siegel D. *The Developing Mind: Toward a Neurobiology of Interpersonal Experience*. New York, NY: Guilford Press; 1999.

25. Wolfe P. *Brain Matters*. Alexandria, VA: Association for Supervision and Curriculum Development; 2001.

26. Marieb E. *Human Anatomy & Physiology*. 4th ed. Menlo Park, CA: Benjamin/Cummings Science Publishing; 1998.

27. Ivry R, Fiez J. Cerebellar contributions to cognition and imagery. In: Gazzaniga M, ed. *The New Cognitive Neuroscience*. Cambridge, MA: MIT Press; 2000:999-1011.

28. Manes F, Villamil AR, Ameriso S, Roca M, Torralva T. "Real life" executive deficits in patients with focal vascular lesions affecting the cerebellum. *J Neuro Sci*. 2009;283:95-98.

29. Jensen E. *Teaching with the Brain in Mind*. 2nd ed. Alexandria, VA: Association for Supervision and Curriculum Development; 2005.

30. Schmahmann JD, Weilburg JB, Sherman JC. The neuropsychiatry of the cerebellum—insights from the clinic. *Cerebellum*. 2007;6:264-267.

31. Parker J, Mitchell A, Kalpakidou A, et al. Cerebellar growth and behavioural & neuropsychological outcome in preterm adolescents. *Brain*. 2008;131:1344-1351.

32. Ravizza S, McCormick C, Schlerf J, Justus T, Ivry R, Fiez J. Cerebellar damage produces selective deficits in verbal working memory. *Brain*. 2006;129:306-320.

33. Shah D, Anderson P, Carlin J, et al. Reduction in cerebellar volumes in preterm infants: relationship to white matter injury and neurodevelopment at two years of age. *Pediatr Res*. 2006;60:97-102.

34. Sousa D. *How the Brain Learns*. Thousand Oaks, CA: Corwin; 2006.

35. Budson AE. Understanding memory dysfunction. *Neurologist*. 2009;15:71-79.

36. Meeter M, Veldkamp R, Jin Y. Multiple memory stores and operant conditioning: a rationale for memory's complexity. *Brain Cogn*. 2009;69:200-208.

37. LaBar KS, Cabeza R. Cognitive neuroscience of emotional memory. *Nat Rev Neurosci*. 2006;7:54-64.

38. Phelps EA, LeDoux JE. Contributions of the amygdala to emotion processing: from animal models to human behavior. *Neuron*. 2005;48:175-187.

39. Daw ND, Shohamy D. The cogntivie neuroscience of motivation and learning. *Soc Cogn*. 2008;26:593-620.

40. Wise R. Dopamine, learning, and motivation. *Nat Rev Neurosci*. 2004;5:1-12.

41. Serrien DJ, Ivry RB, Swinnen SP. Dynamics of hemispheric specialization and integration in the context of motor control. *Nat Rev Neurosci*. 2006;7:160-167.

42. Fernandez G, Tendolkar I. Integrated brain activity in medial temporal and prefrontal areas predicts subsequent memory performance: human declarative memory formation at the system level. *Brain Res Bull*. 2001;55:1-9.

43. Kim JJ, Song EY, Kosten TA. Stress effects in the hippocampus: synaptic plasticity and memory. *Stress*. 2006;9:1-11.

44. van Strien NM, Cappaert NLM, Witter MP. The anatomy of memory: an interactive overview of the parahippocampal-hippocampal network. *Nat Rev Neurosci*. 2009;10:272-282.

45. Gallace A, Spence C. The cognitive and neural correlates of tactile memory. *Psychol Bull*. 2009;135:380-406.

46. Patterson K, Nestor PJ, Rogers TT. Where do you know what you know? The representation of semantic knowledge in the human brain. *Nat Rev Neurosci*. 2007;8:976-988.

47. Muzzio IA, Kentros C, Kandel E. What is remembered? Role of attention on the encoding and retrieval of hippocampal representations. *J Physiol*. 2009;587:2837-2854.

48. Sotres-Bayon F, Cain C, LeDoux J. Brain mechanisms of fear extinction: historical perspectives on the contribution of prefrontal cortex. *Biol Psychiatry*. 2006;60:329-336.

49. Hamm A, Weike A. The neuropsychology of fear learning and fear regulation. *Int J Psychophysiol*. 2005;57:5-14.

50. LeDoux J. *Synaptic Self*. New York, NY: Penguin Books; 2002.

51. Kim JJ, Song EY, Kosten TA. Stress effects in the hippocampus: synaptic plasticity and memory. *Stress Mem*. 2006;9:1-11.

52. Ratey J. *A User's Guide to the Brain*. New York, NY: Vintage Books; 2001.

53. van Stegeren AH. Imaging stress effects on memory: a review of neuroimaging studies. *Can J Psychiatry*. 2009;54:16-27.

54. Phelps E. Human emotion and memory: interactions of the amygdala and hippocampal complex. *Curr Opin Neurobiol*. 2004;14:198-202.

55. Hamann S, Ely T, Grafton S, Kilts C. Amygdala activity related to enhanced memory for pleasant and aversive stimuli. *Nat Neurosci*. 1999;2:289-293.

56. LeBaron SWM, Jernick J. Evaluation as a dynamic process. *Fam Med*. 2000;32:13-14.

57. Bruer JT. Points of view: on the implications of neuroscience research for science teaching and learning: are there any? A skeptical theme and variations: the primacy of psychology in the science of learning. *Life Sci Educ*. 2006;5:104-110.

58. Knowles M, Holton E, Swanson R. *The Adult Learner*. Woburn, MA: Butterworth-Heinemann; 1998.

59. Kensinger E, Corkin S. Two routes to emotional memory: distinct neural processes for valence and arousal. *Proc Natl Acad Sci*. 2004;101:3311-3315.

60. Roozendaal B, McEwen BS, Chattarji S. Stress, memory and the amygdala. *Nat Rev Neurosci*. 2009;10:423-433.

61. Shors TJ. Learning during stressful times. *Learn Mem.* 2004;11:137-144.

62. Joels M, Shenwei P, Wiegert O, Oitzl MS, Krugers HJ. Learning under stress: how does it work? *Trends Cogn Sci.* 2006;10: 152-158.

63. Caron MG, Wightman RM. "To learn, you must pay attention." Molecular insights into teachers' wisdom. *Proc Natl Acad Sci.* 2009;106:7267-7268.

64. McGaugh JL. Memory consolidation and the amygdala: a systems perspective. *Trends Neurosci.* 2002;25:456-461.

65. Uncapher MR, Rugg MD. Selecting for memory? The influence of selective attention on the mnemonic binding of contextual information. *J Neurosci.* 2009;29:8270-8279.

66. Tobias S. Interest, prior knowledge, and learning. *Rev Educ Res.* 1994;64:37-54.

67. Peters J, Daum I, Gizewski E, Forsting M, Suchan B. Associations evoked during memory encoding recruit the context-network. *Hippocampus.* 2009;19:141-151.

68. Hoffman AB, Harris HD, Murphy GL. Prior knowledge enhances the category dimensionality effect. *Mem Cognit.* 2008;36: 256-270.

69. Della Libera C, Chelazzi L. Learning to attend and to ignore is a matter of gains and losses. *Psychol Sci.* 2009; 20:778-784.

70. Pastalkova E, Itskov VA, Buzsaki G. Internally generated cell assembly sequences in the rat hippocampus. *Science.* 2008;321:1322-1327.

71. Riddle DR, Schindler MK. Brain aging research. *Rev Clin Gerontol.* 2007;17:225-239.

72. Sylwester R. *The Adolescent Brain: Reaching for Autonomy.* Thousand Oaks, CA: Corwin Press; 2007.

73. Fick D, Kolanowski A, Beattie E, McCrow J. Delirium in early stage Alzheimer's disease: enhancing cognitive reserve as a possible preventive measure. *J Gerontol Nurs.* 2009;35:30-39.

74. Newson RS, Kemps EB. The influence of physical and cognitive activities on simple and complex cognitive tasks in older adults. *Exp Aging Res.* 2006;32:341-362.

75. Wang H, Karp A, Winblad B, Fratiglioni L. Late-life engagement in social and leisure activities is associated with a decreased risk of dementia: a longitudinal study from the Kungsholmen Project. *Am J Epidemiol.* 2002;155:1081-1087.

76. Colcombe SJ, Erickson KI, Raz N, et al. Aerobic fitness reduces brain tissue loss in aging humans. *J Gerontol A Biol Sci Med Sci.* 2003;58:M176-180.

77. Bijnen F, Caspersen C, Feskens E, Saris W, Mosterd W, Kromhout D. Physical activity and 10 year mortality from cardiovascular diseases and all causes. *Arch Intern Med.* 1998;158:1499-1505.

78. Rebok GW, Carlson MC, Langbaum JBS. Training and maintaining memory abilities in healthy older adults: traditional and novel approaches. *J Gerontol B Psychol Sci Soc Sci.* 2007;62: 53-61.

SECTION II

DESIGNING, IMPLEMENTING, AND ASSESSING EFFECTIVE INSTRUCTION

4

Systematic Effective Instruction
Keys to Designing Effective Presentations

Chapter Objectives

After reading this chapter, you will be prepared to:

- Design effective needs assessments to ensure your presentation meets the needs of your learners.

- Develop appropriate learner-centered objectives in 3 domains of learning to guide your presentation.

- Differentiate between designing single presentations versus presentations linked to a course or a curriculum.

- Create effective motivational hooks and content boosters that capture your learners' attention and maintain it while reinforcing learning.

- Determine how best to sequence a presentation to optimize engagement and learning.

- Select active learning strategies that will engage your learners, reinforce their learning, and enhance their retention.

- Design formative and summative assessments to enhance teaching and learning.

Have you ever had to give a morning presentation to a class when they were having their anatomy midterm that afternoon? Have you ever had to give an in-service to a group of therapists during lunch on a very busy Friday? Have you ever had to do a presentation on Monday at 8 AM after a holiday weekend? Finally, have you ever sat through a lecture and halfway through realized you had been daydreaming and totally missed what the presenter was saying? In this chapter, we will provide you with strategies that will help grab your audience's attention and maintain it throughout your presentation, no matter what the content or when you might be presenting!

Stop and Reflect

You have been asked to put on a presentation about osteoporosis for a community-based women's group. The presentation is set for next month.

- What factors will influence your preparation?

- How will you decide what to teach?

- What teaching-learning activities will you use?

In responding to the scenario presented above, you may have remembered, and reflected on, the various filters that influence the teaching-learning process presented in the first chapter. You may have considered the cultural background and generational status of the audience, as well as learning styles and characteristics of the adult learner. Next, you may have thought about your topic, osteoporosis, and what you know about it. Remembering that any new information must connect to prior knowledge, you may have reviewed some facts about osteoporosis that you learned in school. It is possible that you also remembered that your aunt was diagnosed recently with osteopenia, a precursor to osteoporosis, and that your grandmother had broken several bones due to osteoporosis. Having these episodic or autobiographical memories about your relatives arrive unprompted makes sense to you now that you know how the various memory pathways work together. Certainly your grandmother's story had an emotional

Plack M, Driscoll M. *Teaching and Learning in Physical Therapy: From Classroom to Clinic* (pp 67-116).
© 2011 SLACK Incorporated

Table 4-1. Keys Tasks to Consider in Preparing a Presentation

- Assess the needs of the audience
- Design learner-centered objectives
- Define the specific content
- Create motivational hooks
- Utilize content boosters
  - o Action learning strategies
  - o Guided practice
  - o Independent practice
- Develop formative and summative assessments to check for understanding
- Summarize the key points

Adapted from Hunter M. *Mastery Teaching.* Thousand Oaks, CA: Corwin; 1982; Garmston RJ, Wellman BM. *How to Make Presentations That Teach and Transform.* Alexandria, VA: Association for Supervision and Curriculum Development; 1992; Silberman M, Auerbach C. *Active Training: A Handbook of Techniques, Designs, Case Examples, and Tips.* 3rd ed. San Francisco, CA: John Wiley & Sons; 2006.

impact on you, and you may wonder how you can help your audience connect in a similar way. The topic, osteoporosis, becomes a stimulus for anything you connect with that word.

In addition to reflecting on some of the topics presented in the previous chapter, the first question a novice presenter often wants answered when asked to speak on a topic is, "How much time will I have?" This question may be followed by, "Who will be in the audience?" Although these questions address factors that are important, they are insufficient to determine how to best design an optimal teaching-learning activity. As you can see from this discussion, when asked to do a presentation, intuitively, you may begin to consider many of the concepts presented earlier in this text. You may not yet recognize all of the steps needed in preparing for a presentation, however. Whether you are doing a guest lecture in a doctor of physical therapy class, speaking to a community group, or instructing a patient, there are a number of essential steps to be considered when you are preparing to teach.

This chapter describes a comprehensive, systematic approach to instruction that includes assessing the needs of your audience, gaining their attention, and presenting appropriate content that meets the objectives you have specified ahead of time. This approach incorporates periodic assessments, practice opportunities, and a summary. Because we know that we are more likely to learn and retain information more effectively when multiple memory pathways are engaged, we will emphasize the importance of active learning, using teaching strategies that are multidimensional and interactive. These concepts will be reinforced in later chapters as you begin to see how these very same steps are not only important for classroom or community presentations but effective in planning patient education activities as well.

What to Consider in Preparing to Teach

Critical Thinking Clinical Scenario

Consider these 2 scenarios:

1. You are preparing to teach a class on manual therapy to a group of doctor of physical therapy students.

2. You are preparing to teach your patient an exercise regimen for strengthening his lower back.

Reflective Questions

1. What do you need to consider in preparing to teach in each of the above scenarios? Develop a list for each.

2. How do your lists compare? What is similar about the 2 lists, and what is different?

What did you include in your list of things you need to consider? Most likely, you mentioned the content and the goals or objectives for your topic. Perhaps your list includes providing an opportunity for your participants to practice the skills you taught along with an opportunity for you to observe them practicing to see how well they learned the skills you presented. However, planning for optimal learning, as Fink[1] described, requires us to be even more comprehensive in our approach. We need to consider what the audience already knows about the topic and how to engage the learner's attention, boost content, provide for different types of practice, summarize content, and periodically assess mastery of what we have taught. Table 4-1 contains a list of tasks considered essential to preparing presentations.[2-6]

Knowing Your Audience and Assessing Their Needs

Critical Thinking Clinical Scenario

Revisit the scenario presented at the beginning of this chapter in which you are giving a presentation on osteoporosis to a group of women in your community.

Reflective Questions

1. How would you approach the task if you knew that everyone in the audience had osteoporosis?

2. How would you adapt your talk if you knew that the average age of members in the audience was 20?

3. Would it matter to you if the average age was 60? If so, how? What would you add to your talk? Delete?

4. Would you do things differently if you were told that the audience was composed of health care workers, including nurse practitioners, who were interested in how to incorporate exercise into the recommendations they usually give to women? How would you modify the content?

5. What if your audience was composed of doctor of physical therapy students learning about osteoporosis in an advanced orthopedics course? How might your content differ?

Who Is in Your Audience?

After reflecting on, and responding to, the Critical Thinking Clincal Scenario above, it becomes clear that it is important for you to consider your audience and their needs before planning the content you wish to teach. You might describe different strengthening exercises for 25 year olds than you would for 60 year olds. You might include more information about physiology and kinesiology when presenting to health care practitioners or doctor of physical therapy students than you would for an audience of laypeople. Given what we know about the brain and how neuronal connections are developed based on our prior experiences, it makes sense to learn as much about an audience as possible before designing a teaching-learning experience. In learning about your audience, it will be important for you to recognize and consider the following:

- Learning styles of your audience members
- Level of expertise (ie, novice to expert) of your audience
- Expectations of your audience

What Kind of Learners Are in Your Audience?

Even before conducting an actual needs assessment, we can make some general assumptions about the individual members of the audience. As we learned from our discussion on learning styles in Chapter 1, a presenter should generally expect that all 4 learning styles will be represented in every audience. Without doing a formal assessment of each individual's styles, you can assume from Kolb's[7] work that in any audience, some learners will prefer to watch and listen, whereas others might prefer to be active in the learning experience. At the same time, you will likely have participants who primarily want theory and facts, whereas others might prefer concrete examples, anecdotes, and stories. The optimal teaching-learning experience includes something for each preference, which, if you remember, is the basis for our motto "Teach Around the Wheel"!

Garmston and Wellman[3] provided us with a slightly different view of the audience than Kolb.[7] In any given audience, they too encourage presenters to be cognizant of the presence of 4 different types of learners. They described each type of learner as focusing on a different question. As a presenter, you will want to be sure to answer the questions posed by each. Garmston and Wellman[3] actually gave names to each of the different types of learners:

- The "scientist" wants to know *why* he or she should pay attention to you; what is the personal connection for him or her?

- The "professor" wants to know *what* is important, what are the facts, the objective information you are presenting.

- The "friend" seeks the *so what* or implications of what you are teaching on his or her physical well-being, job, or other relevant factor.

- The "inventor" will listen to your presentation with the perspective of *what if*; how can this information be adapted and reorganized to better meet my, or someone else's, needs?

As you think about your topic, if you can imagine people asking these questions, you can begin to organize your content to answer the questions of the different types of audience members and in this way satisfy the needs of each learner.

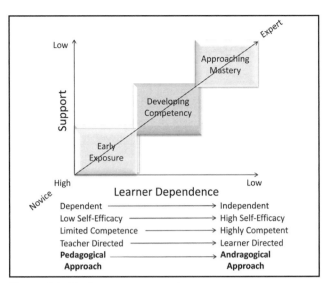

Figure 4-1. Novice to expert continuum.

What Is the Level of Expertise of Your Audience?

The level of expertise of your audience is another factor to consider in determining the actual content you will present. How much does your audience already know about the topic? Will you be introducing a topic to your audience for the first time? Pat Benner[8] is commonly cited in health care literature for her research on the novice to expert continuum. In her seminal work on the development of expertise in nursing, "From Novice to Expert," she first described the Dreyfus Model of Skill Acquisition.[9] Jensen et al[10] used this same model in their study of *Expertise in Physical Therapy Practice*. Dreyfus et al[9] proposed a 5-stage model of skill development:

1. *Novice*—Has no experience with the content, skill, or situation; this learner relies on rules and input from others to guide learning and performance.

2. *Advanced beginner*—Has some exposure to or experience with the content and is just beginning to develop competence; this learner is less rule governed than the novice but still relies on others for guidance; this learner continues to need help in setting priorities and recognizing the important aspects of a given situation.

3. *Competent*—Has some exposure and experience with the content and as a result has developed some degree of competence; with greater experience than the advanced beginner, this learner can begin to rely less on abstract rules and more on applying the information to make decisions in a given context; at this point, the competent learner can prioritize information and effectively apply the information to a variety of situations.

4. *Proficient*—Has the ability to view the situation as a whole; these learners rely on past experiences to help them recognize patterns so they can quickly see when something does not fit the pattern as expected; unlike the learner in the competent stage, the proficient learner has enough experience to determine what aspects of a situation are most important.

5. *Expert*—Has had significant exposure to and experience with the content and no longer relies on abstract rules; this learner can quickly discern a situation and know when to take action; given this learner's depth of understanding and experience, he or she relies to a large extent on intuition.

Understanding where along the continuum your learner's abilities and experiences fall will help you determine how to approach the teaching-learning situation. Figure 4-1 provides a pictorial view of the novice to expert continuum based on the work of a number of adult theorists including Philip Candy,[11] Malcolm Knowles and coworkers,[12] and Daniel Pratt,[13] as well as the work of Pat Benner.[8]

Figure 4-1 demonstrates how learners at the novice end of the continuum (ie, during early exposure) show a low level of competence and self-efficacy in the subject matter and therefore may be dependent upon direction from the teacher and require a great deal of support in their learning. As a teacher, you will likely provide them with significant content information; you may take a more pedagogical approach and provide a great deal of structure, guidance, and supervision. As the learner develops some degree of competence, you may begin to provide less structure and direction and more guidance and feedback; you will want to provide more opportunities for independent practice, complex problem solving, application, and integration. Finally, if you are presenting to an audience of individuals with a high degree of competence, your role as an instructor would be to design a learning situation that requires the learners to actively integrate the information into what they already know. Your presentation may require your learners to be more independent and self-directed in their approach. For example, you may structure your presentation around a complex case study and require your learners to take greater control through independent research and problem solving. You may also ask your learners to reflect on the content, asking them to apply the information to a variety of situations in more creative and novel ways.

For example, the concept of strength training for people in their eighties may be new to someone unfamiliar with the latest research on the benefits of exercise for elderly individuals. If this were the case for your audience, the purpose of your presentation would likely be early exposure to the topic, and you would likely be providing basic information; discussing indications, contraindications, and various types of strength training activities; and using interesting case material to demonstrate the principles discussed. As the instructor, you will need to provide more structure and supervision.

On the other hand, perhaps your audience members have been exposed to the topic of strength training in the elderly already and they now want to develop competence in designing appropriate programs for residents of an assisted-living facility. In your presentation, you will more likely be guiding your learners through interactive discussions and practice with a variety of strength-training activities; you may guide them through a variety of case studies and use guided practice to help them develop exercise protocols for individuals with various health conditions.

Finally, if you are conducting an advanced continuing education course for master clinicians or experts, you may challenge your learners to apply and integrate the information to plan interventions for more complex geriatric patient cases such as adults with intellectual developmental disabilities. You will likely use small group problem-solving activities to draw on the experience and depth of understanding of your audience members.

It is important to remember that you can have learners who have achieved a significant level of expertise in one content area yet still be novices in another. As the instructor, understanding where along the continuum your learners' knowledge, skills, and experiences are relative to the content you will be teaching is critical in designing your presentation.

Key Points to Remember

As learners develop expertise, they will move from novices to experts along the continuum of:

- Early exposure
- Developing competence
- Approaching mastery

At each stage along the continuum, learners have different needs; therefore, teachers have different roles:

- Early exposure
  - *Learner needs:* Looking for details; they are dependent on the instructor for content; they require close supervision and structure.
  - *Teacher role:* Providing information, structure, and needed supervision.
- Developing competence
  - *Learner needs:* Ready to participate and actively engage with the material (eg, guided practice) and can begin applying it to practice.
  - *Teacher role:* Guiding your learner through practice and feedback.
- Approaching mastery
  - *Learner needs:* Interested in integrating the material into daily practice and activities to solve increasingly more complex problems.
  - *Teacher role:* Challenging the learner to independently apply and adapt what has been taught to his or her own practice and to complex and novel situations (eg, problem solving, independent practice, and creative utilization).

What Are the Expectations of Your Audience?

Stop and Reflect

Have you ever gone to a presentation and walked out thinking, "How disappointing, that was not at all what I expected to hear"?

- How did this mismatch occur?
- How might this mismatch have been prevented?

It is also important that your planned presentation and the expectations of the audience are congruent; otherwise, you may very well disappoint your audience and leave unsatisfied yourself. In presenting to any audience of adult learners in particular, it is important to remember that they want to know:

- *What* they will be expected to learn.
- *How* learning will occur and *how* it will be evaluated.
- *Why* it is important for them to learn what you are teaching.
- *Who* the teacher is and what qualifies him or her to teach the content.

Key Points to Remember

Adult learners will want to know:

- *What* they will be expected to learn.
- *How* learning will occur and *how* it will be evaluated.
- *Why* it is important for them to learn what you are teaching.
- *Who* the teacher is and what qualifies him or her to teach the content.

A personal introduction will help the learner understand who you are and what makes you qualified to teach him or her. Creating a plan and goals for your presentation and making them explicit to your audience during the introduction will help them understand the purpose of your presentation and why it is important. It will also give them a sense of what you will expect from them as learners during the presentation. But perhaps most important in designing a presentation is clarifying the needs of your learners. Designing your presentation around their needs will both motivate your learners and add to the success of your presentation.[6]

What Are the Needs of Your Audience?

Once you have considered the audience in general, it is time to get more specific and learn as much as you can about the needs of the individuals who will participate in your learning experience. The needs assessment is the next essential step in developing an effective presentation. Conducting some type of needs assessment will allow you to tailor your presentation to best meet the needs of your learners. The needs assessment can also help you learn more about what people *want* to learn about the topic, their prior exposure to the topic, their preferred methods of instruction, as well as the time of day and location for instruction (eg, staff lounge versus library). The more information you have about the audience, the better you can customize your instructional design.

Ideally, your needs assessment should be done ahead of time. Taking the time to determine the needs of your audience members shows them you care and can help you build a relationship with them before you even

begin presenting. By gathering the information early, you can also obtain specific examples or case material relevant to your audience members, which may also build interest and motivate them to participate in your presentation. Talking with your participants ahead of time may help you refine your content and mode of delivery or even make you decide to change your topic all together. In some instances, the information gleaned from a needs assessment can help determine whether your presentation is even necessary or feasible.[6]

Key Points to Remember

Needs assessments may help you:

- Build relationships with your participants.
- Build interest in and motivation for your topic.
- Obtain specific and relevant case material to support your presentation.
- Determine the feasibility and applicability of your topic.
- Refine your content.
- Refine your method of delivery.

Needs assessments are beneficial in all teaching-learning situations. Clinicians routinely do needs assessments on their patients. For example, when developing appropriate home exercise instructions, the experienced clinician uses knowledge of the patient's daily activities, personal goals and current level of activity, and information obtained formally or informally through prior interactions with the patient. Without labeling it a needs assessment, the clinician uses this background information to design a more effective home exercise program.

How Will You Assess the Needs of Your Audience?

There are numerous approaches to conducting needs assessments prior to meeting with your participants.[4,6,14] Garmston and Wellman[3] recommend an in-person or telephone conversation between the presenter and a number of key participants who may have different perspectives on the topic to be presented. In this era of Internet ease, an on-line discussion about these topics among representative participants and the instructor could easily substitute for an in-person conference or phone call. Table 4-2 provides sample questions you might ask during this phone conversation to determine the needs of your audience.

Wlodkowski[4] and Silberman and Auerbach[6] described a variety of needs assessment techniques. A list of sample strategies, adapted from both Wlodkowski[4] and Silberman and Auerbach,[6] along with an example of how each might be applied in physical therapy or in the health care arena appears in Table 4-3.

Table 4-2. Sample Needs Assessment Questions

- Who are the participants?
- What is the composition of the audience in terms of roles and possible attitudes toward the topic?
- What is the audience's prior exposure to the topic?
- What is their experience with the subject (novice, expert)?
- What is their current level of knowledge? Skill?
- What are their attitudes toward the topic?
- How many participants will be present?
- Do participants believe they have a "need to know"?
- Is attendance mandatory or voluntary?
- What are the participants' expectations about the topic? The presenter?
- What is the context of this presentation? Is it part of a series of presentations? If so, what will come before and after this presentation?
- How might the topic impact their current work activities?
- Are there any underlying problems that I might encounter or needs I should address?
- What is a typical in-service like for them (ie, what types of teaching strategies are they used to)?
- What is the physical environment like?
- Will I have access to resources (eg, Internet, handouts, projector)?
- Are there any possibilities for follow-up?

Adapted from Garmston RJ, Wellman BM. *How to Make Presentations That Teach and Transform*. Alexandria, VA: Association for Supervision and Curriculum Development; 1992; Silberman M, Auerbach C. *Active Training: A Handbook of Techniques, Designs, Case Examples, and Tips*. 3rd ed. San Francisco, CA: John Wiley & Sons; 2006.

Table 4-3. Sample Needs Assessment Strategies

Needs Assessment Strategies	Description	Sample Application in Physical Therapy and Health Care Practice
Observation and experience	Spend time talking with and observing representative people within the organization, preferably engaged in tasks related to your topic	Observe several therapists engaged in performing specific special tests to determine current practice and potential learning needs
Written surveys and questionnaires	Use paper or electronic questionnaires ahead of time to assess reactions, knowledge, attitudes, perceptions, experiences, etc, related to the topic	Develop and disseminate a survey of questions related to your topic and its relevance to the participants
Interview key consultants	In-person or telephone contact with a select number of individuals who know the group you will be working with and can provide essential information relevant to your topic or presentation	Interview program directors, clinical instructors, senior staff, and junior staff to determine the varying levels of expertise and exposure to your topic
Focus group sessions	In a group of 4 to 8 people who are representative of the larger audience, discuss relevant topics to learn more about underlying ideas and issues and to obtain their perspectives on how to design the training for the group	Gather a diverse group of therapists, aides, nurses, physicians, students, etc (individuals who may attend your presentation) and discuss your topic and their perceptions of its relevance to each of the participants. Explore the diverse learning stages of your potential audience
Print materials	Use information (eg, from annual reports, print media, newsletters) to determine the larger context in which presentation will occur	Review recent journals, continuing education advertisements, newsletters, job ads, etc, to determine potential topics for discussion or presentation
Job or task analysis	Using the learner-centered objective established for your presentation, select a number of work activities and analyze them in terms of how they relate to your goals	Complete a task analysis of how patients are scheduled for therapy to determine areas in which educational enhancement or process improvement is needed
Records, reports, work samples	Analyze relevant work samples to determine current levels of expertise and needs for training	Analyze completed documentation to determine potential areas in need of educational enhancement or process improvement
Performance test/tasks	Use standardized measures to assess the knowledge and skills of learners that relate to the topic	Have all members of a given team or staff complete a learning styles inventory to address strategies to enhance team performance

Adapted from Wlodkowski RJ. *Enhancing Adult Motivation to Learn*. Revised ed. San Francisco, CA: Jossey-Bass; 1999; Silberman M, Auerbach C. *Active Training: A Handbook of Techniques, Designs, Case Examples, and Tips*. 3rd ed. San Francisco, CA: John Wiley & Sons; 2006.

Critical Thinking Clinical Scenario

You have a world-renowned expert in women's health coming to a nearby major metropolitan area in May. She would like to offer a continuing education conference on a topic of your choice and wants your clinic to sponsor it. Her fee for the 2 days is $5000 plus hotel, travel, and accommodations. You are personally very excited because that is your area of practice, but how do you decide whether to move forward or not?

Reflective Questions

In completing a needs assessment to determine the feasibility of sponsoring a continuing education conference:
1. What would you need to know?
2. Who would you assess?
3. How would you assess them?

Key Points to Remember

- The more you know about the learners you teach, the better you can tailor your instruction to meet their needs.
- Techniques for conducting needs assessment prior to a presentation include the following:
  - Face-to-face interviews and discussion strategies
  - Paper-and-pencil questionnaires
  - A review of printed material such as case records (de-identified), annual reports, and professional literature
- On-the-spot needs assessment in the form of questions posed at the beginning and throughout a presentation can yield valuable information.
- In assessing the needs of your audience, it is helpful to ask:
  - General questions
  - Content-specific questions
  - Theoretical questions
  - Practical questions

Although needs assessments provide the most useful information when completed ahead of time, this is not always feasible. You can do a needs assessment at the start of your presentation by using judicious questions. Completing a needs assessment ahead of time will give you a general sense of who will be in your audience; completing an on-the-spot needs assessment will give you a better sense of your specific audience. For example, if you are doing a presentation on how to teach skin self-examination to prevent skin breakdown in the diabetic patient, asking your audience, "Who has worked with patients who have had diabetes and diabetic ulcers?" will give you some indication of the audience's experience related to your topic. Garmston[14] provided a framework for the types of questions you might ask at the start of your presentation, including general questions, content-specific questions, theoretical questions, and practical questions. Table 4-4 provides some examples of on-the-spot assessments using this framework in teaching and learning and in health care.

Developing Learner-Centered Behavioral Objectives

Stop and Reflect

You are doing a presentation to physical therapy students on developing patient education materials.
- What do you want your learner to know as a result of your presentation?
- What do you want your learner to be able to do as a result of participating in the presentation?
- How will you determine that your presentation has been effective?

Table 4-4. On-the-Spot Assessment Strategies

On-the-Spot Assessment Types	Sample Application in Teaching and Learning	Sample Application in Physical Therapy and Health Care Practice
General questions	How many of you have had formal training in giving presentations? For how many of you is this content totally new?	How many of you gather evidence on your patients more than once per month? Once per week?
Content-specific questions	How many of you have done needs assessments before? Used motivational hooks? Used formative assessment?	What databases do you most often use for your searches?
Theoretical questions	How many of you agree that active learning strategies increase retention?	How many of you agree that the only evidence that is important enough to consider in patient care comes from randomized controlled trials?
Practical questions	What is the one thing you would really like to learn today?	How many of you have access to the Internet routinely?

Adapted from Garmston R. *The Presenter's Fieldbook: A Practical Guide.* Norwood, MA: Christopher-Gordon; 1997.

When planning any instructional activity, whether it is a verbal presentation or written materials, it is important to think about the outcomes you want your learners to produce before you actually begin designing the presentation. Steven Covey,[15] in *The 7 Habits of Highly Effective People*, discusses the concept of "beginning with the end in mind" whenever you are planning a course of action (p. 98). If teaching someone is the course of action you are planning, you need to think about the end result, the actual outcome the learner is expected to produce. Well-written objectives define the end result of your instruction and provide you with a "road map" to follow throughout both the design and delivery of your presentation.

Key Point to Remember

BEGIN WITH THE END IN MIND!—Steven Covey[15]

In the situation presented at the beginning of this section, you were asked to think about what you might want your learners to be able to do as a result of participating in your presentation on developing patient education materials. If you want your learners to physically create effective patient education materials rather than merely describe what must be considered in developing patient education materials, this outcome needs to be specified ahead of time because this will drive not only the design of the instruction but the expected outcomes of the learner. Developing learning objectives will help you determine the content of your presentation as well as the methods you will use in teaching the content. At the end of your presentation, the learning objectives will also help you determine whether the learner has grasped the critical information and as a result will give you feedback about how effective you were as an instructor. Learning objectives, often referred to as *behavioral objectives*, are specific statements of what you expect your learner to achieve as a result of the presentation.

Key Points to Remember

Well-written learning objectives will help you:
- Define your content
- Determine the teaching methods you will use
- Assess your learners' performance (ie, did your learners learn what you expected them to learn?)
- Assess your effectiveness as an instructor

Benjamin Bloom[16] described 3 distinct domains of learning:

1. The *cognitive domain* refers to the development of knowledge, language-based information, and concepts to be learned. For example, student physical therapists are expected to identify the origins and insertions of various muscles as well as design-appropriate home exercise programs to strengthen certain muscle groups.

2. The *psychomotor domain* refers to the development of motor skills to be mastered. For example, student physical therapists must learn how to transfer patients from a bed to a wheelchair as well as adapt interventions for bedside treatment.

3. The *affective domain* refers to the development of attitudes, feelings, beliefs, and values, which can range from the more simple level of recognizing the importance of something to the more complex level of actually integrating and adopting behaviors that reflect the value. For example, a patient might say, "I know I need to do my exercises more often," demonstrating that he recognizes the value or importance of doing the home exercise program. On the other hand, if your patient says "I am doing my exercises routinely because I know they are important," you know that he has adopted this value personally.

Key Points to Remember

The 3 domains of learning described by Benjamin Bloom[16] are:
- Cognitive: Knowledge
- Psychomotor: Skill
- Affective: Attitudes, beliefs, and values

Critical Thinking Clinical Scenario

The following are examples of learning objectives that might be found in a doctor of physical therapy curriculum:
- After this laboratory session, the student will correctly list 5 contraindications to using ultrasound as an intervention.
- By the end of this clinical internship, the student will integrate the core value of professionalism into his or her daily interactions.
- At the end of this course, the student will safely transfer patients from the bed to a wheelchair.

Reflective Questions

1. Which domain of learning does each objective reflect?
2. How might you change each of these objectives to address a different domain of learning?

Each domain of learning is distinct and should be considered in developing learning objectives. In defining the domains, as can be noted by the examples above, Bloom[16] also developed a taxonomy or hierarchical system of classifying objectives from simple (ie, recall) to more complex (ie, evaluation). Table 4-5 illustrates the taxonomic levels of learning in the 3 domains of learning. Bloom[16] and later Krathwohl et al[17] and Simpson[18] provided sample verbs for each level to enable instructors to write objectives that effectively target each level along the hierarchy. As you move up the hierarchy in creating objectives, you increase the level of complexity and challenge of each objective.

The objectives you establish for any given presentation must meet the needs of the learners. As discussed earlier in this chapter, the level of expertise and learning expectations of your audience will vary from a basic level of exposure to a topic, to a higher level expectation of content mastery and integration of information and skills into one's current practice. If your expectations (ie, learning objectives) do not match those of your audience, both you and your audience will be disappointed. In a classroom, establishing expectations up front by using explicit and detailed learning objectives will help your learners know what your expectations are and will enable them to be better prepared to meet your expectations. Students often ask, "What will be on the test?" Having explicit learning objectives should help to minimize the need for this question.

What follows is a more detailed description of the taxonomies within each of the 3 domains of learning defined by Bloom[16] along with some sample verbs for each level in the taxonomies, which may help you in developing appropriate learning objectives.

Cognitive Domain

If you take a look at your course syllabi, you may see that many of the objectives relate closely to the cognitive domain. The cognitive domain is typically the one domain with which instructors and learners are most familiar. However, just recognizing the domain of learning is insufficient in developing effective objectives. For example, at the end of the unit of instruction, you might want students to explain the various tests and measures that can be used in assessing dysfunction of the knee, or you might want them to develop a decision-making algorithm that will help them decide when to use the various tests and measures presented. These goals are both within the cognitive domain of learning; however, they are at very different levels within that domain. The first objective is at the lower end of the cognitive hierarchy (ie, comprehension), whereas the second is at the higher end of the cognitive hierarchy (ie, synthesis).

The cognitive domain includes 6 levels within the hierarchy. The lowest level is knowledge; as complexity and challenge increase, the cognitive processes move through comprehension, application, analysis, synthesis, and evaluation. Table 4-6 provides descriptions of each level of the hierarchy in the cognitive domain along with sample verbs commonly used in developing objectives that target each specific level, as well as a sample objective for each level of the taxonomy.[16]

Critical Thinking Clinical Scenario

You have recently planned several mini-lectures and have developed several objectives including the following:

- Define *andragogy*.
- Compare action learning to other methods of problem solving.
- Provide an example of how you might use action learning in the classroom.
- Define the elements of reflection.

Reflective Questions

1. Where along the taxonomy of the cognitive domain would you place each one of these objectives?

2. How might you change each one of these objectives to increase the level of expectation and challenge?

Table 4-5. Taxonomies of Educational Objectives

Cognitive Domain[16]	Affective Domain[17]	Psychomotor Domain[18]
Knowledge	Receiving (attending)	Perception
Comprehension	Responding (complying)	Set
Application	Valuing (accepting)	Guided response
Analysis	Organization (integrating)	Mechanism
Synthesis	Characterization (internalizing)	Complex overt response
Evaluation		Adapt
		Origination

Table 4-6 The Cognitive Domain

Level	Description	Sample Verbs	Sample Objective
Knowledge	The learner is expected to observe and recall information like events, dates, places. The capability of doing this implies mastery of basic subject matter	List, label, define, name, describe	After reading the section on behavioral objectives, the student will list the components of a well-written objective
Comprehension	The learner is expected to reproduce or communicate knowledge about the topic in his or her own words without verbatim repetition	Summarize, interpret, estimate, discuss	After discussing the chapter on systematic effective instruction in pairs, the student will summarize the key factors to consider in preparing a presentation
Application	The learner is expected to use information, methods, concepts, and theories in new situations to solve problems	Apply, demonstrate, show, solve, distinguish	After reviewing the chapter on the principles of teaching movement, the student will apply the principles of motor control in designing a treatment plan for a 10-year-old child with spastic diplegia
Analysis	The learner is expected to identify components in the material presented, organize the different components presented, and see patterns in the material	Analyze, order, arrange, connect, classify, separate	After the presentation on developing behavioral objectives, the learner will analyze objectives to determine what domain of learning is being targeted
Synthesis	The learner is expected to use old ideas to create new ones; generalize from given facts and draw conclusions	Combine, integrate, create, design, invent, compose, formulate	After completing the unit on technology in teaching and learning, the learner will develop a patient education module using technology appropriately
Evaluation	The learner is expected to compare and discriminate between ideas, assess value of theories, make choices based on reasoned argument, and verify value of evidence	Assess, decide, rank, grade, recommend, measure	After completing the unit on patient education, the learner will evaluate patient education materials on-site to determine whether they are written at the appropriate literacy level

Adapted from Bloom BS, ed. *Taxonomy of Educational Objectives: Book 1 Cognitive Domain*. New York, NY: Longman; 1956.

Psychomotor Domain

The psychomotor domain refers to skills that require some degree of movement or manipulation. Bloom[16] and Krathwohl[17] never created a hierarchy with subcategories for the psychomotor domain as they had for the cognitive or affective domain. However, others such as Simpson,[18] Dave,[19] and Harrow[20] did create hierarchies to address these behaviors. Simpson[18] described a hierarchy that moved from perception (the learner can use sensory cues to help guide his or her movements) to adaptation (the learner has mastered the activity and can adapt it to meet the needs of the situation). Dave's[19] taxonomy, on the other hand moved from imitation to naturalization (the learner's ability to perform the activity without needing to think about it), and Harrow[20] moved from involuntary reactions to skilled movements. Table 4-7 provides descriptions of the levels of the taxonomy as described by Simpson[18] along with sample verbs and objectives.

Critical Thinking Clinical Scenario

You are developing a presentation on the use of manipulation in managing cervical pain. Your audience is a class of second-year doctor of physical therapy students who are being exposed to manipulation for the first time.

Reflective Questions

1. Write at least 1 goal for your presentation that addresses the psychomotor domain of learning and one goal for the cognitive domain of learning.

2. How would you modify these objectives if your audience was a group of clinicians who have recently begun to use manipulation in the clinical setting and would like to enhance their current level of competence and decision making related to using manipulation?

Table 4-7. The Psychomotor Domain

Level	Description	Sample Verbs	Sample Objective
Perception	The learner has the ability to use sensory cues to help guide his or her movements	Chooses, detects, distinguishes, identifies, isolates, and relates	The learner will distinguish between appropriate and inappropriate interpersonal skills in working with patients from different cultures
Set	Learners at this stage are prepared mentally, physically, and emotionally to take action (Note: This level of the hierarchy is closely linked to the affective domain)	Begins, displays, explains, moves, proceeds, reacts, and shows	The learner can react appropriately in an unsafe situation
Guided response	At this stage, the learner can imitate complex skills	Copies, traces, follows, reacts, reproduces, and responds	The learner will reproduce the steps of preparing for an ultrasound treatment
Mechanism	The learner is expected to perform a complex skill with a degree of confidence and proficiency	Manipulates, performs, measures, and organizes	The learner will demonstrate proficiency in performing all proprioceptive neuromuscular facilitation patterns
Complex overt response	The learner can perform the complex skill with proficiency, accuracy, and speed, with some degree of automaticity	(Note: The key words are the same as the mechanism level, but performance is quicker, better, more accurate, etc)	The learner will accurately perform a complete review of systems within 15 minutes
Adaptation	The learner at this stage has developed proficiency in performing a skill and can now begin to make adaptations to meet the needs of the situation	Adapts, alters, changes, rearranges, reorganizes, revises, and varies	The learner will modify stair climbing activities when faced with a staircase without handrails
Origination	The learner at this stage can develop new and creative movement patterns to meet the demands of a unique situation	Combines, composes, constructs, creates, designs, initiates, and originates	The learner will create a new training program to meet the needs of a patient with a recent below elbow amputation, who would like to return to caring for her newborn infant

Adapted from Simpson EJ. *The Classification of Educational Objectives in the Psychomotor Domain.* Washington, DC: Gryphon House; 1972.

Affective Domain

In 1964, David Krathwohl and Bertram Masia worked with Benjamin Bloom[17] to develop taxonomy of educational objectives for the affective domain. Objectives in the affective domain focus on the learner's level of acceptance of values, beliefs, and attitudes. As with the cognitive and psychomotor domains, the affective domain was developed in a hierarchical manner from simple recognition, attention, and compliance to a situation or phenomenon to internalization of certain values and characteristics. With the affective domain, however, additional transitions occur as you move up the hierarchy of complexity. As complexity increases, there is a transition from concrete to abstract, from an external to an internal locus of control, and from conscious to unconscious internalization of values. Table 4-8 provides descriptions of the levels of the taxonomy along with sample verbs and objectives.[17]

For example, consider the concept of "people-first language." As a new health care professional student, you may be told by faculty that it is very important for you refer to your patients by their names, not their disabilities. It is not, "my knee patient"; rather, it is "Mr. K, my patient who has a knee problem." You recognize the difference (*receiving*) and work hard to correct yourself when referring to patients because you know that is what is expected (*responding*). As you move up the hierarchy, you begin to realize that it is no longer simply an exercise in doing what is expected of you; rather, you begin to recognize how degrading it can be to be referred to as a disability rather than who you are. You now consistently use people-first language and actually begin to correct those around you when they do not (*valuing*). As you progress in your professional development, you not only value the need for using people-first language but you begin to recognize and value the need to place your patient at the center of your care and to view your patient first as a person with needs and second as an impairment that needs correcting (*organizing*). Finally, as your worldview of your patient, your role in the therapeutic relationship,

Table 4-8. The Affective Domain

Level	Description	Sample Verbs	Sample Objective
Receiving (attending)	Learners are expected to recognize that a given situation or phenomenon exists; they will be consciously aware of and can attend to the situation.	Asks, chooses, follows, gives, holds, and identifies	Having completed a unit on different cultures, the student will identify the cultural differences that individuals from the 2 different cultures might display.
Responding (complying)	Learners are expected to move beyond recognition and attention to actively responding to a given phenomenon. They demonstrate a willingness and motivation to respond to and comply with a given situation or phenomenon.	Answers, assists, aids, complies, conforms, greets, helps, performs, discusses, and practices	The learner will select appropriate home exercise activities that demonstrate recognition of the influence of his or her patient's cultural beliefs when designing a plan of care.
Valuing (accepting)	Learners at this level routinely demonstrate overt behaviors consistent with the given phenomenon, such that they are perceived as valuing the given phenomenon (ie, the phenomenon has personal worth to the individual). Value can range from simple acceptance to a strong commitment.	Differentiates, explains, initiates, proposes, and selects	The learner will consistently select culturally appropriate behaviors in working with patients from different cultures.
Organization (integrating)	Learners at this level begin to organize a variety of values into an ordered relationship with one another and synthesize them into a higher-order value complex; can compare values and resolve conflicts between them.	Defends, formulates, modifies, integrates, generalizes, organizes, and synthesizes	The learner will justify the need for culturally sensitive care.
Characterization (internalizing)	The learner has internalized the given phenomenon to the degree that it is an unconscious component of his or her personal philosophy or worldview; demonstrates a predictable and characteristic pattern of behaviors.	Discriminates, displays, influences, qualifies, serves, questions, revises, solves, and verifies	The learner will exemplify cultural competence in working with individuals from all cultures without hesitance.

Adapted from Krathwohl DR, Bloom BS, Masia BB. *Taxonomy of Educational Objectives: Book 2 Affective Domain*. New York, NY: Longman; 1964.

and your role as a professional expand, you begin to internalize the core values of the profession, making people-first language a part of all that you do as a health care provider (*characterizing*).

Critical Thinking Clinical Scenario

You are working with a third-year student on her final rotation in the clinical setting. You noticed that she often arrives to clinic barely 5 minutes before your patients arrive and frequently leaves the clinic before her notes are completed.

Reflective Question

1. To help clarify the expectations you have of your student, write 2 successive goals related to your student's level of accountability. Write your first goal at the level of receiving and your second goal at the level of valuing on the affective domain taxonomy. Indicate when you would expect your student to achieve each of these goals (eg, immediately, within 1 week, by the end of the internship).

These frameworks for developing educational objectives have been in use since their inception with little revision until recently. In 2001, Anderson and Krathwohl[21] revised the framework for the cognitive domain in recognition of the complexity of the thinking process as we now know it. The revision proposed by Anderson and Krathwohl includes 2 dimensions. The first, the cognitive process dimension, similar to Bloom's original taxonomy, has 6 levels (remember, understand, apply, analyze, evaluate, and create). The second dimension is the knowledge dimension, which has 4 categories (factual, conceptual, procedural, and metacognitive). These 2 dimensions create a matrix that can be used to develop objectives across both the cognitive process and knowledge dimensions.

Dettmer[22] also proposed significant modifications to Bloom's taxonomy. She advocates for a framework that is much broader in scope, encompassing 4 domains of learning: cognitive, affective, sensorimotor, and social. She also argues for a unification of these 4 domains, noting that to be a successful learner requires activity in all domains. She describes phases of learning characterized by *realism* (what learners should know), *pragmatism* (what learners can do), and *idealism* (to what learners aspire). Dettmer[22] also suggests that there are 8 phases of learning incorporating all domains that move from basic learning to applied learning and finally to ideational learning. There is much that we still do not know and much left to study. Dettmer[22] notes:

> Educators should never regard frameworks for educational taxonomies as finished and perfect. Research and development must be ongoing and the resulting information shared widely. Much remains to be studied, rethought, created, revised and studied again as teachers teach and learn and students learn and do.

Though our understanding of the complexity of how we learn has grown significantly and some have advocated for change, Bloom's taxonomy remains the most widely recognized and used taxonomy for educational objectives. It is in part because of its widespread use, simplicity, and ease of implementation that we have decided to focus on Bloom's taxonomy in this text, rather than some of the more recent complex iterations. We do encourage those of you who might be interested to use the references provided as a springboard for additional studies about various educational taxonomies.

Finally, before we leave this discussion, it should be noted that though we write objectives specific to each of the 3 distinct domains of learning, as Dettmer[22] suggested, mastery may require some component of the other 2 domains. For example, I could write the following objective: "The student will respond effectively to emergency situations in the clinical setting." The primary focus of this goal is that the student will recognize and respond, which lie in the affective domain. To recognize and respond appropriately, however, assumes that the student already has knowledge of what constitutes an emergency (cognitive domain) and the skills needed to manage the emergency situation (psychomotor domain). In writing goals, it is important to recognize what prerequisite knowledge, skills, and behaviors the student might need in order to successfully achieve the stated goal.

Critical Thinking Clinical Scenario

As a clinical instructor, you are working with a student who is having significant difficulty demonstrating effective interpersonal skills. When interacting with patients, she continually interrupts when they are speaking. Even after asking a question, she does not listen or respond to what the patient is saying. You decide to write some goals to make your expectations more explicit for your student.

Reflective Question

1. Create 1 objective in each of the cognitive, affective, and psychomotor domains that would address this issue.

Stop, Do, and Reflect

Take a look at some of your course syllabi.

1. Can you identify the learning domain for each objective?
2. Can you determine which level of the taxonomy the objective targets?
3. Is each learning domain represented by at least 1 objective on the syllabus? If not, which one is missing? Can you write an objective that addresses that domain?
4. Can you rewrite some of the objectives to reflect a higher level of challenge?
5. Can you develop test questions the instructor could use to assess whether you learned what was expected for each objective?

Using the analogy of objectives serving as a road map to help you stay on course during your presentation, you will want as detailed a map as possible. In developing a presentation, it is easy to go on tangents and add interesting but unnecessary information. Having specific objectives will help you stay focused and on task.

Besides identifying the domain of learning and at what level of the taxonomy you expect your learner to perform, a number of other factors need to be considered in developing a well-written objective. For example, "The student will use active listening skills including rephrasing responses to facilitate effective communication in working with patients." How will you determine whether or not the learner has met the objective? Must the learner demonstrate the desired behavior 100% of the time to be considered adequate? Would you consider 80% of the time acceptable for a novice with the final goal being 100% once he or she has practiced enough? In all teaching-learning situations, in the clinic or the classroom, you will want to consider questions like these when formulating your objectives. The answers to questions like these will help you develop effectively written objectives.

Well-written objectives should specify not only what behavior you expect your learners to accomplish but under what conditions or in what context as well as the degree of mastery you expect. So, a more effective objective than the one above might be, "By the end of this internship, the student will use active listening skills including rephrasing responses to facilitate effective communication in working with patients 90% of the time." A mnemonic device you can use to help you remember some of the components of a well-written objective is "ABCD"[23]:

- <u>A</u>udience; the "Who"
- <u>B</u>ehavior; the "What"
- <u>C</u>ondition; the "When/How"
- <u>D</u>egree of mastery; the "How well/How much"

The following is an example of a behavioral objective written using the ABCD framework: "Following a lecture, the student will describe the physics of an ultrasound machine accurately."

A = The student
B = Will describe the physics of an ultrasound machine
C = Following a lecture
D = Accurately

A number of pitfalls to writing objectives should be considered. For example, instructors sometimes write objectives that describe their plans for the session; that is, they focus on their own behavior rather than on what they expect their learner to achieve by the end of the session (presenter-centered objectives). Objectives should always be learner centered; that is, what you want your learner to achieve. The following are examples of incorrectly and correctly written learner-centered objectives:

- Incorrect: This lecture will review the anatomy of the shoulder.

- Correct: At the conclusion of this session, the student will accurately identify the anatomy of the shoulder.

- Incorrect: The student will be shown how to correctly perform a review of systems.

- Correct: Following a demonstration, the student will correctly perform a review of systems.

Because objectives provide a roadmap for both *teachers* and *learners*, some instructors find it helpful to create objectives for themselves as well as for the learner. These objectives describe what the instructor will do to ensure that the learner achieves the stated outcome objective. Sometimes, working backwards can help. Create the learner-centered objectives, and then decide what you as instructor will do to enable your learners to achieve those objectives. For example, if your learner-centered objective is "The learner will apply the concepts of reflection to practice using questions," your objectives as the instructor might include (1) the instructor will present the elements of reflection, (2) the instructor will

provide a narrative for students to practice identifying the elements of reflection, (3) the instructor will demonstrate the use of appropriate reflective questions, and (4) the instructor will design a clinical role play in which students practice using reflective questions. It is important to distinguish between those objectives that guide the instructor's presentation and those that describe the learner outcomes. Table 4-9 provides examples of presenter-centered versus learner-centered objectives.

Critical Thinking Clinical Scenario

You are working with a student in the clinic on developing an educational presentation for the aides in the clinic on how to transfer a patient from the bed to a wheelchair using proper body mechanics. You have 1 hour to teach her about writing objectives. Your goal is to have your student create the learning objectives for the presentation.

Reflective Questions

1. Write at least 2 learner-centered objectives for your session with your student (ie, what are your expected outcomes for the student?).

2. Write 2 learner-centered objectives you might expect your student to develop for the presentation (ie, what are your student's expected outcome for the aides?).

The focus of effective behavioral objectives is the learner and what behaviors or outcomes you expect from your learner, whether the learner is a student, a patient, an aide, or some other health care provider. An example of an appropriately written behavioral objective for a patient might be, "Following instruction by the physical therapist, the patient will accurately demonstrate the prescribed home exercise program."

A well-written behavioral objective also focuses on the *outcome rather than process*. We cannot directly observe or measure a process. We need to specify the outcome of a process to determine whether the process has occurred. The following is an example of an incorrectly and correctly written objective:

Table 4-9. Presenter-Centered Versus Learner-Centered Objectives

Presenter-Centered Objectives (ie, What Will the Presenter Do?)	Learner-Centered Objectives (ie, What Is the Learner Expected to Achieve?)
During this workshop, the presenter will: - Describe the theoretical perspectives of various reflective theorists. - Present a framework for the development of questions based on the works of Mezirow, Schön, and Bloom that can be used to facilitate reflective thinking. - Provide scenarios for students to practice developing questions through role-plays.	By the end of this workshop, the learners will: - Differentiate between some of the major theorists in reflective practice. - Formulate a variety of questions using the frameworks of Mezirow, Schön, and Bloom. - Ask appropriate questions that facilitate reflective thinking on-the-spot in a role-play situation.

- Incorrect: The student will research iontophoresis.
- Correct: The student will provide a written synthesis of 5 articles on iontophoresis.

We have also observed instructors to write objectives that state the topic for discussion rather than describing what the learner is expected to do as a result of the instruction on the topic (*outcome versus topic*). For example, a clinical instructor might say to a student physical therapist, "Today we'll focus on the biomechanics of the shoulder." We do not know what the clinical instructor expects the student to do at the end of the day. A more effective objective would be, "At the end of today, you will be prepared to discuss the biomechanics of the shoulder with the other physical therapy intern."

Another common mistake in developing objectives is to include more than 1 outcome in an objective. For example, the clinical instructor might tell the student to list and demonstrate the steps necessary to prepare a patient for massage. What if the student can list the steps but cannot demonstrate the steps? Was this objective achieved? It would be better to use one outcome; in this example, you might select the more complex of the 2 behaviors as an outcome or you might split this into 2 objectives: (1) the student will list the steps she will take to prepare a patient for a massage and (2) the student will properly prepare the patient for massage. Note also that the instructor will be assessing 2 different domains of learning with these objectives. The first objective is written to assess the student's cognitive skills, whereas the second is written to assess her psychomotor skills.

Finally, the more *specific, objective, measureable,* and *observable* the objective, the more effective it will be in making the expectations explicit and in determining whether the student achieved the expected outcome. For example, a common goal of clinical education is the development of professionalism in students. Without clear descriptions of desired behaviors, the clinical instructor and students can become frustrated. Your objective for your student might be to interact appropriately with family members and caregivers. What does *appropriately* mean? Is your definition of appropriately the same as the student's definition of appropriately? Or perhaps you have a student who "lacks initiative" or "lacks professionalism." Again, you may have very specific definitions for these terms that may or may not be congruent with your student's definition. By making your objectives specific, objective, measurable, and observable, you will minimize confusion about your expectations and optimize your learner's ability to achieve the desired outcomes. The following are some examples of incorrectly and correctly written objectives related to professionalism:

- Incorrect: The student will use her free time productively.
- Correct: The student will use her free time to collect evidence to support her selected patient interventions.
- Incorrect: The student will demonstrate the core value of accountability.
- Correct: The student will demonstrate the core value of accountability by ensuring that all written documentation is completed before she leaves for the day.

Table 4-10 provides some questions you might ask yourself when writing objectives to ensure that they contain all the information needed in a well-written learner-centered objective.

Table 4-10. Additional Dos and Don'ts to Consider in Writing Learner-Centered Objectives

Dos (Well-Written Objectives)	Don'ts (Common Errors in Writing Objectives)
Does your objective describe: • A behavior you expect the learner to achieve? • A behavior that is specific and not vague? • A behavior that is both measureable and objective? • A behavior that is easily observable? • A single behavior? • The degree to which you expect the learner to master the behavior? • The conditions or context under which you expect the learner to achieve the stated behavior? • An expected outcome, not a topic or learning process?	Does your objective contain: • What you plan to do as a presenter? • What material you will present? • How you plan to present the material? • How you expect the student to learn the content? • Global or vague outcomes? • Multiple outcomes in one objective? • A behavior that is not measureable? • A behavior that is not observable?

Key Points to Remember

Effective behavioral objectives:

- Provide a road map for the instructor and the learner.
- Help define the content of your presentation.
- Help you determine what teaching strategies you will use.
- Help in the assessment of the learner.
- Help guide and assess the efficacy of the instructor.

Effective behavioral objectives include the following:

- A—Audience (who?)
- B—Behavior (what?)
- C—Condition (when?)
- D—Degree (how much?)

Effective behavioral objectives:

- Are learner-centered
- Are specific
- Are behavioral, measurable, objective, and outcome oriented
- Include only 1 outcome per objective

Developing Objectives for a Lecture Versus a Course or Curriculum

The focus of this chapter is on single presentations such as delivering a guest lecture in a doctor of physical therapy program, speaking to a community group, or teaching specific content to a patient. If your presentation is a component of a larger curriculum, it is important for you to understand how your presentation fits within the whole curriculum. You will want to ask many more questions before developing your content, such as how does your presentation relate to the goals and objectives of the course, curriculum, and program? What is the mission of the program? What are the terminal objectives or expected outcomes of the program? Where does your content fit within the overall sequence of courses? What content precedes your lecture, and what comes after? What is the philosophy of the program faculty? What teaching and assessment methods do other faculty members use? What is the curriculum model?

For example, if the physical therapy program where you will teach is built on a problem-based curriculum model, your objectives would need to include language and activities reflective of this problem-centered approach. If you are teaching in a school that emphasizes service learning as a guiding principle for all of its programs, your objectives may very well need to include behaviors that integrate learning in the community. It is important to remember that there are no isolated lectures within a curriculum; all lectures should be linked to the course, the curriculum, and the overall mission, goals, and objectives of the program. In

addition, how you present your content should also be consistent with the philosophy, mission, and goals of the program and its faculty.

Curriculum development and assessment are beyond the scope of this book. If you are being asked to develop an entire course or curriculum, it would be important for you to obtain additional resources related to curriculum design and development before starting.[24] In addition to texts on educational theory and curricular design, in physical therapy, we would strongly recommend that you review professional documents from the American Physical Therapy Association and the Commission on Accreditation of Physical Therapy Education such as *A Normative Model for Physical Therapist Education*,[25] the *Normative Model for Physical Therapist Assistant Education*,[26] *Evaluative Criteria for Accreditation of Education Programs for the Preparation of Physical Therapists*,[27] and *Evaluative Criteria for Accreditation of Education Programs for the Preparation of Physical Therapist Assistants*.[28]

Content

Finally, you are at the point of considering the specific content of your presentation or other instructional activity. You have considered the audience, conducted a needs assessment, and set appropriate learner-centered behavioral objectives. Now, you are ready to organize the information and/or skills to be conveyed to your learner(s). To the layperson, teaching or presenting content is the same as telling the audience what you want them to learn. Knowing what we do about brain function and memory, we recognize how much more complex teaching is than simply presenting information.

We know that people need periodic opportunities to process whatever information they see and/or hear. Without time to process information and make it personally relevant, learners become passive listeners, not engaged learners. Garmston and Wellman[3] emphasized the need to adjust the balance between content and process depending on the goal of your presentation. If the goal is for the audience to integrate and apply the information presented, then the instructor will need to allow a significantly greater proportion of time for processing. If the goal is only to expose the audience to the topic, less time for processing may be necessary. If the goal is for the learner to acquire a certain skill, then the learner will need sufficient time to practice (process) the information being presented. Table 4-11 illustrates different ways you may consider varying the ratio of content and process depending on the goal of your presentation.

Key Point to Remember

Balance content versus process based on your audience and the goals of your presentation.

Table 4-11. Balancing Content and Process in Presentations

If the goal of your presentation is ...	Consider...
Knowledge acquisition	Cycles of content followed by process time should be used throughout the presentation period. Provide a brief presentation of content followed by brief periods of activity to allow the learner to process the material presented, to make connections, and to move what they are learning from short-term to long-term memory. Working in small chunks enhances memory retention. For example: 15-minute mini-lecture, 5-minute activity, 20-minute mini-lecture, 5-minute activity, 15-minute mini-lecture, 10-minute activity, etc
Skill acquisition	As above except the cycles of content are followed by much longer practice periods. For example: 30-minute presentation, 30-minute practice, 15-minute presentation, 30-minute practice, 20-minute presentation 25-minute practice, etc
Attitude development	Begin the cycle with processing time. Have the learner process his or her own attitudes first, and then present material for them to compare and contrast. For example: a 30-minute small and large group discussion of attitudes, followed by a 20-minute presentation of theoretical concepts, end with an activity to compare, contrast, and process content
Application	Begin the cycle with a longer presentation followed by an activity that requires the learner to apply what was presented to practice. For example: 30-minute presentation of theoretical concepts, followed by 45 minutes to apply these concepts to a case scenario

Adapted from Garmston RJ, Wellman BM. *How to Make Presentations That Teach and Transform.* Alexandria, VA: Association for Supervision and Curriculum Development; 1992;

Critical Thinking Clinical Scenario

You are a clinician who is a board-certified sports clinical specialist with advanced training as a biomechanist. You have been invited to do 2 lectures for a nearby doctor of physical therapy program. You will be presenting on the topic of running gait to a class of first-year students and then to a group of post-professional, transitional doctor of physical therapy students. The first-year students have only recently been introduced to gait and gait analysis and want to learn the concept of gait and how gait changes with increasing velocity. The post-professional students all have clinical experience and a keen interest in sports and running injuries.

Reflective Questions

1. How might the goals for these presentations differ?
2. How might the presenter's level of expertise be potentially problematic?
3. Where along the cognitive hierarchy would the goals for the first-year students likely fall? What about for the post-professional students?
4. How might the ratios between content and process differ?
5. If you were in either group, what information about gait would you want?

In thinking about how to sequence the material to allow for the appropriate ratio of content and process time, it is also important to consider how much information to present at a time for optimal learning. Some theorists propose a *"rule of 7."* This is based on the idea that working memory has a limited capacity and can only process 7 items or *"chunks"* of information, plus or minus 2 items at 1 time. Not all theorists agree with the number 7 plus or minus 2. In the literature, this number varies from 2 to 7 chunks of information.[29-31] Regardless of the actual number of discrete items of information that working memory can process, evidence indicates that there are limits. There is no absolute limit, though, because learners differ in terms of the amount of new information each can group or chunk together into a single unit. The more a learner knows about a topic already, and the more experience the learner has related to the topic, the easier it will be for that learner to group larger amounts of information into a single chunk of information. Squire and Kandel[31] suggested that a major difference between experts and novices is the amount of information contained in each chunk to be processed in working memory.

Consider organizing your content in terms of what Garmston[14] described as "containers." These containers help the learner chunk the material, making it easier to remember and retain. Examples of how you might create these containers include saying, "There are 3 key theories," and then cite them or tell the audience, "There are 2 commonly used approaches to the treatment of a specific impairment," and then compare and contrast them. Speakers also may provide acronyms or use the first letter of the first word of several points to help organize content. We provided an example of this when we used the ABCD framework for developing effective behavioral objectives. By including containers such as these, the presenter makes it easier for the information to be considered as 2 to 3 meaningful chunks instead of a larger number of discrete points.[32] Any time you create a mnemonic device or memory aid to help learners organize the new information and embed these mnemonics in your instruction, you are using containers.[33]

Because there are limits in the amount of new information a learner can process, effective instructors use the guiding principle of *"less is more."* It is best to limit the amount of new information you provide at any given time and consider ways to organize that information into meaningful chunks. In addition, because learners need to connect new information to prior knowledge about the topic, they will benefit from frequent processing opportunities. A good rule of thumb would be to consider incorporating an activity to process information every 15 to 20 minutes—less frequently for less content-dense information and more frequently for more content-dense information. This concept will be discussed further later in this chapter under "Active Learning Strategies" on page 90.

Key Points to Remember

Some rules of thumb:
- LESS IS MORE!
- "Chunk" information.
- Incorporate frequent activities (ie, every 15 to 20 minutes) to help learners process information, make it personally relevant, and link it to something they already know.

Another rule of thumb to keep in mind is *"Covering material does not equal learning."* If you listen outside the door of any high school classroom in the weeks before state exams, such as the New York State Regents exams, you may hear comments like, "We have to get through this material before June." Or you might hear a faculty colleague say, "I can't include more collaborative learning activities; I have too much material to cover in this course as it is!" If you agree that learning something is different than *covering it,* again, you will want to limit the amount you present and allow sufficient time for active learning, which is an excellent example of processing.

Key Point to Remember

Covering material **does not** equal learning!

There is one last rule of thumb to consider in determining what content to present and how to present it.

When you are invited to present on a topic, it is usually because you are recognized as having expertise in this area. This can be a double-edged sword; knowing a great deal about a topic makes it more challenging to limit how much you can share effectively. It may be helpful to make the distinction: *need to know vs nice to know.* As an expert, you might think everything is important or necessary for the learner to master. Hearing or reading too much information in the early stages of learning can be ineffective for the novice learner. The sign of an effective presenter is deciding what your learners need to know about the topic to achieve the goals you have set and editing out details that may overwhelm the learner and detract from the essential points.

Key Point to Remember

As an expert, you must distinguish between need to know and nice to know.

Stop and Reflect

Consider the scenario about the topic of gait presented earlier in this chapter.

Reflective Questions

1. Which information might be necessary (need to know) for experienced clinicians?
2. Which information might be potentially overwhelming (nice to know) for first-year students?
3. What factors would help you determine the appropriate information for each group?

Motivational Hooks and Content Boosters

Once you have determined the overall organization of the content you plan to teach, whether you are working with colleagues, students, or patients, you need to think about how you will engage their attention and shift their attention away from whatever other stimuli are available to them in the surrounding environment to what you want them to learn. As we learned in Chapter 3, only a small portion of potential stimuli is attended to at any given time. Two factors that increase the likelihood that someone will pay attention to something long enough for it to enter working memory are personal meaning and emotion. We consider any technique you use to capture your learner's attention to be a *motivational hook,* a term developed by Dr. Nancy

Table 4-12. Motivational Hooks

• A startling or fun fact	• A personal question
• A provocative question	• A relevant video clip
• An interesting picture	• A demonstration
• A puzzling song	• A display of a piece of equipment or a model
• An anecdote	

Aronson and Dr. Beverly Arscht, Philadelphia-based educational consultants. Similar to the *antecedent set*, described by Madeline Hunter,[2] the motivational hook is your "opening line," your opportunity to engage learners long enough to interest them in what you have to teach. Table 4-12 provides some examples of different types of motivational hooks that you might consider depending on your topic and learning goals.

The most effective motivational hooks focus on the topic, build interest, establish rapport, and energize the environment. The best motivational hooks create an emotional connection with the learner, through humor, novelty, or personal relevance, yet do not overwhelm the topic. For example, a group of student physical therapists conducted a classroom presentation on the use of lasers in physical therapy. They chose to begin their talk with a video clip from the first *Star Wars* movie. Had the clip lasted 10 to 20 seconds, it would have been very effective. Instead, the video selection continued for 2 minutes, long enough for the class to become engrossed in the movie and disappointed when the presentation began. What happened in this incident? The length of the motivational hook was too long, and it overwhelmed the topic. It goes without saying that motivational hooks should always be in good taste. Something that strikes you as funny could be offensive to 1 or more people in your audience.

Critical Thinking Clinical Scenario

Recall the scenario presented at the beginning of this chapter about giving a presentation on osteoporosis to a group of women in your community.

Reflective Questions

1. What are 2 possible motivational hooks suitable for a presentation to a group of women who are residents in an assisted-living facility?

2. What are possible motivational hooks for a presentation to a group of female high school athletes?

3. If you chose different motivational hooks for each group, what factors guided your decision?

Now that you have captured your learners' attention, how will you will emphasize the most important points and keep your audience involved? How will you *boost* the content (to use another term coined by Dr. Nancy Aronson and Dr. Beverly Arscht)?[34] *Content boosters* refer to any techniques, materials, and activities that you use to reinforce learning and allow for the processing of information.

Stop and Reflect

- What types of content boosters have you seen used in classrooms?

- What types of content boosters have you seen used in the clinic?

- Do you have preferences regarding the types of content boosters you have personally experienced? Are some more effective for you than others?

Depending on the topic and the specific content you wish to emphasize, you have many options for creating effective content boosters. Table 4-13 lists a variety of frequently used content boosters.

Many of the containers discussed earlier in this chapter could be considered content boosters. For example, the ABCD model for writing effective learning objectives boosts the likelihood that you will remember the essential components of written objectives. As with motivational hooks, your choice of content boosters depends

Key Points to Remember

Motivational hooks are any techniques you use to capture your learners' attention. Personal meaning and emotion increase the likelihood that someone will pay attention to something long enough for it to enter working memory.

- The most effective motivational hooks:
  - Focus on the topic
  - Build interest
  - Establish rapport
  - Energize the environment
- The best motivational hooks create an emotional connection with the learner through:
  - Humor
  - Novelty
  - Personal relevance
- Motivational hooks must not overwhelm the topic.

Table 4-13. Sample Content Boosters

• Handouts	• Demonstrations
• Artifacts and props	• Case studies
• Visual aids (video, PowerPoint, anatomical model, slides, etc)	• Mnemonics
• Flip charts/newsprint	• Active learning strategies
• Stories/songs	• Games, quizzes/role plays
	• Electronic discussion boards/chat rooms

on the topic at hand and the key points you want to emphasize. The same considerations hold for content boosters as for motivational hooks: Select appropriate materials/activities that are in good taste and do not overshadow the key points you wish to reinforce.

There are many similarities among the materials and/or activities listed under motivational hooks and content boosters. In fact, many are the same. What is the essential difference between the two? In 2 words, *timing* and *purpose*—where you place the activity in your presentation and why you chose to use it—If you use a model of the spine at the beginning of a presentation on low back pain and disability, you are using it as a motivational hook, perhaps by asking the group, "What does this model have to do with the cost of various impairments to society at large?" Ideally, you would elicit discussion about, and interest in, your topic if it were about the impact of low back pain and days lost from work. The purpose of the motivational hook is to grab your audience's attention. If, instead, you were teaching students about the anatomy of the spine and you passed around the model of the spine to reinforce what you had taught about vertebrae, you would be using the model as a content booster. The purpose of the content booster is to reinforce the content you are teaching.

Motivational hooks and content boosters also allow you to add activities for the various learning preferences represented in your audience. As noted earlier, without actually assessing everyone's individual learning style, you can assume that there will be "watchers" and "doers" in every group. The watchers prefer to look first, reflect on the task, and then become more active. A motivational hook such as a relevant cartoon or video clip or a startling statistic is perfect for them. Something more active, such as asking your participants to try to go from sitting to standing using only 1 leg, would engage the doers in a presentation about physical therapy with people who have had a leg amputated. Once you have chosen your motivational hook, whether it appeals more to watchers or doers, you can select a content booster that appeals to the other preference. In the prior example that required people to do something physical right at the beginning of the presentation, the presenter might use a PowerPoint presentation as a content booster that appeals more to watchers.

In addition to watchers and doers, remember that there are also people who prefer theory and facts more

than anecdotes, stories, and other content that appeals to the senses, and vice versa. Effective instructors include a number of content boosters to appeal to these varied preferences. A presentation about physical therapy post-amputation might include statistics about incidence of amputation in the target group and reports about the latest, computer-assisted prostheses, provide anecdotal information based on the presenter's clinical experience, and include a case example where participants could work in small groups to adapt and apply what they had learned from the lecture. Watchers and doers would be engaged, as would people who prefer theory, facts, stories, and anecdotes. Overall, the presentation would have something for all 4 learning styles and for all the different types of audiences.

Key Points to Remember

The essential differences between the motivational hook and content boosters are timing and purpose:

- Motivational hooks are used at the start of a component of the instruction to gain attention,
- Content boosters are used throughout the instruction to reinforce learning.

In planning your motivational hooks and content boosters, consider your audience:

- Watchers and doers
- Those who prefer concrete examples versus theory and facts

Critical Thinking Clinical Scenario

Select either the topic of osteoporosis or gait and determine a hypothetical audience and goals for the presentation.

Reflective Questions

1. What content boosters might you choose to use for your presentation?
2. Which learning style and audience type would prefer these content boosters?
3. What other content booster could you add to appeal to other learning preferences?
4. What could you do as a motivational hook to balance your content boosters and expand the appeal to other learning preferences and audience types?

Strategies for Enhancing Memory Formation

The formation and retrieval of memories is the basis for learning. The following are some strategies that may enhance your memory formation and retrieval. You might consider using these same types of strategies in your presentations as well as with your patients to help them learn and retain the information you are providing:

- Rehearsal and elaboration
- Creating context and linking information to prior knowledge and past experiences for learning
- Recruiting multiple memory pathways
- Active learning strategies

Rehearsal and Elaboration

How many times have you been introduced to someone and almost immediately forget his or her name? Has anyone suggested any strategies to help you better remember the name of the person to whom you were introduced? Perhaps they suggested that you might say the name immediately (eg, "Oh, it is so nice to meet you Mary") or maybe try to associate the person's name with something about the person or someone else you know (eg, Mary has the same color hair as my Aunt Mary who also happened to grow up in the same state as Mary). These are examples of 2 key strategies to enhance our memory formation, rehearsal, and elaboration. Rehearsal and elaboration are 2 key strategies we use to manipulate information while in working memory to increase the likelihood that this information will make its way into long-term memory.[32] Repetition is one of the most commonly used types of rehearsal. We literally repeat what it is we need to remember. Any time you needed to remember someone's phone number long enough to punch in the numbers, you probably used repetition. If you were interrupted in the process, however, you probably could not remember the telephone number.

Repetition is not as effective with semantic memory tasks as it is for skill or procedural memory. Repeating or practicing a motor skill over and over generally results in improved performance and enhanced memory of how to execute the movement. For example, at some point in time, you became unconscious of the steps involved in a task such as riding a bicycle, and you began to go through them automatically. Repetition helped you store these movements in your implicit or procedural memory.

Elaboration, or *elaborative rehearsal*, is a more effective strategy for manipulating semantic information while in working memory.[32] Medina[35] and Squire and Kandel[31] emphasized the importance of focusing on meaning when trying to learn new semantic information. One example of an elaborative rehearsal strategy is to create a story to remember a list of items. You are more likely to remember the list of items if you create a story that includes all the items you want to remember in a cohesive narrative, rather than simply trying to memorize the list. The story helps to put meaning to the words in the list, even if it is a silly or fun story.

A mnemonic, as noted above, is a form of elaborative rehearsal as well. For example, how do you remember the names of the planets in order? Have you used a story such as "My Very Educated Mother Just Served Us Nine Pickles" to remember Mercury, Venus, Earth, Mars, Jupiter, Saturn, Uranus, Neptune, and Pluto? We will not tell you how many years ago we learned this "story" but it remains easily recalled as a result of both repetition and elaboration. This strategy is not used solely in grade school; you likely have used the same strategy to learn material in graduate school. For example, how do you remember the cranial nerves? Does this sound familiar: "On Old Olympus' Towering Tops a Friendly Viking Grew Vines and Hops"? How do you remember whether each nerve is a sensory nerve, motor nerve, or both (mixed)? Does this 1-line story/mnemonic have meaning for you: "Some Say Marry Money, but My Brother Says Big Brains Matter More."

There are many other familiar activities that provide opportunities for elaboration although we might not have considered them in this framework. Whenever we engage in a group discussion about newly presented material or we "debrief" after practicing a new physical therapy intervention, we have a chance to increase our connections to the new information and increase the likelihood that we will remember it. Reciprocal teaching, whereby learners "partner up" and take turns using their own words to teach one another the key points presented by the instructor, is an excellent activity to foster elaboration. Even in the clinic, the physical therapist can ask the young patient to describe the key components of her home exercise program and can ask her parent how she might work on it at home before leaving the session as a means of facilitating both repetition and elaboration for the purposes of enhanced recall.

Stop and Reflect

Reflect back on some of the methods you have used to help you recall information.

- What types of repetition and elaborative strategies have you used that have been most successful?
- Can you think of how you might incorporate repetition and elaboration into your current study strategies?

Key Points to Remember

Rehearsal and elaboration can enhance memory formation.

- Rehearsal, or repetition, is most effective for nondeclarative or implicit memory formation (including skill and procedural memory).

- Elaboration or elaborative rehearsal is most effective for declarative memory formation.

- Elaborative rehearsal includes strategies such as:
  - Creating stories
  - Creating mnemonics
  - Discussions
  - Debriefing sessions
  - Reciprocal teaching

Creating Context and Linking Information to Prior Knowledge and Past Experiences for Learning

Medina[35] discussed several guidelines for strengthening the neuronal connections that result in more effective memory formation and retrieval. First, using relevant examples and activities that involve personal reflection fosters deeper meaning of new information. For example, if you are teaching students how to design an effective in-class presentation, first ask your students to think about the best presentation they have experienced in graduate school (personal reflection). Then ask them to identify the behaviors that made this presentation memorable, share these behaviors with a person sitting nearby, and make a list of the most important behaviors to consider (critical thinking). You then proceed to teach the key points about effective instruction, knowing that your students will connect your instruction to their prior experience by making it personally meaningful. You have essentially "primed the pump." In doing so, you make it easier for your students to connect the new information to prior knowledge, making it easier to understand and retain.

Another strategy for enhancing memory retention and retrieval builds on the finding that some of the neural connections made at the time you are first exposed to certain information remain in the area of the cortex where it is first processed. If we can provide students with authentic real-world experiences for learning, it is hypothesized that they may be prepared to more readily retrieve the information when faced with similar circumstance in practice. For example, providing students with multiple opportunities to engage with standardized patients to enhance their communication skills as well as their history and physical skills may enhance the likelihood that they will remember this experience when faced with a real patient in the clinical environment. In addition, recruiting the episodic or more autobiographical process helps. For example, role plays and simulations allow the learner to internalize and act out conceptual information and thus add a personal experience related to the information to be learned.

Is it possible that engaging in these authentic experiences may also elicit implicit memories and explain why a student physical therapist might experience memories of his or her first clinical internship when visiting a hospital years later? The sights, sounds, or odors of the hospital may have triggered a flood of unconscious or implicit memories as he or she entered the hospital again. Field trips to clinical sites, visits to a prosthetist while studying about prosthetics, and volunteering in a facility serving children or elderly people are all multisensory experiences that may enhance learning and retrieval of information related to those places.

Whenever we are actively engaged in learning and applying something new, it is unlikely that we think of neuronal connections forming and becoming stronger. In fact, once we really know something well, it is sometimes difficult to remember how we even learned the information or how the information first connected with something we knew previously. The art of effective instruction lies in helping learners see the relevance of new information to their lives and to what they know already. When new information seems relevant, it is easier to see how connections can be made. In the classroom and the clinic, we can help learners make connections by developing examples based on their experiences and interests. We can ask them questions to prompt reflection about where and how new content might fit into their prior experiences. Throughout this text, we ask you to "Stop and Reflect" so that you have the opportunity to add your own perspective to the content presented. We also provide many clinical examples to make the content as relevant as possible. In the clinic, therapists may incorporate activities of daily living into a home exercise program to make it easier for the patient to learn and perform the new exercises. Whenever and wherever we teach, we want to highlight meaning and encourage learners to connect new information to prior learning.

Key Points to Remember

Creating context and linking information to prior knowledge and past experiences can enhance learning. Examples of how we can create context and link to meaningful experiences include the following:

- Using concrete and relevant examples.

- Fostering reflection through "Stop and Reflect" activities to enable the learner to develop deeper, more personal understanding of the information.

- Using authentic experiences (eg, role plays, field trips, and other simulations such as standardized patients).

Recruiting Multiple Memory Pathways

Because the memory process is distributed throughout the brain, we have the potential to recruit multiple pathways when we teach. In physical therapy and all the health sciences, there is a vast amount of information destined for explicit memory processes. All the theories, rationales for treatment, foundational sciences, and analyses of professional literature depend on semantic or declarative memory, the system thought to be more recently developed and weakest in humans.[29,32] Lack of sleep, stress, and initial misunderstanding are all factors that can interfere with accurate memory formation. One way to optimize the semantic system is to use multiple methods of presentation and provide several different ways to apply the information. As much as possible, use visual aids to support auditory information during lectures. Pictures, especially moving animations, are more effective than the printed word alone.[35] Even adding movement to whatever you are teaching or trying to learn can help recruit procedural memory processes. Something as simple as taking 3 steps while learning the 3 main components of a theory or the 3 components of a particular home exercise program adds a motor element to your learning. Practicing with a partner as though you were actually helping a patient transfer from sit to stand can add both movement and episodic component to preparing for a practical exam.

Recruiting multiple memory pathways is equally important in the clinic setting. For example, as a student physical therapist, when you observe the clinical instructor perform certain interventions with a patient, you begin to make sense of your clinical instructor's actions visually as you activate neuronal connections related to the interventions you learned previously in school. Your ears receive the auditory stimuli created by the dialogue between your clinical instructor and her patient. If the clinical instructor asks you to describe how this intervention is similar to, and different from, other interventions you have used with this patient, the elaborative process is called in, and even more memory pathways are linked. You reactivate prior connections and probably develop new ones as you compare aspects of this observation with past experiences in the classroom and lab situation. Your prior knowledge and memory about this particular intervention will have been strengthened through the multiple types of memory pathways elicited and the elaboration that occurred throughout this encounter.

Providing multimodal input (eg, visual, auditory, kinesthetic) may very well enhance learning and retention more than providing unimodal input (eg, lecture only) alone.

Key Point to Remember

Based on what we now know about brain function and memory formation, in the teaching-learning situation, providing multimodal input (eg, visual, auditory, kinesthetic) will likely enhance learning and retention more than providing unimodal input (eg, lecture only) alone.

Active Learning Strategies

Anyone who has ever watched a baby learn how to eat or manipulate a new toy or try to say the alphabet has observed active learning in its purest form. The baby holds, mouths, drops, grasps, and imitates others as he or she figures out how to do something. When student physical therapists are learning different interventions for various impairments or functional limitations, they too need to watch demonstrations, practice how to position their hands to implement the interventions, and try out these movements on one another in lab sessions before ever working with patients. They are demonstrating one aspect of active learning, the actual doing of something. These hands-on activities are active learning strategies and act as content boosters. Active learning strategies are a particular form of content booster and a critical component of effective instruction.

It would be hard to imagine any other way to teach student physical therapists how to treat patients. On the other hand, it may be more difficult to imagine how to teach a subject like physiology, gerontology, or osteoporosis using active learning strategies. If we consider that active learning also involves actively thinking about, reflecting on, and cognitively interacting with the content being taught, it becomes easier to imagine. Asking learners to think about any associations they have to a topic or requiring them to compare a concept that was learned previously with something being taught currently represents a degree of active learning.

You might ask, "Why should learning be active?" The simplest explanation, based on what we know about how the brain works, is that learning depends on moving information from working memory to long-term memory. The learner needs to do some type of rehearsal or manipulation of the content for this to happen. In other words, the learner needs to actively process information rather than passively receive it. Active learning strategies require the learner to interact with the content rather than simply listen to, or look at, what is being presented. For example, developing a mnemonic or a humorous song about the cranial nerves is 1 way students might actively engage with material that could be considered somewhat "dry." Information about the cranial nerves is more likely to get into, and be retrieved from, long-term memory whenever the student sings that song.

Table 4-14. Retention Rate Based on Instructional Strategies

Instructional Strategies	Retention Rate (%)
Teaching others	90
Practicing by doing	75
Discussion	50
Demonstration	30
Audiovisual presentation	20
Reading	10
Lecture	5

Data from Silberman M, Auerbach C. *Active Training: A Handbook of Techniques, Designs, Case Examples, and Tips.* 3rd ed. San Francisco, CA: John Wiley & Sons; 2006; Sousa D. *How the Brain Learns.* Thousand Oaks, CA: Corwin; 2006.

The benefits of active learning on retention and achievement have been investigated at all grade levels from elementary school through high school, college, and graduate education in the past 2 decades. These strategies were found to result in better achievement than teacher-centered or lecture presentations.[36-38] Fink[1] emphasized the importance of active learning when designing effective college courses. He referred to the creation of "significant learning" as the goal of college instructors, and he included reflection as a key component of active versus passive learning. The use of reflection as a strategy to help learners make sense of their learning and link them to past, present, and future experiences was explored in Chapter 2. Combining active learning and reflection have been shown to enhance all types of learning.[39-43]

Consider the scenario that appeared at the beginning of this chapter. Were you thinking about developing a brief lecture about osteoporosis, perhaps supported by PowerPoint slides? If so, look at Table 4-14, which lists the typical retention rate for a variety of instructional strategies.[6] The percentage of material retained after experiencing the various approaches demonstrates the relative benefits of active approaches such as discussing, practicing, and/or teaching someone else as compared to simply looking or listening. Where would a lecture supported by slides appear? Would you be satisfied with the retention of that percentage of the material you presented?

Silberman and Auerbach[6,44] provided a compendium of active strategies to enhance learning and retention in their seminal book, *Active Training*. Although this book initially targeted corporate trainers, it contains useful activities for many teaching-learning situations. These activities represent content boosters that will appeal especially to the doers in your audience.

As mentioned previously, active strategies allow for more effective learning to occur. If you want your learners, whether they are patients, students, or colleagues, to remember what you are teaching, it is important to plan ways for them to periodically process and manipulate the information presented. Active strategies infuse the learning experience with energy. University students, observed during lectures, have shown predictable patterns of behavior that would distress anyone trying to teach effectively. It has been noted that generally within 5 to 10 minutes students begin to "settle in," getting pens out, etc. After about 20 to 30 minutes, students start fiddling with pens/pencils, looking around, and engaging in tasks other than listening to the speaker. Within 45 to 60 minutes, many students may even begin to exhibit a "trance-like" behavior, and, shortly after that, some students have been noted to fall asleep. This was even observed in medical students, certainly a group of students assumed to be highly motivated.[45] In addition, today's students have cell phones and computers to distract them. If you have ever sat in the back of a large computer lab during a lecture, you may not see trance-like behaviors but you will most certainly see students sending and receiving text messages, checking electronic mail, and surfing the Web. With all of these distractions, keeping students actively engaged in the classroom becomes both more challenging and more critical.

The traditional lecture has a number of limitations, and without modifications, it can foster passivity in students and limit independent thought and problem solving.[1,37,46] Sustained lectures appeal primarily to people with strong auditory preferences and are based on the assumption that everyone in the audience shares this preference. There is also an assumption that when the teacher is talking, the student (patient or colleague as well) is listening to what is being said. You can be the judge of how well this assumption holds up.

Consider this question: During a lecture, have you ever thought about an upcoming event or an argument from the day before? It is common for people to daydream periodically, and these thoughts interfere with attending to what is being taught. But it is also possible to come back to task long enough to get the gist of a presentation. With the goal of teaching as effectively as possible, we want to minimize the frequency of daydreaming and distraction during instruction; we want to minimize the ebb and flow of the learner's attention. We want to optimize the learning experience by helping working memory process information and move this information to long-term memory. Our goal is to promote retention. Listening to lectures without periodic active processing does not foster retention. We want learners to actively engage with the material being presented. We want them to do the work that it takes to gain and retain new knowledge.

Consider this question as well: Who does all the work in preparing and presenting a lecture? Certainly the instructor! With a lecture, the presenter is doing the work of organizing, synthesizing, and learning the material so that he or she can present it with some degree of credibility and expertise. What we want is for the learners to equally engage with the material so they, too, can learn as much as the instructor!

In spite of what we have learned over the years about active learning and effective instruction, the lecture remains a popular instructional methodology.[47] In fact, there are times when lectures are an effective mode of instruction. Lectures can be a time-efficient strategy for pulling information from multiple sources to introduce a new topic to learners. The lecture, or *lecturette*, a brief lecture, can spark interest in, and enthusiasm for, further study. Because the instructor can integrate current research from varied sources in a brief lecture, the lecture can supplement information in a textbook that is typically several years old even at the time of publication. Lectures may be less threatening to learners because they are familiar with them and the teacher is doing almost all of the work. For learners who prefer watching and listening, lectures provide a comfortable and effective format.[46] So, as educators, we do not advocate total elimination of the lecture. Lectures, presented well, can be effective strategies for teaching content. However, punctuating your lecture even for brief periods of time to allow the learner to process information will enhance the efficacy of your presentation and optimize the chances that your learner will retain the information you are presenting. Even taking 60 seconds to ask the learner to write down the key points presented or to share his or her thoughts on the topic with his or her neighbor will engage the learner and facilitate processing of the content.

The length of a presentation may also impact its effectiveness. Sousa[30] described the concepts of *primacy* and *recency*, findings from psychological research first reported in the late 1800s by Ebbinghaus.[48] Briefly, this research demonstrated that people remember best what they hear at the beginning of a learning experience. The second most memorable time in a presentation is at the end. The least favorable spot for information to be remembered is the middle portion of a presentation. Sousa[30] used the terms *prime time* and *downtime* to highlight the most effective and least effective parts of a teaching-learning experience. He noted that a larger percentage of downtime occurs during presentations longer than 40 minutes. In the 40-minute lesson, there are 2 prime times of approximately 15 minutes' duration each, leaving 10 minutes of downtime. In an 80-minute lecture, the downtime constitutes about 30 minutes, a much larger percentage of the instructional period. Given the time needed for working memory to process new information, Sousa recommended using several cycles of 20 minutes of presentation followed by a few minutes of processing time for optimal learning.[30] This is what we refer to as the brief lecturette.

Key Points to Remember

Active learning strategies:

- Give learners an opportunity to rehearse or manipulate the content being presented, which will increase the likelihood of retention.
- Include actively thinking about, reflecting on, and cognitively interacting with the content being taught.
- Infuse the learning experience with energy.
- Encourage the learner to do the work of learning.

Benefits to the traditional lecture:

- It enables the instructor to integrate information from multiple sources to introduce a new topic to learners.
- It can spark interest in, and enthusiasm for, further study.
- It is less threatening to learners because they are familiar with them and the teacher is doing almost all of the work.

We do not advocate total elimination of the lecture; however, punctuating your lecture for even brief periods of time to allow the learner to process information will enhance the efficacy of your presentation and optimize the chances that your learner will retain the information you are presenting. Each 20 minutes of presentation should be followed by a few minutes of processing time (ie, active learning) for optimal learning and retention.

Look at Table 4-14 again, this time in terms of active learning. The 3 strategies that result in at least 50% retention all require learners to be active. Each of the strategies can be considered a content booster. If you want your learners to remember what you have taught, ideally, you will include something active as 1 of your content boosters.

Stop and Reflect

- What types of active learning strategies have you been exposed to throughout your education from grade school through graduate school?
- Have some active strategies been more effective for you than others? If so, which ones, and what made them so helpful?
- How does physical therapy school compare to undergraduate courses in terms of the use of active learning strategies?

There are myriad active learning strategies and comprehensive resources available in book form or online.[30,33] The choice of strategies depends on the content and goals of your instruction. Chances are that you

Table 4-15. Active Learning Strategies

• Think-pair-share	• Role plays
• Reciprocal teaching	• Debriefing—Independent/group
• Gallery review	• Games and simulations
• Jigsaw	• Presentations with group participation
• Action learning	• Fishbowl
• Discussion boards	

Adapted from Silberman M, Auerbach C. *Active Training: A Handbook of Techniques, Designs, Case Examples, and Tips.* 3rd ed. San Francisco, CA: John Wiley & Sons; 2006; Johnson D, Johnson R. *Active Learning: Cooperation in the College Classroom.* Edina, MN: Interaction Book Company; 1991; Millis BJ. Cooperative learning structures. Available at http://www.utexas.edu/academic/diia/research/projects/hewlett/cooperative.php. Accessed June 16, 2009.

engage in more active learning in your physical therapy classes than you did in your prerequisite science or liberal arts classes. Why? Usually, classes that focus on specific motor skills like transferring a patient from a bed to a chair include practice opportunities that are inherently active. Case-based activities, problem-based strategies, simulations, and standardized patients are all examples of active learning strategies commonly seen in the classroom. It may be more of a challenge to integrate one or more active strategies into a class that is traditionally taught in a lecture format, although the literature is replete with examples of active learning strategies being incorporated even into the more traditional classroom setting.[39,49-54] Table 4-15 lists a number of active learning strategies that can be used successfully in almost any class. We will describe a few popular examples here. For a full description of the active learning strategies listed, see Silberman and Auerbach's[6] *Active Training* text.

Most of us have experienced the *think-pair-share* strategy without knowing its name. It requires individuals to reflect on a teacher's question or comment for a minute or so and then turn to a neighbor, someone sitting nearby, to discuss one another's thoughts or responses. The instructor then asks for a few people to share their thoughts or experience with the larger group. It takes only a few minutes in total and can be adapted to respond to anything the instructor thinks is relevant. For example, the instructor might ask individuals to think back over the preceding 20 to 30 minutes of lecture and identify any information or concept that remains confusing for them. When they exchange that information with a neighbor, there is an opportunity for some of the confusion to be clarified by the neighbor. If a number of students have questions about the same concepts, the instructor obtains valuable feedback and can clarify for the group before moving on to other material.

Modifications of this approach that ask students to indicate confusing or *muddy points* periodically during a lecture class have resulted in improved achievement in physical therapy students. Instead of asking pairs of students to discuss or clarify muddy points, other university instructors have required students to solve multiple-choice questions midway through a lecture. Students answered 1 or 2 questions soon after the information had been delivered by lecture. The students responded to the questions as individuals and then in pairs. Achievement in classes where this active strategy was employed was greater than in other physiology classes of equivalent students where straight lecture was the teaching method.[37,54]

Reciprocal teaching refers to any of several techniques that involve learners taking turns explaining to one another what they have learned about a topic, through reading or listening.[6,32,46,49,56] For example, during a lecture about various manual muscle tests, pairs of students periodically could take turns explaining and demonstrating a particular manual muscle test to each other.

Another strategy might be for the instructor to ask the learners to pretend that the person next to them just arrived to class and missed the last 20 minutes of the lecture. The group would be split in half, and half of the group would be asked to summarize the major points and share it with their partners. A variation of this technique can be used in a workshop with a large number of participants who do not know each other.[32] Before the presentation begins, participants are asked to schedule a number of meeting times with different people for specified times throughout the workshop. When each pair meets, someone is designated *A* and the other person is *B*. At the appointed hour, participants are told to meet with their partners for that time slot. Person A is required to teach Person B about one aspect of a topic that had been taught earlier. Person B then has the opportunity to teach another aspect of the topic to Person A. Each person can ask questions, and if any confusing points remain, the instructor of the large group can clarify the information.

Both think-pair-share and reciprocal teaching can be quite brief and interspersed throughout a presentation. They would be appropriate activities to help process information during those periods described by Sousa[30] as downtimes. If participants know that this activity is coming, they will more likely focus on the content being presented so they can teach it to their peer effectively. Requiring learners to move to find their partners can also reenergize the classroom, effectively minimizing the downtime experienced by the participants.

These are both effective ways of keeping the learner engaged in the presentation. A similar strategy can be used at the end of a laboratory class. Students stand in a circle, and one by one the instructor asks each one to explain a certain concept or demonstrate a technique that was presented. If the students are aware that this is going to happen, they will more likely attend throughout the session. Using this strategy can also help the instructor assess how much the students learned. It is important, however, to make this process a learning process. Creating a safe environment where students feel supported if mistakes are made is critical to the learning process.

Stop and Reflect

Have you ever participated in a workshop in which the large group was broken into several smaller groups for discussion and at the end of the discussion each small group was then asked to report their findings? After the third group reported the same findings, what did you do? Did you tune out?

In response to the "Stop and Reflect" box, did you indicate that, by the third report out, you tuned out? This is not an uncommon experience. The *gallery review* is a multistep strategy that has a visual component that serves as an alternative to having small groups verbally report their responses to a question or task. The gallery review omits the repetitive report out while simultaneously facilitating ongoing discussion across groups. There are many variations of this technique.[55]

One variation we have used is to ask small groups of workshop participants to brainstorm how they, as clinical instructors, would create an ideal orientation for a doctor of physical therapy student's first clinical internship. Participants discuss possibilities in their small groups and reach consensus on key components. They write the key components (in detail) on large chart paper, which they post on the wall. After all groups have posted their "ideal orientation," they move from one poster to another and comment on, or raise questions about, the various plans. They view the posters as though they were in an art gallery, and they discuss each as they might discuss the work of various artists.

Another variation we have used is to ask participants to move in their small groups from one poster to another. As they visit each poster with their group, we ask them to discuss it and add a checkmark the each poster with a checkmark if they see something that they had already included in their own poster, a question mark after a comment they had questions about, a triangle or

delta sign if they saw something that made them think differently, and an asterisk after a point they thought was outstanding. This facilitates further discussion and engages the entire group. The instructors can simultaneously view the gallery and then simply summarize the major points of the activity in the large group.

Jigsaw groups are a staple of cooperative learning activities.[46,57] Originally developed to promote improved cross-cultural relationships in college classrooms,[58,59] the jigsaw has several key components and can be used to facilitate growth in the affective, cognitive, and psychomotor domains.[39,46]

- Participants are assigned initially to a base group where they take a few minutes to get to know the members of their group.

- Each group member is then assigned to a second group. Participants in this second group will be considered the "content experts." There will be several homogeneous content expert groups, and each is assigned to master a specific chunk of content. The role of the content expert group is to synthesize the information assigned and develop sufficient expertise on the content so they can teach their peers.

- Once the content expert groups have developed sufficient expertise, they return to their original base group, which now consists of at least 1 member of each content expert group. At this point, group members are expected to take turns and share their expertise by teaching one another what they had learned. In this way, all participants gain expertise in all of the assigned content.

- At the conclusion of this activity, the instructor can choose to summarize the content, have students summarize the content, or assess student learning in a number of other ways.

We have used this technique to present a variety of different topics. For example, we have used this technique in teaching neonatal reflexes. Rather than lecturing on and demonstrating each of the reflexes, a framework is provided, and students are assigned to groups using the jigsaw process to learn and then teach each other the reflexes. The content is then reinforced by quizzing students in a competitive, yet fun, manner. Finally, to summarize and reinforce the content, students watch a videotape demonstrating the reflexes in a typically developing newborn.

The jigsaw activity requires participants to meet in at least 2 different groups and to teach as well as to learn new material. The technique strengthens interpersonal and cognitive skills. It provides a useful alternative to lecturing for hours on a given topic. To ensure success, the material to be learned has to be easily distributed in equivalent amounts to participants. It is helpful to shorten one section of the material to make it more manageable for students whose first language is not English. There needs to be sufficient time for group members to read through their material, discuss the readings with others, and finally to return to their original group to take turns teaching one another.

We have used the jigsaw technique not only to teach new material but as an assessment at the end of a multi-day continuing education course. In this instance, participants bring all their handouts and course material on the final day of the course. They count off and form base groups. They are given time to review quietly by themselves first. They then are assigned to 1 of 4 content expert groups, which represent each of the 4 days of the course. In the day 1 expert group, for example, participants review the key points and concepts presented that day. Other groups are focusing on days 2, 3, and 4, respectively, and are determining the most important points from those days. Once the experts in each of these groups have determined the key points, they return to their base groups. The base group then has approximately an hour to review the key points from each day and to develop a strategy for synthesizing and integrating the essential information from the entire course into a song, skit, poem, or mural. This end-of-course jigsaw culminates in a variety of unique presentations that are novel, fun, and meaningful to the learners. This activity re-engages both meaning and emotion. Students are challenged to distill and synthesize the material in a meaningful way and have fun doing so, again reinforcing retention of the content.

Critical Thinking Clinical Scenario

You are teaching a lab section on bed mobility skills in patients with varying levels of spinal cord injury in a neuromuscular class. You have asked the students to work in pairs to practice these skills. They try the technique once, and tell you they have finished practicing. In your next class session, you ask pairs of students to demonstrate what they learned in the last class. Most students perform the skills incorrectly.

Reflective Questions

1. Why do you think the students did so poorly in the subsequent class?
2. Why do you think the students took so little time to practice?
3. What could the instructor have done to encourage more practice time?

Skills laboratory sessions are active learning activities commonly used in educating students in all of the health professions. Managing skills laboratory sessions effectively represents a challenge for many instructors. On the one hand, laboratory sessions provide wonderful active learning opportunities. On the other hand, making the most of these opportunities requires more structure than many instructors realize. Laboratory sessions require as much planning as, if not more than, your lecture presentation. Students are often noted to consider 1 or 2 attempts at a task sufficient for skill acquisition, or they may limit their practice to those classmates with whom they are most comfortable. Realizing these common student perspectives, it is essential for you to determine the skills you want students to be able to demonstrate and to plan activities that support these goals. Structuring the laboratory session using a variety of active learning strategies can help minimize the "I already did it" response.

It is not uncommon for faculty to struggle to develop strategies to keep all students engaged and accountable throughout the laboratory session. At a recent faculty retreat, we discussed strategies for managing the skills laboratory. Below are some examples of strategies that faculty found effective. These same strategies can be adapted for use in a variety of teaching-learning situations, not just the skills laboratory:

- Providing clear expectations (objectives for each lab).
- Establishing stations for students to rotate through with different activities with measures of accountability at each station.
- Establishing a rotation schedule in which students must work with at least 4 to 5 different partners before they have completed the rotation.
- Dividing the whole group into several pods or clusters. Within each cluster or pod, direct students to perform one activity in pairs. Switch partners for the next activity. At the end of 2 to 3 activities, ask students within each cluster to discuss the strengths and weaknesses of their own performances. Encourage them to practice the more difficult skills with help from their peers.
- Assigning leaders in each pod responsible for managing the pod and keeping students on task at each station. Rotate the leaders periodically throughout the session.
- Using peer or faculty sign-off sheets with a list of skill competencies that need to be practiced. Require each student to have at least 3 people sign off that they observed the student perform the skill accurately.
- Using peer teaching strategies (eg, jigsaw).
- Having the instructor and teaching assistants circulate around the room in a predictable manner so they do not remain with one group for too long, leaving little time for the other groups.
- Asking students to demonstrate a skill or answer a question on-the-spot.

- Using on-the-spot questions as a large group at the end of the laboratory session both as a summary and a means of keeping students accountable.

- Having students call out answers at the end of the session and having students give each other feedback on the answers or demonstration.

- Lining students up in pairs in a line so you can quickly walk up and down and observe them performing a specific technique.

- Having students continually switch partners in an organized manner, not randomly (eg, one student shifts to the right).

- Using index cards with specific tasks, have each student pull a card and demonstrate.

Another strategy that faculty found both important and effective in maintaining student engagement throughout the laboratory session is ensuring that a mechanism of accountability is in place. If students know they will be responsible for demonstrating a skill or answering a question either during the laboratory session or at the end of the session, they are more likely to attend throughout. Some of the activities noted above can function to both keep students on task as well as maintain accountability. Examples of strategies for maintaining accountability in the skills laboratory that faculty have found effective include the following:

- Using "call outs" whereby students are expected to call out the answer to questions related to the day's laboratory session.

- Incorporating worksheets or checklists of activities to be completed by each student during the laboratory session.

- Using peer or faculty assessment checklists or sign-off sheets.

- Using on-the-spot questions either throughout the laboratory or at the end of the laboratory. These on-the-spot questions may also require the students to demonstrate a selected skill.

- Completing self-assessment sheets.

- Assigning 1 person to keep notes of questions or challenging activities that can be raised when it is the group's turn to meet with the instructor.

As noted above, it is critical for the instructor and lab assistants to systematically and predictably circulate among the students, observing, asking questions, answering questions, and providing assistance when appropriate. This is to ensure that all groups receive equal attention. Novice instructors are often caught responding to the groups as they raise their hands or spending so much time with one group that others are missed. This can be frustrating for students who are waiting and have questions. Being systematic and predictable helps you ensure that during the laboratory session, the needs of all students are being met.

It also assures the students that their turn will come. Assigning a student to keep notes of the group's questions and struggles throughout the session can make your session with each group move more efficiently as well. Rotating among each of the groups can provide you with valuable information about the students' skill acquisition as you observe them, thus obtaining an informal assessment of their progress.

Keeping students actively engaged and on task throughout the laboratory session or throughout any active learning activity requires significant planning, structure, and explicit instructions. Just as you create learning objectives and a plan for your presentations, it is important to create learning objectives and a plan for your laboratory sessions.

Key Points to Remember

- Maintaining student engagement and on-task behavior throughout any active learning activity requires significant:
  - Planning
  - Structure
  - Explicit instructions
- Including measures of accountability can help to maintain on-task behaviors.
- Just as you create learning objectives and a plan for your presentations, it is important to create learning objectives and a plan for your laboratory sessions.

Summaries

Just when it seems that you are nearing the end of your instructional design, you have one more important component to consider: the summary. Based on your middle and high school experiences, some of you might think that the conclusion of instruction is when the bell rings! Nothing could be less effective for pulling together the essential points of an instructional period.

What, exactly, is a summary? Wormeli[60] defined summarization as "restating the essence of a text or experience in as few words as possible or in a new, yet efficient, manner." There is evidence that using a summary positively impacts student achievement.[61] Based on a meta-analysis of more than 100 studies that examined the impact of various school and instructional strategies on student achievement, Marzano et al[60] found that the strategies that most affected student achievement after "identifying similarities and differences" were "summarizing and note-taking." Devoting an entire book to summarization, Wormeli[60] related the impact of summaries to the primacy-recency effect described by Sousa[30] and discussed earlier in this chapter. Because we remember best the information presented at the beginning (primacy), and second best the information presented last (recency), it makes sense to teach the most important material first and then to conclude with a summary of the most important points.

The summary, done by the instructor, can take the form of the instructor restating key points or describing the major take-home messages for the day. Learners, too, can create the summary. In a group learning situation, participants can answer quiz questions, share key points with a neighbor, play a class-wide game in the *Jeopardy* game show format, write down the 3 most important things they learned today, or apply key information to a case. These suggestions, or any of the many possible ways described by Wormeli,[60] encourage reflection on the materials presented and foster integration into one's existing neural connections.[30,60]

Critical Thinking Clinical Scenario

You are a student physical therapist and have prepared a 45-minute in-service on the latest approaches to shoulder arthroplasty. You have included 30 minutes of lecture material and a small group activity. Just as you are about to begin, the clinical instructor tells you to finish up in 30 minutes because there are administrative announcements to be made.

Reflective Questions

1. What aspects of your presentation do you consider essential? Why?

2. What aspects of your presentation could you omit? Why?

3. If you are approaching the end of your time and you must choose between presenting the most recent, evidence-based finding or a final summary, which will you choose? Why?

Key Points to Remember

- When choosing your content, consider the purpose of the instruction, the objectives, and the audience.

- Allow sufficient time for presenting and processing content. Tailor the amount of time for processing to goals of the presentation.

- Organize the content by including what Garmston[14] referred to as containers.

- Use the principle of less is more when choosing content and length of instructional period.

- Capture your learner's attention by using the appropriate motivational hooks that are geared toward various learning preferences.

- Be sure to maintain your learner's focus with appropriate content boosters that appeal to various different learning preferences.

- Use active learning techniques to facilitate learning and retention.

- Use a summary to conclude your presentation.

Assessment

Once you have designed the optimal teaching-learning situation, with appropriate behavioral or outcome objectives, motivational hooks, content boosters, active strategies, and a summary, you have one final task. You need to determine how you will know whether your learners learned what you expected them to learn. How do you do this? How will you determine whether or not learners can demonstrate mastery of the expected outcomes? Assessment, in its several forms, provides the answer.

Assessment can occur at several points in the learning experience. You are probably most familiar with summative assessments that happen at the end of a course or a unit of instruction and result in a grade. Summative assessments focus on determining how well the students learned the content presented.[60] Summative assessments provide the evidence you need to be able to make a judgment about student learning.[63]

As we noted earlier, the behavioral or outcome objectives you developed for your presentation, course, or internship provide the basis not only for how you design your learning activities but for how you design your assessment strategies. It is critical to have a direct link from your behavioral objectives to your outcome assessments. If you expect your learner to perform at the analysis level of Bloom's taxonomy, your instruction should be designed to facilitate that level of achievement and your assessments should be designed to assess that level of performance. Similarly, if your outcome objectives are in the psychomotor domain, your assessments should include assessment of psychomotor skills. For example, if your stated objective is "The learner will perform a complete patient history efficiently," it is not enough for you to assess your learner's knowledge of how to perform a compete history; your assessment must include the actual performance of the history itself. Unfortunately, mismatches are not uncommon. We have seen instructors develop outcome objectives related to problem solving and then design fine case-based teaching strategies to facilitate the development of problem-solving skills in their learners; but, when it came to the summative assessment, the instructor used all lower-level factual questions to assess their learners' performance. This type of mismatch often leads to frustration on the part of the learner—particularly if the learner is being graded.[24,64] Keeping the verbs of the behavioral objectives in mind when developing your summative assessment may help prevent these types of mismatches from occurring.

Key Points to Remember

There should always be a direct link between:

- The behavioral objectives and the strategies used for instruction.

- The behavioral objectives and the strategies used for assessment.

Summative assessment is about collecting data on student performance to determine whether the stated behavioral objectives have been met. For data collection to be effective and meaningful, the right type of data must be collected. Data that include direct or observable evidence of student learning will most clearly substantiate the degree to which learning has occurred.[64] Samples of direct evidence of student performance in the physical therapy classroom include scores on multiple-choice and essay exams, practical exams, simulations and standardized patient encounters, electronic discussion threads, portfolios, and student reflections. In the clinic, ratings on instruments such as the *Clinical Performance Instrument*[65] provide further direct evidence of student behavior and learning. Finally, standardized exams such as the National Physical Therapy Exam (NPTE) provide evidence of learning at the end of the curriculum.

Two basic types of data collection methods have been described in educational literature: objective and subjective assessment.[64] *Objective assessments* typically have 1 right answer and require very little professional judgment in actual scoring. A good example of an objective assessment is the multiple-choice exam. *Subjective assessments*, on the other hand, do require some degree of judgment because they often allow for multiple approaches to the problem. Good examples of subjective assessments are essays, reflective writing, portfolios, practical exams, and simulations. Though each student may receive the same case on a practical exam or the same patient in the clinical setting, how they each approach the patient and the process they use to address the problem may be quite variable. Truthfully, even objective assessments have some degree of subjectivity. Professional judgment is required in determining what questions to ask, how to ask them, how they should be interpreted, and how they should be scored.[64] Similarly, we strive to make subjective assessments as objective and fair as possible. As you will read later in this chapter, the objectivity of some more subjective exams and assignments may be enhanced by using rubrics.

Each type of assessment has its advantages as well. For example, objective assessments such as multiple-choice exams generally cover a broad range of content in a short period of time, are easily scored, are efficient, and result in a numerical value. Alternatively, more subjective assessments such as essays and certain types of practical exams can more easily reveal the learner's values and beliefs, thought processes, problem-solving skills, and performance/psychomotor skills. Each has its place in the physical therapy curriculum. Regardless of the type of assessment used, some degree of objectivity is essential to fair and unbiased grading. In addition, it should be remembered that there are no perfect assessments and students have different learning styles, so to obtain an accurate assessment of the learner, we encourage you to use multiple sources of evidence and multiple types of assessment.[66]

Key Points to Remember

The 2 types of summative assessments:

- Objective assessments typically have 1 right answer and require very little professional judgment in actual scoring.
  - Advantages include the following:
    - Cover a broad range of content in a short period of time
    - Easily scored
    - Efficient
    - Result in a numerical value
- Subjective assessments often allow for multiple approaches to the problem and require some degree of judgment in scoring.
  - Advantages include the following:
    - This type of assessment more easily reveals the learner's values, problem-solving skills, beliefs, thought processes, performance skills, and psychomotor skills
- Regardless of the type of assessment used, some degree of objectivity is essential to fair and unbiased grading.
- To obtain an accurate assessment of the learner, multiple sources of evidence and multiple types of assessment should be used.

Entire texts have been written on designing effective assessment strategies, and we encourage you to review some of these texts as you design your own assessments.[24,64,67,68] What we will present here are some of the most common types of summative assessments used in physical therapy education along with a mechanism for fairly and effectively judging performance. Given that the NPTE is a multiple-choice exam, many programs integrate this type of objective assessment throughout the curriculum. Not all content can be assessed easily using a multiple-choice format, however, so more subjective types of assessment such as practical exams, simulations, and standardized patients, written essays, group work, and presentations are also included. To optimize equity and ease of grading, we advocate the use of rubrics when using subjective assessments. Here, we will address the design and development of both multiple-choice questions and rubrics.

Writing Good Multiple-Choice Exams

Effective assessments begin with well-written behavioral objectives or learning outcomes—remember, begin with the end in mind! In developing multiple-choice exams, it is important to start with a blueprint. A *blueprint* is your outline or plan for the design of your assessment.[64,69] Blueprints help ensure that the test you design:

- Assesses all of the expected learning outcomes.
- Appropriately emphasizes the learning outcomes based on their importance (ie, you will want to weigh the importance of each of the learning outcomes).
- Assesses your learner at the level of your teaching and your expected outcome (eg, analysis or application versus knowledge or comprehension).
- Assesses your learner in the domain of your teaching and your expected outcome (ie, cognitive).
- Is comprehensive without consisting of trivial content.[64]

To develop a blueprint, begin with the established learning objectives as outlined in your syllabus. You want to review the objectives along with the materials you presented in class to determine which learning objectives are most important and which ones you emphasized in your teaching. Assign a point value or percentage to each learning objective (ie, the percentage or number of questions that need to be designed for each learning objective) based on your determination of importance. Your blueprint will tell you how many and what types of questions you will need to write to assess each of the expected learning outcomes. From this blueprint, you can begin writing your questions. As you develop your exam, it is important to note that depending on the level of complexity, learners generally can complete 1 to 2 multiple-choice questions per minute.[70] Giving your test blueprint to your students may help them focus their studies as well.[64]

Writing good multiple-choice questions can be challenging, but it is always important to remember that your goal is to assess learning, not trick your students. Some principles to consider before you even begin to write multiple-choice questions can be found in Table 4-16.[64,66,69-72]

Multiple-choice questions consist of the following:

- *Stem*: Which is the direct question or incomplete statement that leads into the answer
- *Responses or options*: Which are the possible choices for the learner
- *Distracters or foils*: Which are the incorrect options
- *Key*: Which is the correct response

In writing the stem, be sure that it does not include extraneous content or grammatical clues that might lead the learner to answer the question without having to fully process it. Avoid negatives, particularly double negatives whenever possible. If this cannot be avoided be sure to capitalize or bold such words as *except* or *not*. Avoid abbreviations and jargon, except where appropriate. The learner should be able to answer the stem question or finish the stem statement without reading all of the options.[64,69] Stems that are complete sentences or questions tend to be clearer and less ambiguous than incomplete sentences or fill-in-the-blanks.[70]

In writing the responses or options and the key, there should be 1 best answer. Responses should be placed in a logical sequence (eg, alphabetical, chronological). Responses should be about the same length and should be similar in format; any discrepancies in length or format may give the savvy test-taker clues. Options should be relatively short; long options tend to be confusing and hard to follow. Be sure that the correct response does not repeat words from the stem and that none of the responses overlap. It is also best to avoid using statements such as "all of the above" and "none of the above."[64,69,73]

Finally, the distracters or foils should all be plausible. The number of options in any multiple-choice exam may vary. It has been suggested that 3 to 5 options is optimal,[70] and on the NPTE most multiple-choice questions have 4 response options. More important than the number of options, however, is the plausibility of the options. If you cannot develop plausible distracters, it

Table 4-16. Principles of Writing Effective Multiple-Choice Questions

- Avoid tricky, grammatically incorrect, or otherwise imprecise language—you do not want your learners to select the wrong answer because of poorly worded instructions or questions.
- Avoid vague, imprecise, or absolute terms such as *always, never, some, few,* etc.
- Avoid overlapping questions (ie, questions that can provide clues to other answers).
- Avoid linking questions (ie, questions that require the learner to know the answer to one question in order to answer another correctly).
- Avoid trivial questions.
- Focus on the content you have identified as important in your blueprint.
- Include as many questions as possible; as the number of questions increases, the variability due to guessing decreases.
- Be sure your blueprint and subsequent exam are comprehensive; otherwise, rather than assessing learning, you may be assessing the degree to which a student determined the "right" material to study for the exam.
- Have a colleague peer review your exam for clarity, grammar, spelling, etc.

is better to use fewer options rather than resorting to implausible or trivial distracters. Implausible, trivial, or otherwise nonfunctional distracters simply waste the learner's time.[74] The best distracters consist of common errors or common misperceptions, not tricky or deceptive answers.[64,69,70]

Stop, Do, and Reflect

Earlier in this chapter, we presented 3 learning objectives that you might typically see in a physical therapy curriculum. For each learning objective or outcome, develop at least 1 well-written multiple-choice question to assess the learners.

1. After this laboratory session, the student will correctly list 5 contraindications to using ultrasound as an intervention.

2. By the end of this clinical internship, the student will integrate the core value of professionalism into her daily interactions.

3. At the end of this course, the student will safely transfer patients from the bed to a wheelchair.

Some multiple-choice exams also include a number of scenario-based questions, also called *context-dependent* or *enhanced* multiple-choice questions.[70] This consists of a patient scenario followed by one or more multiple-choice questions related to that scenario. This requires the learner to interpret the scenario before answering any of the questions. There are advantages to this type of multiple-choice question because it tends to focus on important, realistic concepts and often requires a degree of problem solving and decision making at the higher levels of Bloom's taxonomy.[70] The key to writing these types of questions is to make the scenario realistic. You also do not want the learner to get caught up in reading a very long passage before answering the questions because this can be time consuming, particularly for the slower reader.[64] Context-dependent questions can be developed using items such as x-rays, statistical tables, or pictures of actual patients rather than a long narrative scenario. The following is an example of a well-written context-dependent multiple-choice question that might be found on the NPTE[75]:

A physical therapist treating a patient overhears two of his colleagues discussing another patient's case in the charting area. The therapist is concerned that patients may overhear the conversation. The MOST appropriate action is to

1. Discuss the situation with the director of rehabilitation
2. Discuss confidentiality at the next staff meeting
3. Move the patient away from the charting area
4. Inform the physical therapists that their conversation may be audible to the patients

---

Stop, Do, and Reflect

You have just completed a unit on reflective practice. Your primary goal for the unit was to have students apply the principles of reflective practice to real-world scenarios.

Based on the concepts presented on developing on effective multiple-choice questions, critique the following multiple-choice question:

_____ is NOT one of the elements of reflective practice espoused by Jack Mezirow:

A) Reflection-in-action
B) Premise reflection
C) Content reflection
D) None of the above

Finally, once you have given your exam, it is optimal to complete a post-test analysis. Psychometric analysis of exams is outside the scope of this section because it can become quite complex quickly. What we provide here are a few simple concepts to get you started, and we encourage you to consider this an area of ongoing study if you will be writing and administering tests frequently. Ideally, you will have access to a computerized statistical analysis of your exam. This analysis will allow you to assess each question for 2 key characteristics: difficulty and discrimination. *Difficulty* refers to the number of respondents who answered the question correctly. Although each question must be analyzed independently, in general, an optimal level of difficulty is when approximately 50% to 75% of the learners answer the question correctly.[70] *Discrimination* refers to the degree to which performance on any test question correlates with overall test performance (ie, the degree to which the respondents who answered that particular question correctly also performed well on the exam overall). It describes the degree to which the item distinguishes between more and less knowledgeable students. Discrimination scores range between −1.0 and +1.0 (sometimes described in percentages). Negative scores indicate that students who performed poorly on the exam answered this question correctly more often than those who scored well on the exam. Multiple-choice questions with negative discrimination scores should be revised.[70] Although sources differ on what an ideal score consists of, generally, a score of 0.5 on an item suggests that those who answered the particular question correctly were more often among the top 50% of test performers.[70]

Once you have determined the degree of difficulty and discrimination of each multiple-choice question, you will then want to make some judgments about revising your questions. If a question is too challenging or too easy, you may want to consider revising it. Of course, these decisions must be made in the context of the teaching-learning situation. For example, you may be assessing a question on content that you consider to be very important. The question may have a high level of difficulty but also has a high level of discrimination. In this case, it is a challenging item; however, it also clearly discriminated between the highest and lowest scorers in the class, and you may not necessarily want to modify this question. On the other hand, you may have an item in which a particular distracter was never selected or was often selected. If it was never selected, it is likely that it was an implausible option. If it was chosen often, it suggests that it may actually be a correct answer. In either case, you may want to review and refine your questions.[70,71] Poorly constructed questions unnecessarily add to the difficulty of the exam and present a challenge to a meaningful interpretation of the results of the exam.[70] It is always important to remember that the goal of the exam is to assess learning, not test-taking savvy!

Stop, Do, and Reflect

You are preparing to teach a unit on the prevention of back injuries and repetitive strain injuries to a group of novice sonographers in the hospital.

- Define at least 1 learning outcome for your presentation.
- Based on your expected learning outcome, what teaching strategies might you use?
- Based on your expected learning outcome and teaching strategies, develop at least 1 multiple-choice question to assess your learners.

Key Points to Remember

In writing multiple-choice questions:

- Develop and utilize a comprehensive blueprint.
- Avoid negative and imprecise language.
- Remove all potential cues including any overlapping questions.
- Have someone peer review your exam for clarity.
- Include as many questions as possible but avoid trivia.
- Analyze results of the exam for levels of difficulty and discrimination.

Developing Effective Rubrics

As noted earlier, rubrics provide a mechanism for improving the objectivity of more subjective assessment strategies. Rubrics can clarify your expectations of student performance; can provide more detailed, consistent feedback to students about their performance; and can facilitate ease and efficiency of grading. Essentially, a rubric is a grading tool that consists of clear statements about what you are looking for in terms of content mastery plus criteria for evaluating the degree to which learners demonstrate mastery.[64,68]

Suskie[64] suggests the fist step in developing an assignment should be the development of a rubric. Just as we did earlier in this chapter, she advocates that you begin with the end in mind. Creating a rubric helps you clarify your goals for the assignment and as a result may help you develop a more focused and effective assignment. This may be a challenging task. More often than not, we create our assignments and then determine how to grade them. Using an iterative process may help. That is, determine the learning goals, create the assignment, and finally refine your goals into a more complete evaluation tool or rubric. Once you have designed your rubric you may go back again and refine the instructions to your assignment.

Key Points to Remember

Rubrics can help:

- Improve the objectivity of more subjective assessment strategies.
- Clarify your expectations of student performance.
- Provide more detailed, consistent feedback to students about their performance.
- Facilitate ease of grading.
- Facilitate efficient feedback to students.

Rubrics can also help clarify your goals for your assignments and as a result may help you develop more focused and effective assignments.

In designing a rubric, it is helpful to start with a blueprint based on the main objectives for the course or unit and the desired learner outcomes for a particular assignment, similar to how you design a blueprint for multiple-choice exams. Consider the purpose of the assignment, what outcomes you expect from the learner as a result of completing the assignment, and what level of performance learners are likely to exhibit. You might ask yourself what skills you expect the learners to have or to develop as a result of completing the assignment and what types of evidence would demonstrate that your learners have mastered the content.

Once you have reflected on the purpose of the assignment and how it supports your main objectives, you are ready to specify all the performance indicators or the criteria for determining the degree to which mastery was achieved. As you define the performance indicators, you will group them into similar objectives; for example, clarity, organization, content, originality, creativity. You need to consider all the performance indicators that allow you to assess mastery of the material. Once you have identified the performance indicators, you then need to determine the criteria you will use to evaluate performance and determine the level of competence achieved.[64,68]

Rubrics can vary in format from simple checklists and rating scales to more comprehensive descriptions of performance outcomes and indices of mastery.[64] A checklist rubric might be helpful when you observe students in a laboratory practical exam and you are concerned about

the presence or absence of specific behaviors (Table 4-17). For example, an instructor could simply check off whether or not the following behaviors were present:

❑ Student introduces him- or herself to the patient

❑ Student washes his/her hands

❑ Student asks about past medical history

❑ Student ensures patient safety throughout the treatment session.

Table 4-17. Sample Rubric for a Focused Laboratory Practical

1. Introduces him- or herself	___/	2
2. Explains purpose of interaction	___/	1
3. Previous history of back, leg, or foot pain	___/	2
4. Mechanism of injury	___/	2
Focused Patient History: Pain		
5. Onset	___/	2
6. Location	___/	2
7. Radiation	___/	2
8. Pattern (eg, constant, occasional, intermittent)	___/	2
9. Description (eg, dull, sharp, etc)	___/	2
10. Intensity	___/	2
11. Getting better or worse	___/	2
12. Aggravating factors	___/	1
13. Alleviating factors	___/	1
14. Addresses inconsistencies in patient reporting	___/	2
Blood Pressure Check		
15. Patient's arm is firmly supported	___/	1
16. Cuff placed approximately 1 inch above antecubital fossa	___/	1
17. Locates the brachial artery medial to biceps tendon	___/	1
18. Obtains palpable systolic pressure	___/	1
19. Places stethoscope firmly over brachial artery	___/	1
20. Pumps cuff to 20 to 30 mmHg above palpable systolic pressure	___/	1
21. Deflates cuff slowly, watching manometer	___/	1
22. Obtains accurate reading (accept ±4 systolic and ±2 diastolic)	___/	2
MMT of Appropriate Muscle Group		
23. Chooses appropriate muscle group	___/	2
24. Subject is placed in appropriate position	___/	2
25. PROM checked	___/	2
26. Subject asked to perform AROM	___/	2
27. Resistance is applied in appropriate direction	___/	2
28. Appropriately grades muscle group	___/	2
Total score*		/46

Adapted from a rubric used to grade an OSCE in the Introduction to Examination course at Touro College Doctor of Physical Therapy Program. MMT indicates manual muscle test; PROM, passive range of motion; AROM, active range of motion.
*Note: Any demonstration of unsafe, unprofessional, or unethical behavior will be considered an automatic failure regardless of overall score (eg, does not guard patient, puts patient at risk, or anything deemed unsafe).

Lab practical exams are often a combination of objective and subjective assessment. For example, during a lab practical, one performance criterion might be, "The student washes his/her hands." Some would consider this objective (ie, performed/not performed), requiring little professional judgment. On the other hand, if what you are assessing is the quality of performance, some degree of judgment may be required, and unless a rubric with specific performance indicators is developed, grading may be somewhat subjective (eg, wet hands first, lathered well beyond wrist, washed all surfaces and under fingernails thoroughly for at least 15 to 20 seconds, thoroughly rinsed with clean water, dried hands completely, used towel to turn off water).

Checklist rubrics may be helpful to students before submitting an assignment to determine whether they have included all necessary components. For example, the checklist might include the following expected behaviors for a research proposal:

☐ Citations are written in AMA format

☐ A minimum of 15 references are cited

☐ Completed IRB approval form is attached

☐ Abstract of 75 words is included

A rating scale rubric is similar to a checklist except that it allows the instructor to go beyond noting the presence of a behavior to indicate the degree to which the desired behaviors occurred. The ratings can be written in a variety of formats that include Likert-like scales, where the rater judges the quality of the performance such as

☐ Excellent, Very Good, Adequate, Marginal, Inadequate

☐ Excellent, Adequate, Needs Improvement

☐ Performed Independently, Performed with Cuing, Did Not Perform

☐ Almost Always, Often, Sometimes, Rarely

☐ Strongly Agree, Agree, Disagree, Strongly Disagree

Point values can be used to indicate how well the performance met expectations as well. Rubrics also can be helpful in the peer review process. For example, in an in-class oral presentation, the instructor as well as classmates could use a rating scale rubric with assigned point values such as the one presented in Table 4-18.

Table 4-18. Rating Scale Grading Rubric for a Group Oral Presentation

| Rater's Name: | Students' Names: | 1. | | 2. | | |
| | | 3. | | 4. | | |

Complete this review, using the following scale: N/O = Not observed; 1 = Unsatisfactory; 2 = Marginal; 3 = Meets Requirements; 4 = Exceeds Requirements; 5 = Exceptional

Process	1	2	3	4	5	N/O
Speaks clearly and succinctly	☐	☐	☐	☐	☐	☐
Participation of all group members	☐	☐	☐	☐	☐	☐
Rapport with audience	☐	☐	☐	☐	☐	☐
Pace and time utilization of delivery	☐	☐	☐	☐	☐	☐
Content	1	2	3	4	5	N/O
Needs assessment (designed and implemented)	☐	☐	☐	☐	☐	☐
Motivational hook (relevant, engaging, appropriate)	☐	☐	☐	☐	☐	☐
Objectives (clearly stated in behavioral terms and appropriate number)	☐	☐	☐	☐	☐	☐
Content and sequence (well organized, logical sequence, appropriate amount of content for allotted time)	☐	☐	☐	☐	☐	☐
Content booster (appropriate, supports content, reinforces learning)	☐	☐	☐	☐	☐	☐
Summary (clearly stated; appropriately placed)	☐	☐	☐	☐	☐	☐
Active Learning Strategies	1	2	3	4	5	N/O
Active learning strategy (consider participation of all audience members)	☐	☐	☐	☐	☐	☐
Overall score						/55

Identify 1 or 2 strengths of this presentation._____
Identify 1 aspect of this presentation you suggest this group or particular individual improve upon._____

Adapted from a rubric used in the Teaching and Physical Therapy Practice course at the George Washington University Doctor of Physical Therapy Program.

Descriptive rubrics go beyond checklists and rating scales to provide clearly delineated performance expectations; rather than simply checking off "outstanding" or "needs improvement," each rating has a full description of the expected level of achievement. Although time consuming to develop, descriptive rubrics allow the instructor to make the standards for student performance very clear. These descriptions can provide useful feedback to students, minimize confusion about the grade received on an assignment, and make it more likely that grading is consistent across students and over time.[64,68] Because descriptive rubrics clearly specify the performance expectations, they can facilitate critical thinking in students. For example, performance indicators for an "adequate" rating might include the student presents a thesis statement, provides supportive data from a variety of sources, and demonstrates analysis of multiple points of view. A discussion about these performance indicators before students work on the assignment can encourage them to complete a paper or project with a deeper level of analysis than they might have provided without the discussion or descriptive rubric. Descriptive rubrics are well suited for more complex assignments such as research papers and essays. An example of a descriptive rubric for a research paper appears in Table 4-19.

Table 4-19. Descriptive Grading Rubric for an Evidence-Based Teaching Assignment

	Meets/Exceeds Requirements	Gets By/Needs Work	Unacceptable/Not Observed
Summarizes major points of the research poster presentation or article	Summarizes key points including background, purpose, methodology, participant(s) selection, methods, data analysis, results, discussion, and conclusion	Summarizes most key points logically	Limited or inaccurate summary of key points
	10-8	**7-5**	**<5**
Critical analysis of the research methods and conclusions	Evidence of original thought and critical evaluation of the research methods and conclusions. Evaluation is accurate	Evidence of some original thought and evaluation of the research methods and conclusions. Less visible/logical links made between assertions and evidence	Limited or inaccurate evidence of original thought and critical evaluation of the research methods and conclusions; limited or inaccurate links between assertions and evidence
	10-8	**7-5**	**<5**
Relates information presented to the teaching and learning course	Strong links made between poster/article and information presented in this course	Good linkage made between poster/article and information presented in this course	Little to no linkage made between poster/article and information presented in this course
	10-8	**7-5**	**<5**
Relates information presented to future practice in PT (applies the theory to practice drawing logical conclusions based on supporting evidence)	Strong evidence of application of theoretical concepts to physical therapy practice	Good evidence of application of theoretical concepts to physical therapy practice	Little to no evidence of application of theoretical concepts to physical therapy practice
	10-8	**7-5**	**<5**
Overall: clarity and organization of submission; selected an appropriate article/poster and followed instructions	Logical sequence and transitions throughout; well written and easy to follow; article/poster related to teaching/learning. For the article review: no older than 2007; no more than 400 words, original article included in submission	Logical sequence and transitions; some spelling/grammatical errors; follows most instructions	Inconsistencies; hard to follow; multiple spelling/grammatical errors; poster/article did not relate to teaching/learning; did not follow instructions
	10-8	**7-5**	**<5**
Total points earned			/50

Adapted from a rubric used in the Teaching and Physical Therapy Practice course at the George Washington University Doctor of Physical Therapy Program.

Critical Thinking Clinical Scenario

The following is an assignment you created for class. The purpose of the assignment is for your learners to prepare for future job interviews by engaging in an authentic interview process.

Assignment

To facilitate your continued professional development and preparation for career placement, you will be participating in standardized interviews with local clinicians who routinely interview new graduates. You are to prepare for this interview by reflecting upon your ideal job and preparing some thought-provoking questions. This assignment has 3 parts.

Part I—Preparation: Given what you currently know about yourself and your chosen profession, describe your ideal job. Be as detailed as possible. In considering what you are looking for in a position and in preparation for your standardized interview

1. Develop 5 questions you anticipate being asked by your interviewer plus your response to each.

2. Develop 5 thoughtful questions you plan to ask your potential employer. These questions should go beyond the mundane such as things like salary and benefits (although these are questions that you will ultimately want answered).

Part II—The Interview: During the standardized interview process, you will observe and be observed by 2 peers. While observing your peer, you will be asked to provide effective feedback to each interviewee. Your feedback should address: appropriateness of dress; greeting; verbal communication; nonverbal communication; evidence of active listening skills; responses to interviewer's questions posed (complete, accurate, etc); complexity of the questions posed by the interviewee; closure; interpersonal skills.

Part III—Post-Interview Reflection: After completing your standardized interview:

1. Reflect on your performance and the feedback you received from your peers and from your interviewer. Self-assess and describe what you did well and what you would like to improve upon. Describe your reaction/response to the feedback you received.

2. Reflect on your initial job description. This time, consider the classroom discussion, your own personal research, and any new insights gained. What have you added? Deleted? Modified? If nothing, what alternatives have you either considered or rejected?

Reflective Activity

1. Create a rubric that will be used by peers to assess each learner's performance during the interview.

2. Create a rubric to use in assessing the learners' written assignments.

3. Compare the rubrics you designed to the assignment, and refine both your assignment and your rubric.

Key Points to Remember

Effective rubrics:

- Reflect course and unit objectives
- Clearly state the expected performance outcomes
- Allow for objective assessment across students
- Can include checklists, rating scales, and comprehensive descriptions
- Include a list of performance indicators for checklist rubrics

Rating scale rubrics include the following:

- A list of performance indicators
- A scale showing the level of achievement (eg, Excellent, Adequate, Needs Improvement)

Descriptive rubrics include the following:

- A list of performance indicators
- A scale showing the level of achievement (eg, Excellent, Adequate, Needs Improvement)
- A description of the performance expectations required to attain each level of achievement

Because periodic summative assessments are necessary throughout a curriculum, and we know that students with different learning styles may have different strengths, it can be useful to expand our repertoire of summative techniques. In addition to written and practical exams and term papers, Table 4-20 provides a number of options for you to consider.[64] Regardless of the strategy you select to assess your learners' performance, it must match the established behavioral objectives and the teaching strategies used and must include a mechanism for fairly and effectively judging performance.

Another type of assessment, *formative assessment,* refers to an ongoing process that allows instructors and

Table 4-20. Summative Assessment Alternatives to Written and Practical Exams

- Portfolios/work product
- Case reports/presentations
- Abstracts
- Graphic organizers, models, illustrations
- Poster presentation
- Reflective essays
- Self-assessments
- Self-selected projects
- Action plans
- Videotapes of skill performance
- Objective structured clinical skills exams and standardized patient exams

learner(s) to adjust instructional practices based on student feedback and performance.[62,76] Formative assessment indicates progress toward the accomplishment of the various objectives while there is still an opportunity to make adjustments in both teaching and learning strategies. Another purpose of formative assessment is to provide feedback to the instructor about teaching or presentation skills. Areas for improvement can be identified and strategies implemented. Because formative assessment, according to Popham[62] and others, is a planned, ongoing process, a variety of techniques can be used in the classroom and clinic.

Angelo and Cross[77] described a number of classroom assessment techniques that provide formative assessment in the classroom. We have adapted many of the classroom assessment techniques presented by Angelo and Cross[77] to assess different aspects of student learning in the clinical setting as well. Table 4-21 provides a number of these techniques, along with examples of how they can be adapted for use in the clinical setting. Each of these formative assessment approaches can provide valuable information that can be a useful adjunct to the final, summative assessment of performance in a particular clinical internship.

Table 4-21. Sample Formative Assessment Techniques With Adaptations for Use in the Clinic

Level of Assessment Using Bloom's Taxonomy	Name of Assessment Technique	Purpose	Description and Classroom Use	Clinical Example
Knowledge	Focused listing	To assess how well your learners can identify the most important terms or concepts of the presentation.	Ask your learners to take 2 to 3 minutes to make a list of the most important concepts related to the presentation.	In planning for an evaluation of a patient with complaints of dizziness, ask your student to list the essential components of the evaluation.
	Misconceptions/ preconceptions	To assess whether your learners hold any preconceived notions about a topic that may interfere with learning.	Create a questionnaire to obtain your learners' perceptions on a particular topic in which misperceptions are often noted.	Given a particular diagnosis, and before entering a patient's room, ask your student to list his or her assumptions about the patient's current presentation and expected outcomes.
Comprehension	One-minute paper	To assess what your learners understand of the major concepts presented.	At the end of your presentation or during the last few minutes of a class, ask your learners to write down answers to these 2 questions: What is the most important point you learned today? What important question remains unanswered for you?	Before your student leaves clinic for the day, ask him or her to write down 3 new things he or she learned today and what questions remain for him or her. You can take it one step further and ask your student to research answers to what remains muddy when he or she goes home and be prepared to discuss it in the morning. Consider minimizing the intimidation factor by letting your student know you too will research the topic to ensure that you both learn from the questions raised.
	Empty outlines	To assess how well your learner captured the major points of the presentation.	Provide your learners with a partially completed outline of the presentation and ask them to fill in the rest.	Prior to starting a new patient evaluation, give your student a brief outline of the components of a history and review of systems. Ask him or her to complete the outline based on the initial evaluation he or she is observing. In a hand therapy clinic, give your student the diagnosis and patient history, and have him or her fill in the blanks to problem solve the type of splint that is appropriate for your patient. Give your student a brief outline of the components of a patient interview, history, and review of systems. Ask your student to observe your initial evaluation with a patient and complete the outline based on his or her observations.

(continued)

Table 4-21. Sample Formative Assessment Techniques With Adaptations for Use in the Clinic (continued)

Level of Assessment Using Bloom's Taxonomy	Name of Assessment Technique	Purpose	Description and Classroom Use	Clinical Example
Comprehension	Muddiest points	To assess what remains confusing for your learners.	Ask your learners to take a minute and write down "what is the muddiest point?" or "what remains confusing or unclear?"	After your student observes a pediatric evaluation, ask him or her what he or she thought was the most confusing or difficult part of the evaluation, and then review or give resources to augment knowledge. Have your student keep a list of diagnoses seen during the day. At the end of the day or week, discuss the salient aspects of those diagnoses with which he or she is least familiar. Ask your student to research a number of possible interventions for these diagnoses. Have your student do a chart review and take a history of the patient. Then, discuss what remains muddy and offer knowledge and resources.
	Directed paraphrasing	To assess whether your learner fully understands the information and can put it into his or her own words (jargon-free). This may be particularly helpful when the learner needs to translate technical information to patient-friendly information.	Identify the audience for whom you want your learners to paraphrase information (eg, patient, family, community members). You can also ask the same learner/other learners to paraphrase the information for different audiences (ie, patient, family, consulting professional, etc).	Before presenting the results of a complex evaluation to your patient, discuss the findings with your student. Then, have your student repeat the information in her own words to you as if she were speaking with the patient and his or her family. Have your student practice translating an MRI report sentence-by-sentence into laymen's terms so your student has practice explaining to a patient or family member what the radiology report means. Your student can look up any terms he or she is not familiar with to increase learning. Ask your student to review the patient's chart and summarize what the physicians and nurses reported in the past 24 hours as if he or she were speaking to a patient.
Application	Application cards	To assess your learner's ability to see the relevance of the information presented. It assesses his or her ability to link the theoretical concepts to real-world application.	Ask your learner to provide 3 possible applications, indicating that the goal is for him or her to come up with his or her own ideas of how the principle or procedure can be applied to practice.	After discussing a new treatment technique with your student, ask him or her to come up with 2 to 3 other applications for the same technique. *(continued)*

Table 4-21. Sample Formative Assessment Techniques With Adaptations for Use in the Clinic (continued)

Level of Assessment Using Bloom's Taxonomy	Name of Assessment Technique	Purpose	Description and Classroom Use	Clinical Example
Application	Concept maps	To assess your learner's ability to link the information together and make sense out of it. This may be particularly helpful in encouraging the learner to explore all possible diagnoses and interventions related to particular symptoms before narrowing the differential diagnosis.	Ask your learner to brainstorm terms and phrases related to a particular concept. Have your learners place the concept in a circle at the center and then draw lines to the different terms, demonstrating the relationship of the term to the concept. Ask your learner to link more than one concept together.	Have your student map out some alternative plans of care for your patient who recently had a stroke. Have your student consider the following possibilities at discharge: that he or she will be going home with limited family support, going to a nursing home with access to weekly therapy, or going to a rehabilitation setting. Have your student list all the findings of his or her evaluation and draw a map linking them to potential diagnoses.
Analysis	Pro and con grid	To assess a learner's ability to objectively analyze a decision, an issue, a policy, etc.	Ask your learner to write out a list of pros and cons related to the issue. Have him or her provide the rationale or evidence for his or her responses.	Have your student list the pros and cons for home health versus skilled nursing facility based on insurance limitations. Have your student list the pros and cons for which modalities may be most effective for treatment of a particular diagnosis. Have your student list the advantages and disadvantages of various orthotic devices for your patient who have neurological impairments. Have the student brainstorm as many interventions he or she can think of for the next patient, then write a list of pros and cons of each before deciding which ones to use.
	Categorizing grid	To assess the learner's ability to sort or categorize information.	Select several different categories useful for organizing information covered and the identify subordinate terms for each category. Scramble a list of terms under each category and ask your learner to categorize them appropriately.	Take 3 or 4 different screening tools that you use for your older adult with neurologic impairments, and scramble the different components of the tools. Then, ask your student to categorize them into balance, motor control, reflex testing, cognition, etc. Then, ask your student to look at the tools as a whole and determine which tools screen for what components of neuromuscular function. Have your student organize a list of statements into the subjective/objective/assessment/plan (SOAP) format. *(continued)*

Table 4-21. Sample Formative Assessment Techniques With Adaptations for Use in the Clinic (continued)

Level of Assessment Using Bloom's Taxonomy	Name of Assessment Technique	Purpose	Description and Classroom Use	Clinical Example
Analysis	Analytic memos	To assess the learner's ability to problem solve and communicate his or her decision-making processes	Select a typical problem and the provide the necessary background information. Ask your learner to prepare a memo describing the steps he or she took in analyzing the problem.	After evaluating a complex patient, ask your student to determine what type of assistive devices might be necessary for your patient. Ask him or her to write an analytic memo describing how he or she made these decisions. Your patient has an amputation with skin breakdown. Have your student outline how this may have happened; how it may affect the current plan of care including prosthetic wear and ambulation; how it might be corrected/prevented; and how the patient's level of cognition might play a role. Have your student write a letter to the insurance company justifying the type of wheelchair system your young patient with cerebral palsy spastic quadriplegia might need. Be sure the analysis includes why less costly alternative systems might be inappropriate.
Synthesis	Documented problem solving	To assess the learner's reasoning process in developing solutions. It also encourages self-assessment and self-awareness of problem-solving abilities. This may be particularly helpful in developing a differential diagnosis.	Select a problem, case, etc. Ask your learner to write down all the steps he or she took to solve the problem—all of the decisions he or she made and why he or she made those decisions.	Give your student a history of a patient with a complex neurological problem and limited family support. Tell him or her that your patient is being discharged home and ask him or her to determine what needs to be accomplished to enable him or her to be safe at home. Ask him or her to document his or her solution and include rationale for whatever he or she decides. Review the lab values of a patient in ICU. Ask your student to articulate how he or she might modify the current plan of care based on these lab values. Have him or her justify his or her decisions. Patient with increased blood pressure is "on hold" by nursing. Have your student list why/how increased blood pressure impacts activity and what is the safe range.
	Invented dialogues	Helps assess a student's ability to synthesize his or her knowledge into a structured dialogue. This may be helpful for learners preparing for challenging communication issues (eg, speaking to a physician or insurance company, providing feedback).	Select a problem, issue, or theory that lends itself to a dialogue format. Ask your learner to write a short dialogue between 2 people (eg, doctor and patient; therapist and family member) on the topic. Have your learner practice the dialogue. Assess its completeness and the quality of the reasoning (learners can do this in small groups, assessing each other).	Tell your student that the insurance company has just denied your patient's claims for further reimbursement and you would like him or her to call the insurance company to explain why additional sessions are necessary. Have him or her create the dialogue he or she envisions will ensue. Develop a scenario where an MD, orthotist, and PT all have different opinions on a patient's case. Have your student create a dialogue that presents each of these differing views in preparation for a team meeting. In preparation for contacting a physician to recommend an MRI for your patient, ask your student to create a dialogue that considers the doctor's perspective and how the student might respond to an adverse response.

(continued)

Table 4-21. Sample Formative Assessment Techniques With Adaptations for Use in the Clinic (continued)

Level of Assessment Using Bloom's Taxonomy	Name of Assessment Technique	Purpose	Description and Classroom Use	Clinical Example
Evaluation	Self-confidence surveys	To assess the learner's level of confidence in his or her skills or abilities. The more confident a learner is, the more likely he or she will follow-through.	Create a list of competencies that are important to having a successful performance, and ask your learner to rank how confident (ie, 0 = not at all confident to 5 = very confident) he or she feels in applying his or her knowledge and skills.	During orientation, provide your student with a list of treatment techniques typically used in the clinic, and ask him or her to rate his or her level of confidence in performing each (0 = not comfortable, 5 = performed in past without difficulty). This will help you determine how much guidance and supervision you might expect to provide early on.

Adapted from Angelo TA, Cross KP. *Classroom Assessment Techniques: A Handbook for College Teachers*. 2nd ed. San Francisco, CA: Jossey-Bass; 1993. With input from Ellen Goldman, EdD, and Jennifer Halvaksz, PT, DPT, George Washington University, Washington, DC. MRI indicates magnetic resonance imaging; PT, physical therapist.

Critical Thinking Clinical Scenario

You are preparing to provide a full-day workshop on both effective instruction and assessment. You will be presenting some information about classroom assessment techniques. You would like to include at least 2 formative assessments to determine whether the audience has grasped the major concepts and whether they can apply them to their own practice when they leave the workshop.

Reflective Questions

Review the examples provided:
1. Which 2 assessment techniques might you consider using?
2. Why did you select those 2 techniques?
3. What other techniques might you consider?
4. Which ones would not be appropriate in this context? Why?

Finally, providing feedback to the audience can be beneficial both to you as the instructor and to your learners. As a means of formative assessment, we often ask our audiences to respond to the following questions regarding the teaching strategies being used: What is most helpful to your learning? What is least helpful to your learning? We then compile a list of the most and least helpful and report back to the audience. Inevitably some of the strategies learners listed in the "most helpful" category are also seen in the "least helpful" category. Knowing what we know about the typical audience (ie, the 4 different types of learners in every audience), this makes sense. It is also quite surprising to the learners when they see that what they dislike about the teaching strategies someone else finds helpful. This feedback helps learners understand why we use a variety of strategies when we teach—some they may find most effective and some they may not.

Effective formative assessment can provide valuable feedback to everyone involved in the teaching-learning situation. Formative assessments should be ongoing throughout a course, a workshop, a clinical internship, or any teaching-learning situation. In designing effective formative assessments, you will want to consider your learning objectives and where along the taxonomy you expect your learner to perform. You will want to identify what it is they learned and what they thought was important as well any areas of difficulty or confusion. Some equate formative assessment with feedback, and for feedback to be effective, it must be both diagnostic and remedial. That is, feedback should be designed not only to help your learners understand their weaknesses but to provide them with strategies for improvement. As noted, assessment should also be a reciprocal process. It is equally important for you as the instructor to ask for feedback on your teaching strategies to know whether you are meeting your goals as well as the needs of your learners.

Key Points to Remember

There are 2 types of assessment:
- Summative
- Formative

Summative assessments occur at the end of a course or a unit of instruction and result in a grade.
- Focuses on determining whether the student learned the material and whether the instruction was effective.

Formative assessment occurs throughout the course and allows instructors to adjust their instruction along the way, based on student feedback and performance.
- Indicates progress toward the accomplishment of the objectives while there is an opportunity to make adjustments in both teaching and learning strategies.
- Provides feedback to the instructor about teaching or presentation skills.

The previous examples of formative assessments have emphasized classroom assessments that could be modified for use in the clinic. There are also some formative assessments that clinicians use specifically in the clinical setting to assess their students' progress toward the specific objectives for the various internships. Frequently used tools in physical therapy practice include[77]

- *Weekly Planning Form*: These forms require students to assess what they did well during the previous week, identify their areas of weakness, and develop goals for the upcoming week. In addition to ensuring that ongoing formative assessment occurs and assisting the clinical instructor in planning the learning situation for the student, these forms also promote the following:
  o Self-directed learning
  o Self-assessment
  o Reflective practice
- *The Anecdotal Record and Critical Incident Report*: The anecdotal record is used to document both positive and negative incidents. The advantage of this report is that it separates fact from opinion and interpretation. Essentially, it requires the clinical instructor to objectively document the student's behavior and then identify the results of that behavior. The critical incident report is typically used to document a series of events. Similar to the anecdotal record, the critical incident objectively documents the student's behavior and the results of that behavior. What differentiates the critical incident is that it also identifies consequences if the behavior should persist.
- *Learning Contract:* Learning contracts are usually developed in response to a series of incidents often documented by critical incidents. The contract makes the expectations of appropriate performance explicit and clarifies both expectations and consequences of specific student behaviors. Learning contracts generally require students to sign the contract and include a timeframe for achievement.
- *Midterm Clinical Performance Instrument:* This form is used by many physical therapy programs across the United States. The form requires both the clinical instructor and the student to independently to rate the student's performance on 18 cognitive, psychomotor, and affective behaviors along a continuum from beginner performance to entry-level performance and beyond. In addition to the clinical instructor assessing the student's performance, the student is expected to complete a self-assessment both at the midpoint and endpoint of the clinical internship. The student and clinical instructor then compare student assessment to clinical instructor assessment and discuss any discrepancies. Besides being an effective assessment instrument, it is an excellent opportunity for clinical instructors to provide direct feedback to students and for students to hone their self-assessment skills.[64]

As you reflect back on factors to consider when you are preparing to teach, you probably realize how much more complicated it is to plan an effective instructional experience than you first thought. From needs assessment through learning expectations, objectives, motivational hooks, content and content boosters, summary, and assessments, there are so many important components. Still, there is more to consider when planning truly optimal instruction.

Timing and Sequence

Depending on the time period allotted to your presentation, you can include more or less lecture, more or less active techniques, and more or less small group activities. The key point to remember is that certain factors are essential regardless of the amount of time:

- Motivational hook
- Objectives
- Content
- Content booster
- Summary

You realize that you need a motivational hook to pull your learners' attention from the environment to your instruction. Behavioral objectives begin to provide context for the learners so they know where you are planning to take them. Because both the motivational hook and objectives occur at the beginning of your instruction, they benefit from the primacy effect. The information presented in the early moments of instruction is most likely to be remembered. Interesting content boosters and active strategies help maintain focus and engagement during the middle of the instructional period when attention is most likely to wane. The summary allows you to rely on the recency effect to emphasize the key points at the end of the instructional period, the second most powerful position for learning.

You also want to allow some time for questions throughout or at the end of the instructional period. You do not want to speed up your delivery in hopes of finishing everything in the allotted time. You want participants to be engaged and to have time to process and integrate the information. How do you know how long something will take? The obvious answer is often overlooked: you time it! Practice your instructional activities, and time your presentation. Do a "walk-through" of your active strategy with a stopwatch running. When you participate in various activities in school or at conferences, time them and begin to keep track of how long things take. A common mistake of the novice instructor is too much content/activity for the time allotted. Remember, a good rule of thumb is that any active learning strategy you design will likely take longer than you initially anticipate. We will discuss how you can modify and adapt presentations for different settings and time frames in Chapter 5.

Although you, as the expert on your topic, will determine how best to sequence the content you are presenting, there are a few general guidelines to maximize your effectiveness. As a general rule, present the "big picture" first and then the details.[29,32] This provides context for your learner and makes sense when we consider what we discussed in Chapter 3 about the importance of meaning in grabbing a learner's attention. If we create a context, the big picture, then the details that follow have a place to connect. It is also important to consider the natural, logical sequence of material, if there is one. For example, in this chapter on optimizing instruction, the content followed the logical progression found in effective presentations. We began with a scenario about designing a community-based presentation. We then proceeded to describe the essential elements in the same order as they would occur in the actual design and delivery of an effective presentation.

Room Arrangement and Resources

There are 2 final factors to consider when designing optimal teaching-learning experiences. The physical environment, which includes room arrangement, chairs, tables, space for movement and/or small group work, will influence your presentation. If you are conducting an in-service on spinal mobilizations and you plan to have participants demonstrate these techniques in pairs on each other, you need plinths and adequate space. If you are teaching about conflict-resolution techniques and plan for small groups of participants to do role plays, you will need moveable chairs. The more you know about the setup, and the earlier you obtain this information, the easier your preparation will be. Finally, you want to consider technology and other educational resources. Will you have access to the Internet connection, PowerPoint, a liquid crystal display (LCD) projector, newsprint pads, markers, white boards, handouts, and/or instructional models, etc?[3,5,6] It is important to develop a list of resources you will need to support your presentation, and it is equally important to develop a plan B in case those resources are not available or are not working properly. Though room arrangements can at times be limiting, a little planning and creativity may help you overcome any less than desirable accommodations.

Regardless of the topic, room arrangement, and selection of instructional supports, the key to a successful teaching-learning experience is planning and practice. Test the equipment, photocopy the handouts, visit the room where you will teach, test out your technology, and obtain all necessary materials before the day you present. Practice your instruction, time the complete presentation, and time the active strategies.

Critical Thinking Clinical Scenario

You have been asked to conduct an anatomy review of the shoulder, hip, and knee for student physical therapists assigned to your facility. Many of the patients they will treat have had surgeries in these areas. The students range from first-time interns to students on their final internship. You have a total of 3 hours, divided as you choose, to present the information.

Reflective Questions

1. What goals/expectations might the learners have in terms of exposure, acquisition, or integration?

2. How will you divide the time? What factor(s) influence your decisions?

3. What motivational hooks and content boosters might you use?

4. What active strategies could you use to facilitate learning?

5. What summary strategy could you use?

Summary

In this chapter, we provide strategies to help you develop effective presentations that will grab your audience's attention and maintain it throughout. Table 4-22 provides a summary of the essential elements of effective presentations along with questions you might ask yourself to ensure that your design includes knowing your audience; assessing their needs, creating well-written behavioral objectives to help focus your content, balancing content and process to allow for information processing, providing motivational hooks to grab your audience's attention, using content boosters and active learning strategies to maintain attention and reinforce the content, developing formative and summative assessments to optimize teaching and learning, and providing summaries to capitalize on the recency principle.

Table 4-22. Keys to Developing Effective Presentations

Elements of an Effective Presentation	Why They Are Important
Knowing your audience	Remind you to consider that most audiences include "watchers and doers" as well as those who prefer theory and concrete examples; knowing where along the continuum from novice to expert your learners fall will help you determine the appropriate teaching strategies to use
Needs assessments	Help you determine the specific needs of your audience
Behavioral objectives	Help you "begin with the end in mind"; they provide context and help you create a focused presentation
Focused content	Less is more and covering is not learning
Information processing	Rules of thumb Chunk content Balance content and process time
Motivational hooks	Grab your audience's attention
Content boosters	Reinforce the learning
Active learning strategies	Engage your audience and enhance retention
Formative assessments	Help you determine whether your learners are learning what you planned to teach and help you refine your teaching to meet the needs of your learners
Summative assessments	Help you determine whether the behavioral objectives established at the start of the presentation were achieved
Summaries	Help to ensure your learners retain the key points from your presentation by taking into consideration the concept of primacy and recency

Key Points to Remember

Questions to help guide effective teaching:
- Motivational hook
  - Does it have relevance, emotion, and meaning?
- Objectives
  - Are they observable and measureable?
- Content
  - Is the sequence from general to specific and logical?
- Content boosters
  - Do the content boosters engage watchers and doers? Is there something for the people who appreciate anecdotes and examples? Are theory, concepts, and references included?
  - For your learner at the exposure stage, are you providing sufficient and balanced content and process?
  - For your learners who are developing competency, are you guiding them through practice and feedback?
  - For your learners approaching mastery and expertise, are you challenging them through independent application of the content/skills being taught?
- Formative assessment
  - Do you have a way of monitoring or checking for understanding, such as asking questions about or requesting a demonstration of material presented?
- Summative assessment
  - Does the strategy that you selected to assess your learners' performance match the established behavioral objectives/learning outcomes?
  - Does the strategy you selected to assess your learners' performance match the teaching strategies used?
  - Does the assessment follow a comprehensive blueprint?
  - Does the assessment include a mechanism for fairly and effectively judging performance?
- Summary
  - Do you provide an opportunity to highlight the key points of instruction at the end of the instructional period?

References

1. Fink LD. *Creating Significant Learning Experiences.* San Francisco, Calif: Jossey-Bass; 2003.
2. Hunter M. *Mastery Teaching.* Thousand Oaks, CA: Corwin; 1982.
3. Garmston RJ, Wellman BM. *How to Make Presentations That Teach and Transform.* Alexandria, VA: Association for Supervision and Curriculum Development; 1992.
4. Wlodkowski RJ. *Enhancing Adult Motivation to Learn.* Revised ed. San Francisco, CA: Jossey-Bass; 1999.
5. Shepard KF, Jensen GM, eds. *Handbook of Teaching for Physical Therapists.* 2nd ed. Boston, MA: Butterworth-Heinemann; 2002.

6. Silberman M, Auerbach C. *Active Training: A Handbook of Techniques, Designs, Case Examples, and Tips.* 3rd ed. San Francisco, CA: John Wiley & Sons; 2006.

7. Kolb D. *Experiential Learning: Experience as the Source of Learning and Development.* Englewood Cliffs, NJ: Prentice-Hall; 1984.

8. Benner P. From novice to expert. *Am J Nurs.* 1982;82:402-407.

9. Dreyfus HL, Dreyfus SE, Athanasiou T. *Mind Over Machine: The Power of Human Intuition and Expertise in the Era of the Computer.* New York, NY: Free Press; 1986.

10. Jensen GM, Gwyer J, Hack LM, Shepard KF. *Expertise in Physical Therapy Practices.* Boston, MA: Butterworth-Heinemann; 1999.

11. Candy P. *Self-Direction for Lifelong Learning.* San Francisco, CA: Jossey-Bass; 1991.

12. Knowles M, Holton E, Swanson R. *The Adult Learner.* Woburn, MA: Butterworth-Heinemann; 1998.

13. Pratt DD. Andragogy as a relational construct. *Adult Educ Q.* 1988;38:160-181.

14. Garmston R. *The Presenter's Fieldbook: A Practical Guide.* Norwood, MA: Christopher-Gordon; 1997.

15. Covey S. *The 7 Habits of Highly Effective People.* New York, NY: Simon and Schuster; 1989.

16. Bloom BS, ed. *Taxonomy of Educational Objectives: Book 1 Cognitive Domain.* New York, NY: Longman; 1956.

17. Krathwohl DR, Bloom BS, Masia BB. Taxonomy of Educational Objectives: Book 2 Affective Domain. New York, NY: Longman; 1964.

18. Simpson EJ. *The Classification of Educational Objectives in the Psychomotor Domain.* Washington, DC: Gryphon House; 1972.

19. Dave R. Psychomotor levels. In: Armstrong RJ, ed. *Developing and Writing Behavioral Objectives.* Tucson, AZ: Educational Innovators Press; 1970.

20. Harrow AJ. *A Taxonomy of the Psychomotor Domain: A Guide for Developing Behavioral Objectives.* New York, NY: David McKay; 1972.

21. Anderson L, Krathwohl DA. *A Taxonomy for Learning, Teaching and Assessing: A Revision of Bloom's Taxonomy of Educational Objectives.* New York, NY: Longman; 2001.

22. Dettmer P. New Bloom's in established fields: four domains of learning and doing. *Roeper Rev.* 2006;28:70-78.

23. Heinrich R, Molenda M, Russell J, Smaldino S. *Instructional Media and Technologies for Learning.* 7th ed. Englewood Cliffs, NJ: Prentice-Hall; 2001.

24. Diamond RM. *Designing & Assessing Courses & Curricula: A Practical Guide.* 3rd ed. San Francisco, CA: Jossey-Bass; 2008.

25. *A Normative Model of Physical Therapist Professional Education: Version 2004.* Alexandria, VA: American Physical Therapy Association; 2004.

26. *A Normative Model of Physical Therapist Assistant Professional Education: Version 1999.* Alexandria, VA: American Physical Therapy Association; 1999.

27. *Evaluative Criteria for Accreditation of Education Programs for the Preparation of Physical Therapists.* Alexandria, VA: Commission on Accreditation of Physical Therapy Education; 2006.

28. *Evaluative Criteria for Accreditation of Education Programs for the Preparation of Physical Therapist Assistants.* Available at http://www.apta.org/AM/Template.cfm?Section=PTA_Programs2&CONTENTID=62536&TEMPLATE=/CM/ContentDisplay.cfm. Accessed December 6, 2009.

29. Jensen E. *Teaching with the Brain in Mind.* 2nd ed. Alexandria, VA: Association for Supervision and Curriculum Development; 2005.

30. Sousa D. *How the Brain Learns.* Thousand Oaks, CA: Corwin; 2006.

31. Squire L, Kandel E. *Memory: From Mind to Molecules.* 2nd ed. Greenwood Village, CO: Roberts and Company Publishers; 2009.

32. Wolfe P. *Brain Matters.* Alexandria, VA: Association for Supervision and Curriculum Development; 2001.

33. Sprenger M. *Differentiation Through Learning Styles and Memory.* 2nd ed. Thousand Oaks, CA: Corwin; 2008.

34. Aronson N, Driscoll M, eds. *Classroom Management and Student Self-Discipline.* Springhouse, PA: Learning Institute; 1987.

35. Medina J. *Brain Rules.* Seattle, WA: Pear Press; 2008.

36. Lake D. Student performance and perceptions of a lecture-based course compared with the same course utilizing group discussion. *J Phys Ther Educ.* 2001;81:896-903.

37. Cortright RN, Collins HL, DiCarlo SE. Peer instruction enhanced meaningful learning: ability to solve novel problems. *Adv Physiol Educ.* 2005;29:107-116.

38. James D. Are four minds better than one? A study on the efficacy of group work. *Coll Univ.* 2005;80:47-48.

39. Wong CK, Driscoll M. A modified jigsaw method: an active learning strategy to develop the cognitive and affective domains through curricular review. *J Phys Ther Educ.* 2008;22:15-23.

40. Dunfee H, Plack MM, Driscoll M, Rindflesch A, Hollman J. Assessing reflection and higher order thinking in electronic discussion threads in the clinical setting. *J Phys Ther Educ.* 2008;22:60-66.

41. Plack MM, Dunfee H, Driscoll M, Rindflesch A, Hollman J. Virtual action learning sets: a model for facilitating reflection in the clinical setting. *J Phys Ther Educ.* 2008;22:33-41.

42. Blatt B, Plack MM, Mintz M, Simmons S. Acting on reflection: does student performance on a standardized patient examination improve with reflection and revisiting the "patient"? *J Gen Intern Med.* 2007;22:49-54.

43. Plack MM, Santasier A. Reflective practice: a model for facilitating critical thinking skills within an integrative case studies classroom experience. *J Phys Ther Educ.* 2004;18:4-12.

44. Silberman M. *101 Ways to Make Training Active.* 2nd ed. San Francisco, CA: John Wiley & Sons; 2005.

45. Johnson D, Johnson R. *Active Learning: Cooperation in the College Classroom.* Edina, MN: Interaction Book Company; 1991.

46. Johnson DW, Johnson FP. *Joining Together.* 7th ed. Boston, MA: Allyn and Bacon; 2000.

47. Lammers WJ, Murphy JJ. A profile of teaching techniques used in the university classroom. *Active Learn High Educ.* 2002;3:54-67.

48. Youdas JW, Krause DA, Hellyer NJ, Hollman JH, Rindflesch AB. Perceived usefulness of reciprocal peer teaching among doctor of physical therapy students in the gross anatomy laboratory. *J Phys Ther Educ.* 2007;21:30-38.

49. Ghosh S. Combination of didactic lectures and case-oriented problem-solving tutorials toward better learning: perceptions of students from a conventional medical curriculum. *Adv Physiol Educ.* 2007;31:193-197.

50. Bressmann T, Martino R, Rochon E, Bradley K. An action learning experience for speech-language pathology students: on the experience of having dysphagia for a day. *Can Lang Pathol Audiol.* 2007;31:127-133.

51. McNeil HP, Hughes CS, Toohey SM, Dowton SB. An innovative outcomes-based medical education program built on adult learning principles. *Med Teach.* 2006;28:527-534.

52. Heidari F, Galvin K. Action learning groups: can they help students develop their knowledge and skills? *Nurs Educ Pract.* 2003;3:49-55.

53. Rao SP, DiCarlo SE. Peer instruction improves performance on quizzes. *Adv Physiol Educ.* 2000;24:51-55.

54. Millis BJ. Cooperative learning structures. Available at http://www.utexas.edu/academic/diia/research/projects/hewlett/cooperative.php. Accessed June 16, 2009.

55. Palinscar AS, Brown AL. Interactive teaching to promote independent learning from text. *Read Teach.* 1986;39:771-777.

56. Slavin SR. *Cooperative Learning: Theory, Research, and Practice.* 2nd ed. Boston, MA: Allyn and Bacon; 1995.

57. Aronson E, Blaney N, Sikes J, Stephan G, Snapp M. *The Jigsaw Classroom.* Beverly Hills, CA: Sage; 1978.

58. Williams D. Improving race relations in higher education: the jigsaw classroom as a missing piece to the puzzle. *Urban Educ.* 2004;39:316-344.

59. Wormeli R. *Summarization in Any Subject.* Alexandria, VA: Association of Supervision and Curriculum Development; 2005.

60. Marzano RJ, Pickering DJ, Pollack JE. *Classroom Instruction That Works.* Alexandria, VA: Association for Supervision and Curriculum Development; 2001.

61. Popham WJ. *Transformative Assessment.* Alexandria, VA: Association for Supervision and Curriculum Development; 2008.

62. Taras M. Assessment—summative and formative—some theoretical reflections. *Br J Educ Stud.* 2005;53:466-478.

63. Suskie L. *Assessing Student Learning: A Common Sense Guide.* San Francisco, CA: Jossey-Bass; 2009.

64. *Physical Therapist Clinical Performance Instrument for Students.* Alexandria, VA: American Physical Therapy Association; 2006.

65. McCoubrie P. Improving the fairness of multiple-choice questions: a literature review. *Med Teach.* 2004;26:709-712.

66. Banta TW, Jones EA, Black KE. *Designing Effective Assessment: Principles of Good Practice.* San Francisco, CA: Jossey-Bass; 2009.

67. Stevens D, Levi A. *Introduction to Rubrics.* Sterling, VA: Stylus Publishers; 2005.

68. Bridge PD, Musial J, Frank R, Roe T, Sawilowsky S. Measurement practices: methods for developing content-valid student examinations. *Med Teach.* 2003;25:414-421.

69. Collins J. Education techniques for lifelong learning: writing multiple-choice questions for continuing medical education activities and self-assessment modules. *Radiographics.* 2006;26:543-551.

70. Bush ME. Quality assurance of multiple-choice tests. *Qual Assur Educ.* 2006;14:398-404.

71. Tarrant M, James W. Impact of item-writing flaws in multiple-choice questions on student achievement in high-stakes nursing assessments. *Med Educ.* 2008;42:198-206.

72. Ascalon ME, Meyers LS, Davis BW, Smits N. Distractors similarity and item-stem structure: effects on item difficulty. *Appl Meas Educ.* 2007;20:153-170.

73. Swanson DB, Holtzman KH, Clauser BE, Sawhill AJ. Pyschometric characteristics and response times for one-best-answer questions in relation to number and source of options. *Acad Med.* 2005;80: S93-S96.

74. Giles SM. *PT Exam: The Complete Study Guide.* Scarborough, ME: Scorebuilders; 2007.

75. Baroudi ZM. Formative assessment: definition, elements and role in instructional practice. *Post-Script.* 2007;8:37-48.

76. Angelo TA, Cross KP. *Classroom Assessment Techniques: A Handbook for College Teachers.* 2nd ed. San Francisco, CA: Jossey-Bass; 1993.

77. *Physical Therapy Clinical Instructor Educator Credentialing Manual.* Alexandria, VA: American Physical Therapy Association; 1997.

Design Considerations
Adapting Instruction for Varied Audiences and Formats

Chapter Objectives

After reading this chapter, you will be prepared to:
- Define the non-negotiable elements of systematic effective instruction.
- Apply the non-negotiable elements to a variety of presentation formats.
- Use the non-negotiable elements to problem-solve a variety of common instructional mistakes.
- Identify additional variables that influence instructional design.
- Adapt presentations to meet the demands of various formats and time frames.

Stop and Reflect

What do you think of when you think about "teaching and learning in physical therapy"?
- Who do physical therapists teach?
- What do physical therapists teach?
- Where do physical therapists teach?
- When do physical therapists teach?
- How do physical therapists teach?

In the introductory chapter, we asked you to "Stop and Reflect" on what you think of when you think about teaching and learning in physical therapy. From there, we explored what the learner brings to the learning situation and the characteristics of our learners; we examined the reflective process and discussed how to facilitate critical thinking on the part of our learners (students and patients); we described the structure and function of the brain and the potential implications of current brain research on teaching and learning; and we presented a systematic approach to designing effective teaching-learning situations.

By now, you recognize the complexity of your role as educators. You know that teaching is much more than simply telling your patients what is important and expecting that they will do it or relying on the old mantra "see one, do one, teach one." Teaching requires a systematic and comprehensive approach to understanding your learners, focusing their attention, presenting materials in a manner that meets their needs, and continually reinforcing the learning so they can achieve behavior change and/or knowledge retention. By now, you also recognize just how much teaching is an integral part of being a health care practitioner and how each teaching-learning situation is unique.

In the previous chapters, we presented the principles behind effective teaching, whether in the classroom or clinical setting. However, as we said, each teaching-learning situation is unique, and as health care professionals, we engage in a great variety of teaching activities. For example, you may be asked to present at a community fair or a national meeting; you may want to present your scientific findings in a poster or platform presentation format; you may be invited to do a workshop that lasts 3 hours or a continuing education course that lasts 3 days; or you may be called to participate in a panel discussion. How can you use the principles discussed in the previous chapters to prepare for the variety of teaching-learning situations in which you may be expected to engage in physical therapy practice?

Plack M, Driscoll M. *Teaching and Learning in Physical Therapy: From Classroom to Clinic* (pp 117-132).

This chapter is designed to build on the principles presented in the previous chapter as you think about how you might adapt your presentation to meet the demands of different presentation formats and different audiences. Which components of the principles of systematic effective instruction are non-negotiable and which ones can be modified or deleted depending on the situation? What else must you consider in trying to meet the demands of the requested presentation format? What will you do if you arrive and find that your audience is much more knowledgeable than you anticipated or the room setup is not what you planned? What will you do if your presentation is taking much longer than you planned? Will you be ready? To begin this chapter, we would like you to take some time to ponder the following scenarios:

Critical Thinking Clinical Scenario

MJ is presenting at a national conference for the first time. She is eager to share her recently developed curriculum model for teaching effective communication with challenging patients. She is speaking to an audience made up of experienced academicians and clinicians. Out of respect for her audience's expertise, she decides that it is important to provide solid background information including the history of, and an evidence-based rationale for, the curriculum. She prepared 120 PowerPoint slides for the 30-minute presentation. The presentation did not go well. People looked distracted and no one participated when given the opportunity to ask questions. Because of the time constraints, MJ had to rush through some of the curricular components. The written evaluations were awful.

Reflective Questions

1. What do you think went wrong?
2. What might have been the expectations of the audience members?
3. How might the presenter's goals have differed from the audience's goals?
4. What might have helped this situation?

Critical Thinking Clinical Scenario

Being a reflective practitioner, MJ stopped to reflect on her presentation and on the feedback she received from the participants. Fortunately, she was given another opportunity to present her curriculum at a different national conference. She was given a 45-minute time frame. This time she decided that she wanted to draw on the expertise of the audience and engage them more in her presentation. Rather than a PowerPoint presentation, she decided to plan a less structured, more conversational approach to her presentation. MJ wanted the audience members to feel valued and an integral part of the workshop, so she decided to begin the presentation with introductions. She asked participants to walk to a central microphone and introduce themselves to the rest of the audience, one at a time, by telling their names, where they worked, and why they were there. When approximately half of the 30-member audience had completed this activity, MJ was upset to realize that more than 20 minutes had elapsed and they were not finished yet! There would be no time for the small group tasks; there would barely be time to go over the handouts.

Reflective Questions

1. What do you think went wrong?
2. What could the presenter have done differently?
3. How could the goal of the presenter to have participants feel valued have been accomplished in a different, more timely way?
4. How might she have engaged the audience differently?
5. How might she have better managed to incorporate the expertise of the participants?

Critical Thinking Clinical Scenario

TR has been invited to do an introductory lecture in the doctor of physical therapy program from which she graduated 3 years ago. During the intervening years, she worked in the physical therapy department at a large hospital, became certified as a lymphedema specialist, and conducted extensive patient education programs on this topic. She has planned a 2-hour class on lymphedema and the role of patient education with small group activities, handouts, a PowerPoint presentation, and photographs that demonstrate the outcomes of effective lymphedema treatment. The class did not go as well as she had planned. Students seemed overwhelmed yet asked very few questions. Written evaluations revealed their appreciation for her expertise but there was confusion about what they were supposed to have learned.

Reflective Questions

1. What do you think went wrong?
2. What do you think the goals of the presenter were?
3. What could the presenter have done differently?

In the first scenario, MJ was excited about her topic and wanted to convey as much information as possible in a 30-minute time frame, so she designed a highly structured and extensive PowerPoint presentation, taking care to ensure that all of the information she planned to present was included. Given the expertise of the audience, MJ also wanted to make sure she appeared credible, so she spent a great deal of time making sure that the audience recognized the steps she took in creating the curriculum and how it was based in evidence and grounded in theory. The problem was that she spent so much time on the background information that she had to rush through the curricular design, which is what the audience really wanted to hear. To her credit, MJ reflected on her presentation and the feedback she received. Given another opportunity, she reframed her presentation. So, now what went wrong? This time, she wanted to be sure that she fully understood who was in her audience and what each hoped to take away from her presentation; however, getting to know a large audience one by one is time consuming and may be boring for many of the participants. Again, she used so much time getting to know her audience that she ended up rushing through the content that was relevant and meaningful to her participants.

In the third scenario, TR was excited to have been asked back to her alma mater to share her expertise. She was anxious to do an excellent job and wanted to provide the students with as much information as she could because she knew she had not received this information when she was in school. The problem here was 2-fold: (1) the more expertise you have on a topic, the harder it is to know what is a "need to know" versus "nice to know" and (2), again, TR did not stop to gauge the expertise (or lack of expertise in this case) of her audience. Giving too much information without time to process can be overwhelming to an audience. The end result might be that students shut down and disengaged altogether from the learning situation.

Each of the previous scenarios would have benefited from a plan B, a modified plan of action that would allow the presenter to make a few changes based on direct observations and information obtained from, and about, the audience early on (ie, an on-the-spot needs assessment). In the first scenario, had MJ included an *on-the-spot needs assessment*, she would have realized how knowledgeable the audience was, could have omitted much of the background rationale and theory, and could have spent more time discussing the curriculum itself. For those in the audience with less knowledge, she may have provided handouts and used a few minutes in small groups during which time audience members with greater expertise may have been able to answer questions of the more novice participants. This same solution may have benefited in the second scenario as well and would likely have taken much less time to accomplish than individual introductions. The small group activity would

have enabled participants to both introduce themselves and share their expertise with their group members and would have provided background information for the novice audience members. In TR's case, a discussion with a member of the faculty who is familiar with the students' level of knowledge as well as the expectations of an entry-level practitioner may have helped TR determine what to include and exclude from her presentation. In addition, sequencing her presentation in a way to provide sufficient processing time would have engaged the learners and enabled them to ask questions along the way.

How do you know what to consider when planning a modification to your original plan? As a novice presenter, you may be overwhelmed by the idea of planning more than one way to conduct your presentation. Start with simple modifications, such as differentiating between background or basic information and more advanced information. Or, if you discover through a few questions at the beginning that your audience participants are more knowledgeable or experienced than you expected, plan to skip over the extra background information and make the extra information available for audience members who are less familiar. As described in Chapter 4, active learning strategies can also help everyone learn more effectively. You can design an activity in which participants discuss (review) basic information to be sure that everyone is at the same level. In this way, those with expertise can share their knowledge with novice participants, and the novice participants will have enough information for you to be able to move through your presentation without having to first review all of the basic information needed. These active learning strategies can be as brief as a few seconds or much longer, and the duration of each activity can be modified to meet the needs of the group. In general, we recommend planning at least 2 activities of different lengths for even brief presentations of 30 minutes' duration. If time is going by more quickly than you anticipated, you can eliminate or spend less time on one activity.

In all 3 scenarios, a solid *needs assessment*, refined *learning objectives*, and some *active learning strategies* could have enhanced the presentations greatly. Each of the scenarios presented above is different and required specific design considerations; however, in any presentation, there are still some non-negotiables to consider.

The Non-Negotiables of Systematic Effective Instruction

In each of the 3 preceding scenarios, a well-intentioned presenter experienced disappointing results. In this chapter, we will consider a variety of presentational formats that require different design considerations. To optimize your teaching, regardless of the instructional situation, we consider certain components of systematic effective instruction to be *non-negotiable*. The components or elements of systematic effective instruction were presented in detail in Chapter 4. Table 5-1 summarizes those elements that are considered non-negotiable.

Let us consider the non-negotiables as they apply to the opening scenario. In attempting to ensure credibility of her presentation, MJ used 120 slides to convey as much as possible about her model for teaching communication. There was a mismatch between her goals and the audience's expectations. In this instance, the presenter could have done an on-the-spot needs assessment and asked participants whether they were clinicians or academicians and whether they had encountered challenging patients with whom it was difficult to communicate. The presenter might have asked the participants to think about any questions or concerns they hoped would be addressed during the workshop. Once the participants had spent 30 to 60 seconds thinking about their questions/concerns, they could turn to a person nearby to exchange their questions/concerns. Lastly, the presenter could have asked for questions/concerns from the larger group and written these on a flip chart, or digital white board. Within 2 to 3 minutes, the presenter could have learned something about the audience's expectations and could have clarified the extent to which the planned presentation would address their concerns. Audience members also would have learned quickly whether to stay in this workshop session or to leave and find another session more appropriate for them. Asking audience members to reflect on questions and concerns they hope will be addressed and responding to these expectations can serve both as a needs assessment as well as a motivational hook. It will help focus the participants' attention on the topic of the presentation. Personal connections to relevant concerns also help establish context for the workshop material. In describing the purpose of the workshop, the presenter has the opportunity to present the specific goals of the session as well.

Assuming that this workshop was not, in fact, a workshop and that it was a presentation about a recently developed program for improving communication, it would be important to consider ways to engage the audience (active learning) as much as possible and to boost the content in a meaningful way. The presenter might have shown video clips of students engaged in clinic-based role-plays before they learned the new techniques. These video clips could be followed by an opportunity for audience members to speak with participants nearby to critique the student-patient role-play scenarios. Several comments about the student performance from the audience could be shared in the large group. This brief discussion could be followed by a brief lecturette (10 minutes) about the new communication training program. Following this lecturette, a second video clip showing students using the new communication techniques could have been presented. Once again, audience members could comment on the student role-plays, with instructions to compare and contrast the different communication approaches they had observed (2 to 3 minutes). Based on observations and comments from the audience, the instructor could review the key points of the new communication training program and highlight the different outcomes observed in the role plays. This 2- to 3-minute encapsulation could serve as a summary of the presentation. This interactive presentation could be done within the same 30-minute time frame originally allotted for the lecture plus PowerPoint presentation. The adapted version contains all the components necessary for effective instruction and is much more likely to engage learners.

Table 5-1. The "Non-Negotiables" of Systematic Effective Instruction

- Needs assessment (interest/knowledge)
- Motivational hook
- Learning objectives
- Content boosters and active learning strategies
- Summary

Key Points to Remember

- Good teaching requires good planning.
- Good planning requires having a plan B and being prepared to adapt to the needs of your audience and the constraints of your environment.
- Good planning means including all of the non-negotiables of systematic effective instruction:
  - Completing a needs assessment either beforehand or on-the-spot.
  - Incorporating motivational hooks to grab your audience's attention.
  - Developing well-written objectives to help guide your presentation.
  - Utilizing content boosters such as active learning strategies to maintain your audience's attention and enable the participants to process the information you are presenting.
  - Summarizing the major points to reinforce retention.

Critical Thinking Clinical Scenario

Consider the 2 teaching scenarios presented earlier: (1) the less structured, more conversational conference presentation on communication curriculum, and (2) the guest lecture about lymphedema.

Reflective Questions

1. Using the non-negotiable components of systematic effective instruction, what kind of suggestions would you have for these 2 presenters?

2. What kind of goals might be appropriate for these 2 presentations?

3. How might your suggestions differ in view of the different time frames, 45 minutes versus 2 hours?

4. How might these 2 presentations compare with any presentations you have done?

Beyond Systematic Effective Instruction: Variables to Consider in Designing Effective Instructional Experiences

Although we emphasize the importance of incorporating certain components of effective instruction regardless of the teaching-learning situation, these are not the only variables to be considered when designing your instruction. Additional variables appear in Table 5-2. Creating optimal teaching-learning experiences requires you to consider both the non-negotiable components of effective instruction and the unique characteristics of your situation. These unique characteristics or variables may include but may not be limited to the audience, timeframe, situation, format, room setup, and the equipment available.

Table 5-2. Variables to Consider in Designing Effective Instructional Experiences

- Audience
- Time frame
- Format
- Room setup
- Equipment and other resources context

Audience

The people who comprise your audience definitely influence your instructional plan. As discussed in detail in Chapter 1, the participants may have different expectations of your presentation depending on their level of experience, current knowledge of the topic, cultures, generational differences, learning styles, and purpose for using the content you are presenting. What about participants of different ages or literacy levels? For example, if you are presenting information on the benefits of aerobic conditioning to a high school health class versus a group of senior citizens at the local community center, you will likely need somewhat different pacing (ie, ratio of content and process), content boosters, and active learning strategies. Even in a setting where you assume a more homogeneous audience in terms of education and experience, such as when you present at a conference of professional peers, it is important to consider the specific audience in your session. Are these participants clinicians or academicians or a combination of the two? Are they expecting a lecture or a workshop format? How familiar are they with your topic? More often than not, you should expect a fair amount of diversity in your audience.

The key is to make the presentation as relevant as possible for the audience. If you discover that most of the group is familiar with key background information needed in your presentation but a handful are not, you may provide less of the background information you prepared and frame it as "review for many of you and new information for some of you." Clearly stating that you are aware of, and accommodate for, these differences in baseline knowledge indicates that you recognize and value the characteristics of this specific audience.

Critical Thinking Clinical Scenario

Imagine that you have been invited to give a presentation for 40 minutes on the topic of aerobic conditioning to 2 groups in your community: 25 adolescents in a high school health class and 15 senior citizens at a local community center.

Reflective Questions

1. How does the composition of your audience influence your expectations of their active participation?

2. How will your selection of content boosters differ? What boosters might you select for each group?

3. How might your pacing (ratio of content and process) differ?

Time Frame

Earlier in the chapter, we presented scenarios where the topic was the same and the time frame was different. This situation is common. Imagine that you have conducted research on the benefits of specific interventions for individuals who have sustained lower-extremity amputation. Many of the patients lost their limbs as a result of diabetes, motor vehicle accidents, and war injuries. In addition to your expertise in orthopedics, you have developed competence in diabetes management, patient education about skin care, and selection criteria for various prosthetic sockets. You have the potential to teach a number of topics to a variety of audiences including physical therapists, student physical therapists, patients, and caregivers in a variety of settings, formats, and time frames. Let's look at how the time frame can influence your instructional design. Table 5-3 describes various design options you might consider for the 2 different time frames.

Stop, Do, and Reflect

Using the non-negotiable components of systematic effective instruction, design 2 presentations on the topic of physical therapy interventions for patients with lower-extremity amputations, given the following parameters:
- 30-minute presentation in-service for a physical therapy department
- 2-hour presentation for third-year students in a local doctor of physical therapy program

---

In the examples in Table 5-3, note that there are several important differences in design based on the different time frames and audiences. After assessing the needs of the audience, it was determined that the in-service presentation for the experienced physical therapists need not include objectives and content related to background information and anatomical changes due to the different types of amputations. Given the expertise of your audience, you could assume that they will remember key information on basic anatomy or that they could retrieve this information with little difficulty. If you were unsure of the audience's immediate recall of pertinent anatomy, you might consider using one of the content boosters described for the doctor of physical therapy (DPT) class (eg, anatomy review sheet). You could distribute an unlabeled diagram of the relevant anatomy and ask participants to label all or selected parts and then compare them with someone nearby. Within minutes, participants would be "up to speed" on the pertinent anatomical information. This activity could also serve as a motivational hook if it were done at the beginning of the presentation. The anatomy review would be completed in a few minutes in an interesting, active way and would eliminate the need for including an in-depth review of the anatomy in your presentation.

Stop and Reflect

Review the designs for the 2 different presentations described in Table 5-3.
1. Given the 2 different time frames and audiences, why were multiple motivational hooks included in the longer presentation?
2. What else could have been chosen for motivational hooks in each presentation?
3. How did the differences in audience and time frame influence the choice of content boosters?
4. What other content boosters would have been appropriate?
5. How else might you conduct the summary in each presentation?

Notice also in Table 5-3, we included approximate time frames next to each of the components of the presentation. This is particularly helpful in planning your content to meet the demands of different time frames. Keeping this handy during your presentation can also help you determine whether you are on track to meet your stated objectives. If certain aspects of the presentation are taking longer than anticipated, having this timeline in front of you can help you quickly make adjustments to your presentation and still meet the stated objectives (eg, which components of my presentation can I modify on-the-spot? Is there content that I can omit? Can I modify, shorten, or omit the next small group activity so I can stay on time?).

In fact, preparation for a professional conference usually begins with the submission of a written proposal, which goes through a competitive, peer-review process before being accepted for presentation. Typically the abstract is accompanied by an outline of the content and listing of proposed activities with the amount of time designated for each activity as suggested in Table 5-3. Table 5-4 provides a sample of a proposal submitted for a 2-day continuing education course. If you look closely, you will realize that a 2-day continuing education course essentially consists of several iterations of motivational hooks, brief content lecturettes, content boosters, and active learning strategies. We consider these elements to be the building blocks of effective presentations. The non-negotiables of systematic effective instruction can help you design presentations of any length from as little as 15 minutes to as much as 15 weeks of course content and more!

Table 5-3. Design Options Based on Audience and Time Frames

Non-Negotiable Components	30-Minute In-Service in a Physical Therapy Department	2-Hour Presentation for a Doctor of Physical Therapy Class
Needs assessment	1. On-the-spot questions (2 minutes)	1. Key consultation with course coordinator about current knowledge of amputation, interventions for patients with amputation, and experience adapting PT interventions, (2 weeks prior) 2. On-the-spot Qs (1 to 2 minutes)
Goals/objectives	1. Compare/contrast physical therapy interventions for this population 2. Discuss precautions and contraindications (1 minute)	1. Discuss the causes and prevalence of lower extremity amputations. 2. Describe the anatomy of lower extremity amputations. 3. Explain precautions and contraindications for various exercises. 4. Adapt exercises for individuals with lower extremity amputations.
Motivational hook(s)	1. Pictures of 2 patients with different levels of amputation, doing different exercises. Question to group, "How could exercise A be modified for patient B? (1 to 2 minutes)	1. First hook: pictures of people doing physically challenging tasks (eg, skiing and sky diving). Question: What physical impairment do these people share? (1 to 2 minutes) 2. Second hook: diagram of leg with muscles/tendons/ligaments/skeletal components indicated and *not* labeled, ask the students to correctly label all anatomical features, individually, and then compare and correct in pairs. (5 to 7 minutes) 3. Third hook: demo a PT exercise on an able-bodied student and ask the group how it could be modified for someone with lower-extremity amputation. (3 to 5 minutes)
Content booster(s) and active learning strategies	1. PowerPoint presentation of key points (10 minutes) 2. Paired discussion of a case scenario handout with 2 precautions and 2 contraindications embedded in the patient's chart notes (4 to 6 minutes) 3. Paired practice of 2 exercises, each partner adapting an exercise for a patient with an amputation and certain precautions or contraindications (5 to 7 minutes)	1. PowerPoint presentation of key points related to the increased incidence of people with amputations due to diabetes, MVAs, and war injuries (10 minutes) 2. Paired correction of anatomy review sheets (5 to 7 minutes). 3. PowerPoint presentation describing the most common anatomical changes due to amputation and the impact of these on function (10 minutes) 4. Demonstration of adapted exercises (5 to 10 minutes) 5. Paired practice of various exercises, with presenter and course coordinator circulating among students (15 to 20 minutes) 6. A PowerPoint presentation about precautions and contraindications to certain exercises (15 minutes); 7. Handouts with simulated patient information including a contraindication and a precaution embedded; paired discussion and modification of exercises (10-15 minutes)
Summary	1. Q&A (2 minutes) 2. Presenter reviews 4 key points (3 minutes) 3. Presenter asks the group to think of any new information, shift in perspective, or reaffirmation of previously learned information that occurred for them as a result of this presentation	1. Q&A (2 to 4 minutes) 2. Presenter reviews key points (3 minutes) 3. Activity: the presenter asks the group to call out a total of 5 things they learned that were new for them (2 minutes)

PT indicates physical therapist; MVA, motor vehicle accident; Q&A, question and answer.

Table 5-4. Sample Proposal Accepted for a Two-Day Continuing Education Course at the American Physical Therapy Assocation Combined Sections Meeting

PRESENTATION TYPE: Two-day preconference instructional course

SESSION SUMMARY
TITLE: Systematic Effective Instruction: Grabbing Your Audience's Attention and Maintaining It Throughout Your Presentation

AUTHORS/INSTITUTIONS: M.M. Plack, Physical Therapy, the George Washington University, Washington, DC; M. Driscoll, Physical Therapy, Touro College, New York, NY

PARTICIPANT LEVEL: Multilevel

DESCRIPTION: Have you ever been faced with an instructional challenge—for example, being asked to present at a mandatory in-service—at lunchtime or at the end of the day on Friday? Have you ever tried to teach first-year DPT students about professionalism—just before an anatomy midterm? How can we grab our audience's attention, maintain it, and be sure that they learned what we wanted them to learn? This 2-day workshop will present a systematic approach to designing effective presentations. Participants will experience a broad array of instructional strategies, apply them to topics of their choice to enhance their own presentations and consult with one another to develop optimal methods of delivery. This workshop will present a systematic method of instruction and will engage the whole learner in a time-efficient and effective manner. Whether you are a presenter or evaluator, this model provides a 7-step framework that will help you plan, implement, and assess effective presentations. From the needs assessment to the summative assessment, this model utilizes a variety of active learning strategies that incorporate learners' past experiences and learning styles. Participants will learn about motivational hooks, content boosters, active learning strategies, and practical formative and summative assessment techniques. Strategies for gauging attention and changing the energy of the group to maintain focus will be modeled. Participants will experience a variety of active learning strategies that can easily be incorporated into a continuum of educational designs that range from brief in-services to semester-long courses. Participants are encouraged to bring a topic or presentation to work on throughout the day. Participants will work in small groups to apply, practice, and fine-tune the methods discussed. This presentation will culminate in an enjoyable summative activity that will allow participants to integrate what they have learned while enabling the instructors to assess whether learners have assimilated content sufficiently for use.

OBJECTIVES
Upon completion of this course, you will:
1. Apply the elements of systematic effective instruction including needs assessments, motivational hooks, content boosters, active learning strategies, summaries, formative and summative assessments to a presentation.
2. Plan an effective presentation that incorporates active learning strategies.
3. Evaluate the efficacy of a summative experiential activity that engages the whole brain and reinforces integration, application, and deeper learning.
4. Critique and provide feedback to enhance the effectiveness of future presentations.
5. Develop summative activities for assessment purposes.
6. Apply the lessons learned to future educational presentations through the development of individual action plans.

KEY WORDS: *Instructional strategies, presentation strategies, active learning strategies*

Course/Session Format

DAY 1
AM
20 min: Lecturette—Overview of systematic effective instruction
10 min: Small group activity—Factors to consider in designing a presentation
30 min: Lecturette—Audience and instructor characteristics
30 min: Small group activity—Characteristics of the adult learner and motivating instructors
15 min: Break
45 min: Lecturette—Learning styles
45 min: Small group activity—Self-assessment of personal learning styles

60 min: Lunch

PM
20 min: Lecturette—Needs assessment
20 min: Small group activity—Needs assessment
30 min: Lecturette—Determining content and behavioral objectives
20 min: Small group activity—Behavioral objectives
15 min: Break
20 min: Lecturette—Reinforcing content
30 min: Small group activity—Motivational hooks and content boosters
15 min: Newsprint gallery review—Share motivational hooks, behavioral objectives, content boosters that were developed by the individual small groups
30 min: Individual work sessions and peer consultation

(continued)

Table 5-4. Sample Proposal Accepted for a Two-Day Continuing Education Course at the American Physical Therapy Assocation Combined Sections Meeting (continued)

DAY 2
PM
20 min: Lecturette—Active learning strategies, guided practice, and independent practice
60 min: Small group activity—Active learning strategies
20 min: Small group activity—Application of active learning strategies to individual topics
15 min: Break
20 min: Lecturette—Check for understanding, formative and summative assessments
20 min: Small group activity—Develop appropriate formative and summative assessments
20 min: Individual work sessions and peer consultation

60 min: Lunch

PM
20 min: Lecturette—Summaries
20 min: Small group activity—Develop a summary for each individual topic
20 min: Newsprint gallery review—Share active learning strategies, summaries, and formative and summative assessments that were developed by the individual small groups
10 min: Debrief—Newsprint gallery review
5 min: Muddiest points, summary, questions, and answers
15 min: Break
50 min: Small group activity—Participants will engage in a jigsaw integrative activity to reinforce, integrate, and summarize the content presented
15 min: Summary of the 2 days
10 min: Muddiest points, critique, summary, questions, answers, and summarize
30 min: Open work sessions and peer consultation

Teaching methods: Case study, question and answer, small and large group discussions
Evaluation method: Question and answer, small group discussion
Participant limitations: 35-50

Course/Session Management
Audio/visual equipment: AV set (LCD, AV cart, screen, Lavalier microphones, laser pointer)
Unique considerations: Round tables; no stage (one of the presenters has a physical disability); newsprint

REFERENCES
1. Fink D. *Creating Significant Learning Experiences*. San Francisco, CA: Jossey-Bass; 2003.
2. Jensen E. *Teaching with the Brain in Mind*. Alexandria, VA: Association for Supervision and Curriculum Development; 1998.
3. Lujan HL, DiCarlo S. Too much teaching, not enough learning: what is the solution? *Adv Physiol Educ*. 2006;30:17-22.
4. Silberman M, Auerbach C. *Active Training*. San Francisco, CA: Jossey-Bass/Pfeiffer; 2006.
5. Wolfe P. *Brain Matters: Translating Research Into Classroom Practice*. Alexandria, VA: Association for Supervision and Curriculum Development; 2001.
6. Tileston DW. *10 Best Teaching Practices: How Brain Research, Learning Styles, and Standards Define Teaching Competencies*. Thousand Oaks, CA: Corwin Press; 2000.
7. Walker S. Active learning strategies to promote critical thinking. *J Athl Train*. 2003;38:263-270.

FACILITATORS' BIOGRAPHIES
Margaret Plack, PT, EdD, is the chair of the Department of Health Care Sciences and director of the Physical Therapy Program at the George Washington University, Washington, DC. Dr. Plack received her EdD in adult education from the Department of Organization and Leadership at Teachers College, Columbia University, New York. Dr. Plack co-authored and taught a course entitled "Teaching in Physical Therapy Practice." She has implemented the strategies to be discussed in this workshop in a number of teaching and learning conferences including the CSM and APTA Annual Conference. She has been involved in ongoing research related to adult learning principles and educational outcomes and has published several manuscripts on topics related to this workshop. Dr. Plack twice received the Stanford Award from the *Journal of Physical Therapy Education* for her writing.

Maryanne Driscoll, PhD, is an educational psychologist and associate professor in the Doctor of Physical Therapy Program at Touro College, New York. Dr. Driscoll received her PhD in educational psychology from Teachers College, Columbia University, New York. Dr. Driscoll consults with schools and hospitals throughout the metropolitan New York region on effective instruction. With Dr. Plack, she co-authored and taught a course entitled "Teaching in Physical Therapy Practice" for 2 post-professional DPT programs and also teaches similar content in 2 professional DPT programs. She has implemented the strategies to be used in this workshop in a number of teaching and learning conferences including CSM and APTA Annual Conference. Dr. Driscoll has been involved in ongoing research related to adult learning principles and educational outcomes and has published several manuscripts on topics related to this workshop.

Stop and Reflect

Review the sample proposal presented in Table 5-4.
1. Modify the proposal to be given in a half-day time frame. Consider:

    a. Objectives
    b. Content-process ratio
    c. Active learning strategies

The preplanning required by professional conferences helps you think through your design. In addition, the handouts that you might have planned to distribute at the presentation may need to be submitted to the conference planning committee months in advance so they can be available to participants online. Conference attendees often expect detailed handouts, references, and a PowerPoint presentation. Increasingly, they expect a combination of lecture, small group activities, and practical application of the content presented.

In contrast to the formality surrounding a professional conference, the invitation to speak at a nearby high school may have occurred through a casual invitation. The same detailed planning is needed. Handouts and references will likely be expected, but there may or may not be equipment to support a PowerPoint presentation, and access to a photocopier may not be possible a few minutes before the presentation. In this, as in any effective teaching-learning situation, you need to be prepared before you arrive at your presentation and always have a plan B in mind.

Format

The specific format you are considering is another factor that may influence your instructional design. In the previous scenarios, we focused on formal and informal lecture-style presentations. If you have ever been to a professional conference, you may have noticed that there are a variety of other presentation formats, including panel discussions, platform presentations, and poster presentations. Each one of these requires special design considerations.

Panel Discussion

Some keys to optimizing the panel discussion format are planning and clear guidelines. Consider the number of members on the panel, the length of time allotted for each panelist, the order of the presenters, and the amount of time set aside for questions and audience participation. In addition, will there be a facilitator to introduce the topic and the panelists or a discussant who will respond to the key points raised by all the panelists? Before agreeing to participate, find out as much information as you can. What is the topic? Who are the other panelists? What is your role?

Often, program planners get excited by the concept of multiple speakers discussing different aspects of the same general topic. Incorporating multiple perspectives often enhances the discussion and elicits more comments from the audience. If not planned well, however, the panel can become a passive learning activity for audience members as they listen to a series of mini-lectures with little opportunity to actively engage with the content.

What can you do to make the panel a more effective learning experience? As a program planner, consider the non-negotiables we discussed earlier. Be sure that your goals and objectives are clear and are clearly communicated to your panelists. Be realistic about the number of panelists and the time frame allotted for the program. If you have an hour for your presentation, consider no more than 3 panelists, and tell them they have 10 to 12 minutes each to speak. Remind them that there is limited time. Keep everyone on time by providing a detailed timeline and by giving them a 2-minute warning near the end of their turn. Prior to the first panelist's presentation, ask a few on-the-spot needs assessment questions to learn something about the audience and their familiarity with the topic. Present the objectives of the session. Ask each panelist to include some type of motivational hook and an opportunity for participants to at least turn to a neighbor to share a reaction or summarize a few key points. Allow time after each panelist for audience participation (ie, comments/questions). Provide time for the panelists to interact and offer thought-provoking questions of one another and of the audience.

Ideally, there will be a facilitator to present the objectives, keep the group on task and on time, and summarize the major points discussed. If there is no facilitator and you are the first panelist, be sure to ask the on-the-spot questions and present the objectives. If there is no facilitator and you are the last panelist, be sure to summarize the key points and/or questions raised by the entire panel and the audience at the end of the presentation. A well-designed panel discussion can be invigorating and thought-provoking for the learner; a poorly planned or executed panel discussion can be a passive and often redundant series of lectures that do not engage the learner.

Platform Presentation

A platform presentation consists of a brief, formal presentation generally accompanied by PowerPoint slides. It is typically a means of sharing current research or curricular innovations with colleagues. As with other presentations at professional conferences, you must submit a written abstract about the topic that will be peer reviewed before being accepted for presentation. Other characteristics of this format are strict time limits of 15 to 20 minutes with little or no audience interaction, except for a short question-and-answer period at the end. Even in this tightly scripted format, you can include a motivational hook, objectives, content booster, and summary. Your motivational hook could include a few questions to the audience to assess their knowledge of your topic or a thought-provoking picture in your PowerPoint presentation that can promote curiosity about your topic. Your objective might be for the participants to be able to explain key points of your research design or apply your research results or curriculum model to their academic or clinical setting. The PowerPoint slides and handout serve as content boosters, and your take-home message should summarize the key points of your presentation.

Poster Presentation

Unlike the preceding formats, the poster presentation is not primarily spoken; rather, it is a graphic depiction of research results that are presented in a gallery-style format at local, state, and national conferences. Again, abstracts generally are submitted for peer review before being accepted for presentation. The content of these poster presentations can range from innovative programs and case studies to pilot data of research not yet disseminated. Though not a spoken presentation per se, the non-negotiables may apply. For example, the title of your poster and its visual appeal, including pictures, graphs, and tables, can serve as a motivational hook to attract the attention of conference attendees who are walking throughout the poster displays. The objectives of the poster may be written as the purpose or goals of the study. Additional visuals such as photographs of equipment used in the methods and graphs that display results can serve as content boosters. Finally, a written summary of the findings would be included in the poster design. In addition to the poster itself, the lead researcher(s) involved in the study usually stands next to the poster and is often expected to succinctly present an overview of the content of the poster, answer questions, and discuss the content with people who are viewing the posters.

Besides presentations, workshops, panel discussions, platform presentations, and poster presentations at professional meetings, you may very well be involved in community health and wellness fairs or advocacy days. These are designed for professionals to provide important information to the community and the lay public about physical therapy and the role of the physical therapist and physical therapist assistant in health care. During these fairs, your role may be to identify and disseminate information about community resources that may be important to a certain patient population. It may also be a time for you to discuss the importance of health and wellness and the role of the physical therapist in fitness and prevention.

Health and Fitness Fairs

Similar to the poster presentation previously described, the emphasis of a presentation at a community health fair is on the visual display that will draw people to your table or booth. Poster-size displays (2 feet by 3 feet) that contain accurate, relevant information clearly written in layman's terms are helpful. In addition, you might provide handouts that contain accurate illustrations and include key points that are written at the fifth- to sixth-grade level in English and any other language that is commonly spoken in your community. Providing information about community resources relevant to your topic shows that you know your audience. Motivational hooks might include pictures or narratives of particular patients. Adding a hands-on screening (eg, blood pressure screening, posture screening, range-of-motion screening) can be considered a motivational hook and is an excellent opportunity to demonstrate your skills as a physical therapist while engaging your participants in a brief informal one-on-one conversation about the importance of wellness and prevention. Hands-on activities are excellent content boosters; participants may very well remember what you did with them and why, much more readily than simply viewing a poster display or reading about it in a pamphlet. Still, providing handouts as your participants leave may serve as an additional content booster. Particularly in situations such as this, where you may engage your participants for just a few brief minutes, having a 1- or 2-line summary bulleting the major message you want your participant to hear is crucial. Keep in mind the concept of less is more that we described in Chapter 4.

Advocacy Day

Though most often health fairs are local events targeting the local community, at times, they may target local or national politicians and policy makers as a way of advocating on a larger scale for the needs of particular patient populations (eg, speaking to politicians about the needs of children with developmental disability), the needs of students (eg, loan repayment), or simply to help them understand the breadth and depth of the profession. Lobby Day is a good example of an advocacy day. Lobby Day is when physical therapists en masse go to the state capitol or to Capitol Hill in Washington, DC, to advocate for important issues for the profession. After a briefing from members of the professional organization, you will participate in meetings with your congressional representatives to advocate for issues that are of particular importance. Combining this type of information/advocacy session with a health, wellness, and prevention fair has been effective in teaching policy makers about the physical therapy profession. During these fairs, physical therapists volunteer to assess different aspects of fitness for policy makers and their staff members. Again, this is an excellent opportunity to hone your teaching skills while simultaneously advocating for the profession!

Clinical Scenario Critical Thinking

You have done a fair amount of research related to childhood obesity. In fact, you have published several articles on the topic and are considered the local expert in fitness and childhood obesity. You are frequently called upon to do presentations to both community members as well as other health care professionals. In fact, recently you were called to testify in front of Congress on the role of physical therapists in the prevention of childhood obesity.

Reflective Questions

Considering the non-negotiables of systematic effective instruction, how might you design your next presentation* if it were:

1. A poster presentation on your most recent research findings at a national professional meeting?
2. A panel presentation to a group of elementary school students and their parents?
3. A full-day workshop for obese teens?
4. A community health fair?
5. A congressional hearing followed by a fitness fair for staffers on Capitol Hill?

*Include goals/objectives, motivational hooks, content boosters, summaries, and time frames for each.

Having considered a variety of presentation formats and venues, there is 1 final set of variables to be considered: the room setup and equipment.

Room Setup

Even the most carefully designed instructional programs may be helped or hindered by the physical environment in which you are presenting. Small group activities are difficult, although not impossible, if you find yourself in an auditorium with fixed seats. You may have to modify how you do certain activities if there are no tables when you had planned for people to work together in groups of 6 to 8 at round tables. Your plan B might include having participants work in pairs instead of groups and periodically switch partners with those in other parts of the room to obtain multiple perspectives. Sometimes you expect a more formal classroom setting, and you arrive at a conference room with a single large table and chairs all around it. Small group discussions are more difficult in this setting unless you get comfortable early on asking people to work with people on either side of them and then asking them to switch seats with people in places around the table. If you are invited to present an in-service in the physical

therapy department of a local hospital, be prepared to work with an audience seated on any available surface, low plinths, high plinths, mats piled on the floor, as well as the occasional chair. Setting up a LCD projector becomes a special challenge when you try to find a spot where everyone can see it. The key is to get to your room early so that you can modify the setup to optimize the learning environment, and if you cannot modify the setup, be prepared with a plan B. Fortunately, most audiences are flexible and willing to shift positions to accommodate a friendly presenter.

Equipment

Sound systems, video systems, computer systems, and Internet access are all variables to be considered when planning effective teaching-learning experiences. Seamless use of technology is essential to a seamless presentation. We prefer wireless, clip-on microphones because they allow the most movement and flexibility when presenting, allowing you to more effectively engage with the audience. The least effective although commonly used setup is the podium microphone, which limits your movement and opportunity to connect more directly with the audience. If you plan to use PowerPoint, find out ahead of time whether you need to bring your own laptop computer. Make sure that you have the appropriate wires to connect to the computer and that you have access to the appropriate software. Even asking for written instructions on how to turn the machinery on can make for a smoother start to your presentation. If you are not bringing your own computer, check to be sure that the software you used to create your presentation is compatible with the software on the equipment you will be using. If you need sound, are speakers available? If you need video, can you connect through the computer or do you need some other source? If you require access to the Internet, is it available? Is there a technician on site should things go wrong? If so, do you know who it is and how to contact that person? Technology can be challenging and needs extra attention to detail in the planning and execution stages of a presentation. When the technology fails, no matter the source of the problem, your credibility as a speaker may suffer, so be prepared to function without technology if necessary.

Finally, consider every piece of equipment you plan on using in your presentation. Will you need flip charts, markers, tape, Post-it notes, index cards, and/or name tags? Double check their availability at the site and bring extra supplies.

Context

When you think of the context surrounding your presentation, it may be important to consider the following questions: What time of day is your presentation? Is it first thing in the morning, during lunch, on a Friday afternoon? What time of year is it, and how are the participants getting to your presentation? Do you need to consider the potential of weather-related delays? Will you be presenting for the full time or are you expected to provide breaks? If so, what is customary? Are you the only presenter, or are there competing or complementary presentations? Should you expect participants to be coming and going at different times, or will the same participants be there throughout your presentation? Is attendance mandatory or voluntary? Is there technical support on site in case anything goes wrong, or should you be prepared to bring additional technology or handouts for backup?

The more you can anticipate, the more prepared you will be with your plan B. For example, if you are told that you have a 60-minute timeslot within which to present, but you anticipate a potential delayed start because of weather conditions, you will be prepared to alter your presentation to meet the demands of a shortened session. If you are presenting an in-service to a group of clinicians at 7:30 am, consider bringing coffee and a light breakfast to help maintain their attention. On the other hand, if you are presenting at lunch time when people are eating, first, anticipate a delay as your participants settle in with their food, and, second, consider presenting a bit more information up front (ie, while they are eating) with more active engagement (ie, discussion and active learning strategies) toward the latter half of your presentation. If you are one presenter in a series of presenters, be sure to ask what the other presenters will be presenting. There is nothing worse than being at a full-day conference when a speaker just repeated essentially what the previous speaker said. Though you cannot anticipate every eventuality, the more prepared you are, the more comprehensive your plan B will be and the more effective you will be as an instructor.

In addition, the more information you obtain ahead of time, the more relaxed you will be when you arrive at your presentation site. We recommend arriving at least 30 to 60 minutes before the scheduled start of your session to allow time to rearrange chairs, modify placement of the LCD projector, conduct an equipment and sound check, set out any materials that you plan to use during the workshop, and greet your participants as they enter the room. Greeting your participants as they walk in the room immediately creates a connection between you and your audience members, places you at ease, and may likely increase the willingness of your audience members to participate.

Any number of things can go wrong in a presentation. The more you reflect on your own experiences—good and bad—the more prepared you will be to manage your teaching situation. Careful planning is essential for creating optimal teaching-learning experiences. More than anything, you want to *practice, practice, practice!*

Even then, be prepared to adapt. Table 5-5 provides examples of situations that have caused presentations to go awry along with suggestions for how to improve the final outcomes. Table 5-6 provides examples of behaviors that can be challenging to a presenter along with suggestions for dealing with these challenges. We then consider some of the key concepts that were discussed in this chapter and in the previous chapter on systematic effective instruction and draw on our own experiences to offer some potential solutions.

Stop and Reflect

- Consider some potential answers to the questions raised under the "context" section of the text. What might you do to optimize your readiness to adapt as necessary?
- What other issues might arise? How might you troubleshoot those issues?

Critical Thinking Clinical Scenario

You have been invited to present a 3-hour workshop on the topic of your choice (and expertise) at the annual state conference for physical therapists. You have a choice of formats and physical settings. You can have any audio-visual technological support you want.

Reflective Questions

1. Identify a topic that you would like to present and then decide:
   a. What format (eg, interactive workshop or lecture) do you prefer and why?
   b. What physical setting would be best to accomplish your goals? Why?
   c. What audio-visual technological support would enhance your presentation? Why?
2. If you chose a different topic, would your responses be different? If so, how so?

Table 5-5. Problematic Presentations

Problem	Key Concepts to Remember	Potential Solutions
The Lecture With Too Many Slides and Too Little Time! *(the presenter planned to present 120 PowerPoint slides in only a 20-minute timeframe)*	Remember: *Less is more* and *need to know versus nice to know.* There is too much information for this short timeframe.	• Assess your audience. • Distill key information; need to know versus nice to know. • Provide a handout on the way out or ahead of the talk. • Highlight key points for discussion.
Repetitive Panel *(each panel member repeated the problem and purpose of the talk)*	Remember: *Motivational hooks and content boosters* help grab your audience's attention and maintain it throughout even panel discussions. Repeating the objectives will not grab or maintain your audience's attention.	• Know your content, your objectives, and your role as well as that of the other panelists. • Ensure that each panelist considers a motivational hook and brief active strategy. • Use a facilitator to introduce the panelists, state the objectives, keep the program moving, engage the audience, and summarize the key points.
The 3-hour Lecturer *(the presenter presented a 3-hour lecture with no time for processing)*	Remember: *Covering material does not equal learning.* Remember: It is critical to *balance content and process time.* The goal is to move information from working memory to short-term memory and ultimately to long-term memory. Active learning strategies enable the learner to process the material and move it out of working memory.	• Pause for the audience to process the information being presented by incorporating an activity at least every 20 minutes.
The 30-person Ice-Breaker *(the presenter asked each of the 30 participants to introduce themselves and tell why they decided to come to the presentation)*	Remember: The concepts of *primacy* and *recency.* If you spend the first 20 minutes on introductions, you lose the value of this principle.	• Personal introductions work if the group is small or if the group will be working together for an extended period. • Introduce each other at your table. • Have participants use index cards to say what questions they hope will be answered. • Realistic allotment of time for various activities. For example, an ice-breaker activity where 30 participants stand up and introduce themselves and state where they work and why they are taking this workshop could take up at least 30 to 40 minutes. This would not be appropriate for a 2- to 3-hour workshop. It might work, in a small group format, for a multiday program.
The Repetitive Report-Out *(following an excellent small group active learning strategy, the presenter asked 1 person from each table to report the results of the group's discussion to the larger group)*	Remember: *Active learning strategies* require some debriefing; however, just as it is ideal to engage each participant in the activity, it is equally ideal to engage each participant in the debriefing.	• Try a newsprint gallery review where the groups post their results and each participant—either alone, in pairs, or in their small group—reviews the written results of each group and comments on whether there was any new information or shifts in perspective. • The instructor can then summarize some of the themes from the groups and then ask if there are any questions or comments from the large group.
The Wandering Lecturer *(the presenter was interesting but went off on numerous tangents, leaving the audience confused about the goal of the presentation)*	Remember: *Well-written objectives* provide a roadmap for your instruction. Remember: *Formative assessments* help you stay on course.	• Create objectives as a roadmap. • Create a minute-by-minute schedule to keep you on track. • Use a periodic formative assessment to help determine whether your audience is learning what you expected.
The Lecturer With Too Much Background/Baseline Information* *(the lecturer felt compelled to provide the audience with basic information in great detail despite the fact that the audience was comprised of experienced clinicians)*	Remember: A good *needs assessment* (either beforehand or on-the-spot) can help you determine the needs of the audience. Remember: Always have a *Plan B*; be prepared to modify your planned presentation if you find out that your audience is more knowledgeable than you anticipated	• Complete a needs assessment. • If you find that much of the group is at least minimally familiar with your topic, rather than reviewing baseline content, try to use a handout with questions, pictures, etc, to elicit small group discussion that would require the audience to review and discuss the content.

*Note: This may be the case when students do in-service presentations for clinicians, particularly because they are being graded. The clinical instructor can forestall this by giving the student permission to leave out the basic information.

Table 5-6. Challenging Audience Behaviors

Challenging Audience Behaviors	The Problem	Potential Solutions
Controversies that get too heated	Other audience members may become uncomfortable and disengaged.	Remind participants that people have strong feelings about the topic. For now, people need to agree to disagree. Summarize key point(s) of each perspective and then move on to your next topic/activity.
Questions or discussion that take you off topic	This may cause the lecturer to lose focus of the stated objectives, takes extra time, and may prevent you from meeting the stated objectives.	Let the participants know that you will use a "parking lot" (piece of chart paper) to hold all questions not directly related to the topic and if there is time at the end you will address the topics as raised.
The discussion hog	When 1 person dominates discussion, other participants may tune out or become distracted. It is not uncommon to observe other audience members roll their eyes or look to one another when this individual raises his or her hand or begins to speak.	Wait several seconds before calling on someone to respond to a question. This may give other individuals time to formulate a response and raise their hands Acknowledge that the learner is clearly interested in and familiar with the topic but that you would like to give others an opportunity to speak up.
The persistent unanswered question (ie, you explained it several times but the student persists with questions)	In attempting to help a single student understand the concept, the instructor may lose the attention of the rest of the group.	Take a break (if appropriate) and meet with the student separately to clarify the point. After 1 or 2 attempts to rephrase the response, suggest that the learner take a few minutes to think about the concept and if he or she still has questions, meet after the presentation. Indicate that you are available after the presentation to discuss this concept further.
Sidebar conversations	Sidebar conversations may be a sign that participants are confused or have questions about something you have presented, need to be more active, or need a break.	Ask the group if there are questions about the material presented, and, if there are, answer them. Inject an opportunity to actively process material or tell people when the break will occur.

Summary

Regardless of the teaching and learning situation there are certain essential components of instructional design that must be considered. There are certain non-negotiable elements of systematic effective instruction that must be considered regardless of the format of your presentation. These non-negotiables include completing a needs assessment either beforehand or on-the-spot to make sure that you know your audience and can design your presentation to meet their needs; developing objectives to focus and guide your presentation; using motivational hooks and content boosters—including active learning strategies—to grab your audience's attention and maintain it throughout your presentation; summarizing the key points to take advantage of the concept of recency in memory formation.

In addition to these non-negotiable elements, unique variables must be considered in designing any presentation: Who is in your audience? How much time do you have to present? What presentation style or format will you be required to use? What type of room will you be in? How is the room set up? What kind of equipment will you have available to you? The answers to each of these questions and more will help you refine your presentation design. Finally, always prepare a plan B. Be prepared for unanticipated events such as speaking to an audience that is much more knowledgeable about your topic than you anticipated; a room setup that is not conducive to some of your planned active learning strategies; technology problems that prevent you from using the technology you had planned; or needing to manage challenging audience behaviors. Planning and practice are critical to designing and implementing effective presentations, no matter what the format.

Key Points to Remember

- Regardless of the type of presentation you are planning, try to include the following non-negotiable components of systematic effective instruction:
    o Needs assessment (interest/knowledge)
    o Motivational hook
    o Learning objectives
    o Content boosters and active learning strategies
    o Summary
- Always consider the unique variables of any teaching-learning experience:
    o Audience
    o Time frame
    o Format
    o Room setup
    o Equipment and other resources
    o Context
- Plan ahead, and ask as many questions as you need to find out about the specific characteristics of your teaching-learning situation.
- Plan your presentation right down to the minute, and if you think you have enough, remember that presentations most often take more time than you anticipate, so less is more.
- Plan longer presentations and workshops as if they were several iterations of shorter presentations.
- Always have a plan B and be prepared to modify your plan based on the needs of the audience and environment.
- To keep your audience engaged, it is important to be able to manage challenging audience behaviors.
- Practice, practice, practice!

References

In this chapter, we apply the principles of systematic effective instruction to a variety of presentation formats. For a list of references, see Chapter 4, "Systematic Effective Instruction: Keys to Designing Effective Presentations."

6

Strategies for Teaching and Learning Movement

Joyce R. Maring, PT, EdD

Chapter Objectives

After reading this chapter, you will be prepared to:

- Describe the influence of theories on motor control to the application of teaching motor skills.

- Identify the stages of motor learning and the focus of each stage in skill development.

- Discuss taxonomies and classifications of motor skills.

- Describe the conditions and variables that influence how motor tasks are processed.

- Relate the conditions of prepractice and practice to outcomes in motor performance and motor learning.

- Consider the role of providing feedback in effectively teaching motor skill acquisition.

- Apply the principles of motor learning to clinical case scenarios to enhance the effectiveness of teaching and learning and patient/client performance.

In this chapter, we transition from presentations to designing environments and conditions that encourage learning through active engagement and practice. We focus on teaching and learning movement, a topic integral to physical therapy patient care. We will explore our role as movement educators and describe how theories of motor control and motor learning inform practice. We examine various types of movement, task characteristics, and movement taxonomies. Humans as information processors are discussed and linked to concepts such as attention, interference, response alternatives, and accuracy demands, all essential to teaching

and learning about movement. We examine conditions of practice, types of practice, practice schedules, and how each can be used to optimize learning given the individual, the task, and the environment. The various forms of feedback are introduced and linked to effective learning. The chapter concludes with a discussion of differences across the life span.

The Role of Theory in Practice and Theories of Motor Control

Physical therapists are considered movement specialists. We analyze movement and movement dysfunction and then work with individuals to establish or re-establish movements that lead to improved function and quality of life. Therefore, we are also movement educators and need to effectively apply clinical practice to all of the principles of teaching and learning discussed in this book. We need to know what strategies, patterns, and types of practice will lead to the most effective motor learning in the populations that we serve. What are those internal and external processes associated with practice and experience that contribute to motor learning or the acquisition of a motor skill?

Motor learning is usually inferred by changes in motor performance. Throughout this chapter, we will be distinguishing between *learning* and *performance* because they are not the same. For example, it is possible for someone to demonstrate an improvement in motor performance for a short period of time without demonstrating learning.

Plack M, Driscoll M. *Teaching and Learning in Physical Therapy:*
From Classroom to Clinic (pp 133-156).
© 2011 SLACK Incorporated

Critical Thinking Clinical Scenario

You are working with a patient who is practicing mat-to-wheelchair transfers. The session is 30 minutes long. By the end of the session, the patient is performing the skill independently (eg, without any verbal or physical cues).

Reflective Question

1. Has this patient learned the motor skill? How would you be able to tell?

Even though a patient *performs* the movement fairly well at the end of the session, he or she may not have *learned* the new motor skill. For us to assess whether the patient has really learned the transfer, we would have to evaluate whether he or she could demonstrate the skill several weeks in the future or apply what he has learned about transfers to a new situation in which he was required to perform a transfer (eg, between a bed and commode). We call the ability to perform a movement over time *retention* of movement and the ability to use that movement in a new situation the *transfer* of learning. Both retention and transfer are evidence of learning.

Questions surrounding *motor learning* cannot be separated from questions of *motor control*, the study of the nature of movement and how it is regulated. Understanding the neural, physical, and behavioral aspects that control movement provides the background from which to establish effective motor learning strategies. That is why we spend so much time in school studying the basic sciences and why we must become lifelong learners of the factors that contribute to the successful production of functional movement. It is up to us to remain informed and participate in updating motor control theory to help us make sense of what we see.

Theories are sets of assumptions we use to explain and predict behaviors. They provide a framework for our intervention strategies and therapeutic approaches. Theories drive practice. Theoretical assumptions should not be randomly selected but chosen as a result of careful, systematic testing and observation. As the systematic testing of assumptions in motor control and learning progressed over time, the theories also evolved, and this evolution has had a tremendous impact on the way we practice physical therapy. Just as your assumptions about culture influence your practice, the conjectures you have about how we control movement influence how you intervene when working with an individual with movement dysfunction. Physical and occupational therapists

have been referred to as "applied motor control physiologists."[1] That is why, although an in-depth discussion of current theories of motor control is beyond the objectives of this chapter, we need to include a brief discussion in order to meet the objectives related to motor learning and teaching patients new motor skills.

Theories of Motor Control

Historical theories of motor control were based on assumptions of hierarchical and stimulus-response control of movement.[2] Sensory input dictates motor output. According to this theory, if we are trying to improve the way someone walks, our best treatment strategy would be to provide the person with optimal sensory feedback that would result in a better walking pattern. For example, if we are working with a child with cerebral palsy who uses excessive hip adduction and internal rotation and is having difficulty getting full hip extension when walking, we might facilitate his movements by giving tactile and proprioceptive input (ie, placing our hands on) to his gluteus medius and gluteus maximus muscles to facilitate hip extension and inhibit the adduction. Traditionally, therapists viewed movement dysfunction, secondary to a neurological lesion, as an interruption of the ability of the higher levels to inhibit or control the lower level primitive reflexes. In this context, our primary role as therapists was to use sensory feedback (such as facilitation and inhibition) to help the higher centers recover control over the lower centers of the nervous system.

Systems Theory and Beyond

Today, we have moved beyond stimulus-response and hierarchical control theories of *movement control*. Current theories of motor control suggest that there are many complex factors that may influence the control and learning or relearning of movements. Much of the early work in this area was conducted by Russian scientist Nicolai Bernstein. Bernstein hypothesized that movement control was distributed among interacting systems and all of these interactions must be considered in accounting for the control of movement. This is referred to as a *distributed model of motor control*.[3] Today, that model continues to evolve and expand to take into account the many parameters of movement that must be considered. For example, theories of motor control must explain factors such as the initiation of movement, the pattern and timing of muscle recruitment, and the influence of environmental variations and task requirements on movement production. There is a lot to consider.

Stop and Reflect

You are working with a patient who recently sprained his ankle, and you want to teach him how to walk up stairs using crutches. Think about all of the factors that must be considered in trying to teach a patient how to walk up stairs using crutches. Consider the following:

- Task factors (eg, handling the crutches, keeping the leg out of a weight-bearing position, etc)
- Individual factors (eg, muscle strength, range of motion, etc)
- Environmental factors (eg, depth of step, handrail or no handrail, etc)

Shumway-Cook and Woollacott,[4] among others, described the *dynamic systems model* in which movement emerges from the interaction of 3 primary factors: the environment, the task, and the individual. Each of those factors has the ability to both constrain and enable movement possibilities. To focus on only one factor (eg, the processes within an individual) excludes the contribution of the demands of the task and environment to the control and production of movement. As physical therapists, we have been well trained to identify the movements we want to facilitate, and we can describe in detail the musculoskeletal components required to produce those movements. But that is only one piece of the puzzle. To be effective teachers of movement, we need to pay attention to the attributes of the tasks we are asking the individual to learn and the environmental contexts in which those tasks will be performed. Movements that may serve an individual well in one environment may need to shift in response to a change in a key parameter. For example, imagine you are walking on a treadmill. As the velocity increases, your gait pattern will dramatically change as you transition from walking to running to meet the increasing velocity demands.

This evolving theory of motor control impacts how we examine and intervene with patients who are learning or relearning how to accomplish a functional skill. Theory impacts practice. Current theories of motor control and learning stress the organization of practice and movements around a behavioral goal so that retraining becomes "task oriented."[4] All practice sessions should be centered on an established goal or task valued by the participant.[5] As you know by now, this is a concept important to all teaching and learning strategies. The added purpose of a goal-directed task enhances motor learning in all contexts.[6]

Given the earlier example, evolving theories require the therapist to consider the goal of the task (eg, independent and safe ambulation in a specific environment) in addition to the process of ambulating. Potentially, the therapist can think of ways to change the task or modify the environment to improve the pattern of movement and therefore the outcome. This allows the therapist and patient to focus not only on individual factors, such as strength and range of motion, but on task and environmental factors when designing an intervention designed to achieve movement goals.

Critical Thinking Clinical Scenario

A physical therapist is working with a patient who has had a stroke. The patient is unable to initiate any movement at all with her right arm. The goal of the session is to improve the patient's independence in bed mobility (especially rolling onto the uninvolved side).

Reflective Question

1. How might the therapist's approach differ if the therapist primarily used a reflex or hierarchical control of movement to influence therapy versus a system's approach that considers factors related to the environment and task in addition to the individual?

Critical Thinking Clinical Scenario

A child is able to climb the stairs independently in the therapy gym.

Reflective Questions

1. How does the task change if the child is climbing stairs in between scheduled classes with her classmates?
2. What are some of the different individual and environmental attributes that will come into play in this new scenario that were not as important in the therapy gym?

Key Points to Remember

Considering how movement is controlled is important to considering how movement is learned.

- Theory drives practice!

Motor control theory continues to evolve.

- Dynamic systems theory considers the influence of the environment, the task in addition to individual factors in movement control.
- Movement is increasingly viewed as goal- rather than process-oriented.

Motor Learning and Types of Movement

Although knowing about motor control is important to understanding how our patients learn new movements, it is motor learning and the therapist's role in teaching movement that is the focus of this chapter. *Motor learning* refers to the acquisition of skilled movement. We have reflexive movements that are predictably produced with the right stimulus and do not require any experience. For example, withdrawal from a painful stimulus and scratching an itch are movements that take place without practice and learning. Our discussion focuses on the types of movements that take place only as learning occurs, the type of movements that can be consistently reproduced as a result of practice and experience. A tennis serve, a corner kick in soccer, and the use of a 4-point gait pattern with crutches are examples of learned movements that required practice.

Although we measure learning by measuring performance, we have already talked about how learning and performance may not be the same thing. *Performance* is the actual demonstration of skill, and its parameters can be clearly described and measured. Accuracy, velocity, range, and power are all attributes of motor performance that are relatively easy to quantify. Though improved performance is likely associated with learning, it is possible to perform well without learning and learn without performing well. Consider the athlete who learned a task well but is fatigued, stressed, or nervous. Although the task is well learned, it may be poorly performed under those conditions.

Do you remember the first time you had to take a practical exam? Perhaps you learned how to perform a manual muscle test with a lab partner and felt that you had learned it quite well. Yet, when it came time to perform it on the practical exam, you may not have performed it as well thanks to the added stress from your instructor watching. Someone may also practice a skill several times in a row in a single session and perform it well on the last trial. Yet, a week later, the performance may be back to the baseline level because the improvement was temporary and motor learning did not occur. Remember the distinction between learning and performance because we will come back to it later in this chapter. As a teacher of movement, you will need to distinguish between strategies that will enhance someone's performance versus approaches to improve motor learning.

Stages of Motor Learning

Through practice, the acquisition of skilled behavior moves through several stages of learning: *cognitive, associative,* and *autonomous* (Table 6-1). These were described by Fitts and Posner[7] quite some time ago but still provide a useful framework today.

Cognitive Stage

At this stage of learning, the individual is seeking to understand what it takes to perform the skill and develop a cognitive map. The learner will perform a series of trials and discard the strategies that are not successful. The learner at this stage usually relies heavily on feedback (especially visual cues) and practices best in a stable or closed environment. A *stable* or *closed environment* is defined as a predictable environment in which everything is the same each and every time a person does the task.

For example, you may be working with a patient who had a recent amputation and has a new prosthetic limb. Initially, the patient may want to practice walking using the parallel bars (a stable and closed environment) and receive lots of feedback. The patient may experiment with shifting his or her weight in different directions over the prosthetic limb and moving the prosthetic limb in all planes of motion. A mirror could be set up to provide visual input.

As a therapist working with patients who are in the cognitive stage of motor learning, you may want to provide the following:

- A safe, closed environment
- Opportunities for trial-and-error practice of the movement
- Opportunities for feedback (particularly visual cues)

Associative Stage

This is the middle stage of learning a new motor task. The movement begins to look more organized and coordinated than it did during the cognitive stage. There is greater consistency and fewer errors or "extra" movements except when he or she is distracted or is asked to perform more than one task at a time. At this stage of practice, the patient is able to successfully walk with the prosthetic limb in a closed environment (ie, within the parallel bars) and reliably moves in all directions as long as he or she is able to "concentrate" on what he or she is doing. The patient tells you he or she is beginning to get the feel of it. Errors in gait pattern and problems with balancing on the new limb emerge when the patient is unexpectedly distracted or if he or she has to do too many things at once, such as answer a question and turn a corner at the same time.

Autonomous Stage

This final stage generally happens after much practice and the task no longer requires cognitive effort. The individual can now concentrate on other demands at the same time as performing the task and can readily perform in a predictable or a dynamic and changing environment. Research in cognitive neuroscience supports that performing a skill in the autonomous stage is associated with less cortical effort, especially for the parts of the brain that have to make decisions.[8]

Building on the previous example, now the patient is able to walk successfully using his or her prosthetic limb in most environments. He or she is able to shift directions and maintain conversation simultaneously. Moving from linoleum to carpet is not a problem. He tells you he sometimes forgets he is even wearing a prosthetic limb. At this point, your patient may be able to perform a certain task independently without thinking. As a therapist, you may begin to introduce new tasks to your patient so that he can begin to manage more than one task at a time (ie, dual-tasking), which is consistent with the demands of day-to-day life.

As a therapist working with patients who are in the autonomous stage of motor learning, you may do the following:

- Continue to provide opportunities for practice in increasingly more complex and challenging environments
- Provide challenges and distracters within the environment to increase the demand

Critical Thinking Clinical Scenario

You are working with an 8-year-old girl with cerebral palsy and spastic diplegia who is learning to negotiate the stairs independently. One of the classes she attends during the school day requires her to ascend/descend the stairs one time each day with her class.

Reflective Question

1. Apply the framework of learning to teaching a patient a new skill. Consider the type of practice, environment, and feedback you would provide during learning in the following stages:
   - Cognitive stage
   - Associative stage
   - Autonomous stage

Types of Movement

Given the interaction we described between an individual, a task, and the environment, it likely comes as no surprise that tasks and movements can be classified and that each type of movement may be controlled

Table 6-1. Characteristics and Teaching Strategies for the Stages of Motor Learning

Stage	Characteristics	Teacher's Role	Learner's Role
Cognitive	The learner is seeking to understand what it takes to perform the skill and develop a cognitive map. The learner will perform a series of trials and will discard the strategies that are not successful.	• Provide opportunities for feedback (especially visual cues); reinforce correct performance • Provide opportunities for practice in a stable or closed environment • Model the task • Provide purpose and relevance • Link back to similar tasks they have performed • Provide manual guidance • Avoid too much verbal cuing	• Utilize trial-and-error strategies • Utilize feedback to determine effective movement strategies
Associative	The movement begins to look more organized and coordinated. There is greater consistency and fewer errors or "extra" movements.	• Add complexity to the environment • Increase unpredictability of the environment (open environment) • Utilize authentic environments (ie, outside of the therapeutic setting) • Provide feedback (emphasizing proprioceptive feedback/internal cues) • Decrease manual cuing • Use mental imagery	• Identify the typical challenges they face in daily life • Focus on proprioceptive feedback of the task at this stage of practice • Perform the skill or task in a predictable environment
Autonomous	The task no longer requires cognitive effort.	• Give the patient maximal control • Focus on patient education • Identify strategies the patient can use to embed practice into his or her daily routine • Work toward patient discharge	• Focus on other demands at the same time as performing the task • Perform the skill or task in a dynamic and changing environment • Incorporate dual task demands • Vary the environment to increase the challenge; increase distractions

and learned differently. This is an important point. As therapists, we are required to analyze the task the individual is trying to learn so we can help him or her select a strategy with the best chance of success. Tasks can be classified in many different ways. Movement scientists have created groupings and taxonomies based on a variety of organizing principles. Some of the ways tasks can be classified include the following:

- Movement taxonomy along 3 continua
- Open versus closed tasks or skills
- Discrete versus continuous tasks or skills
- Stability versus mobility tasks or skills

Movement Taxonomy

Gentile[9] created a taxonomy that looked at movement along 3 continua simultaneously:

1. A stationary versus variable environment
2. A stable versus dynamic body
3. No manipulation versus maximum manipulation demands.

Figure 6-1 illustrates Gentile's taxonomy of tasks.[10]

Critical Thinking Clinical Scenario

You are working with a patient who has had a stroke affecting the cerebellar region and has impaired balance in all positions.

Reflective Question

Apply the taxonomy of movements by planning a progression of activities that move the patient from learning to stand without support to managing activities of daily living (eg, eating and brushing his or her teeth) while in the upright position. Set up a progression of activities that considers:

- Moving the demands from a stable to a dynamic body position
- Moving the demands from a closed or stable environment to a variable environment (How can you vary the environment so that the task becomes more demanding?)
- Moving the demands from no manipulation to reasonably complex manipulation (Consider how to progress the patient in terms of holding an eating utensil or comb to using for eating or grooming, all while maintaining balance).

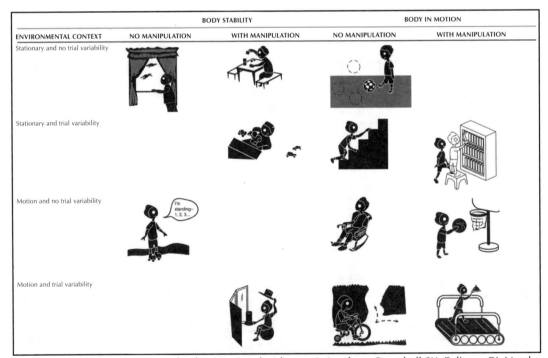

Figure 6-1. Gentile's taxonomy of tasks. (Reprinted with permission from Campbell SK, Palisano RJ, Vander Linden DW. *Physical Therapy for Children*. 3rd ed. Philadelphia, PA: WB Saunders; 2006:144.)

Open Versus Closed Tasks

This classification considers the interaction of the task and the environment. Closed tasks are characterized by fixed environmental demands and can be produced with minimal variations each time. Open tasks occur under variable conditions, requiring instantaneous adaptation. Most tasks fall along a continuum of open or closed depending on the role of the environment. Sometimes, we use the terms open and closed to refer to the environment itself. The closed environment is stable and predictable; the open environment is constantly changing. Table 6-2 describes the characteristics of open versus closed tasks and provides examples of each.

Discrete Versus Continuous Tasks

Intuitively, you know that the type of skill required to perform a specific task such as picking something up from the floor from a standing position is very different than the type of skill required to go for a walk. Tasks can be classified as to whether they are discrete tasks with a recognizable beginning or end versus a continuous task, which does not have an inherent beginning and end. Table 6-2 describes the characteristics of discrete versus continuous tasks and provides examples of each. Sometimes, a series of discrete movements can be performed in a sequence. We refer to those as *serial movements*, and they are composed of discrete movements strung together. Many activities of daily living are serial movements (eg, dressing in the morning requires a series of discrete tasks performed together).

Stability Versus Mobility Tasks

As previously described in Gentile's[9] taxonomy (stable vs dynamic body) movement requirements can vary depending on whether the base of support is in motion. Table 6-2 describes the characteristics of stability versus mobility tasks and provides examples of each.

Table 6-2. Characteristics of Movement Variables

Type of Task	Examples	
Open Versus Closed Tasks	Closed Tasks	Open Tasks
Tasks can be classified based on the interaction of the task and the environment. For example, closed tasks occur in a constant environment and can be produced with minimal variations each time. Open tasks occur under variable conditions, requiring instantaneous adaptation.	• Throwing a bowling ball, where the weight of the ball, the distance of the lane, and the required strength to throw the ball do not appreciably change between trials • Kicking a soccer ball from a stationary position a specific length on an empty field • Teaching a patient to walk in the parallel where the distance, surface, height, and length of the bars remain constant	• The typical soccer game requires the player to kick the ball under extremely variable conditions, adapting instantaneously to the position of other players and the speed and direction in which he or she is moving • Walking in the busy corridor of a hospital where the patient must constantly be adjusting the trajectory and velocity of his or her path to accommodate carts and other people moving at varying speeds and directions
Discrete Versus Continuous Tasks	Discrete Tasks	Continuous Tasks
A discrete task has an inherent beginning and end point. Conversely, a continuous skill has no inherent beginning or end; the performer arbitrarily decides when to begin or end the task.	Kicking a ball or a tennis serve is a discrete task. Setting the brakes on a wheelchair is a discrete skill.	• Driving a car or riding a bike do not have an inherent beginning and end, you decide when to start and stop the task based on factors not related to the motor performance • Propelling a wheelchair
Stability Versus Mobility Tasks	Stability Tasks	Mobility Tasks
The demands of tasks requiring a stable base of support can be distinguished from task demands associated with a mobile base of support. In between those 2 ends of the continuum are movement transitions that occur over a modified base of support such as coming to a stand from a sitting position or a supine position to a sitting position.	• Lying down • Sitting • Standing	• Running • Jumping

Stop, Do, and Reflect

List one task you have completed today that was:

- Continuous
- Discrete
- Serial

Label each of the following tasks your patient likely has to perform every day as continuous, discrete, or serial.

- Walking
- Brushing his or her teeth
- Eating a meal
- Turning on a light switch
- Combing his or her hair
- Transferring from the bed to the toilet

Which of the above tasks would you consider open? Why? Which of the above would you consider mobility task? Why?

It Matters!

We have talked about how therapists need to consider the taxonomy of tasks and environments so that they can intentionally increase the complexity and demands of the task. This building process helps our patients perform necessary skills at an autonomous level. Performing necessary skills autonomously means they can be performed safely in real-life scenarios. The individual can walk independently but can also cross a street while monitoring other pedestrians and the color of the traffic light. We have now described several characteristics intrinsic to a task. We will soon tie those characteristics into ways the tasks should be practiced to maximize successful learning. For now, file that information in your memory bank and move on!

Key Points to Remember

- Motor learning should be distinguished from motor performance. Motor learning occurs in stages, and therapists should adjust the type and environment of practice to reflect the patient's stage of learning.

- There are several ways to classify movement. This is useful to know because:
  - Therapists should consider the type of functional task the patient needs to perform in order to design the best practice.
  - The classification may be viewed as a way to progress the complexity and demands of a task.

Factors That Influence How We Process Motor Tasks

Historical concepts of motor control emphasized human beings as reflexive. In a reflexive model, sensory input drives the motor output. In a similar fashion, educational psychologists and behaviorists described associative learning and operant conditioning as primary principles governing how we learn and what behaviors to expect based on the stimulus received. Through experience, we associate 2 stimuli, and it is theoretically possible to predict an individual's behavior based on the stimulus he or she has received. We do not need to know much about the inner workings of the individual's mind, only the stimulus received and its associated behavioral output.

Human Beings Are Complex Information Processors

There is a significant body of evidence that we exert far more control over our responses than such a perspective would indicate. We are much more than a "black box" that receives input and subsequently drives the output. A number of factors influence what stimuli we attend to, how quickly we can filter the stimuli and select possible response options, and then how we implement the output we selected. Schmidt and Lee[11] described human beings as complex *information processors*. After the stimulus is received from the environment, we process it in a number of ways before acting upon it. As information processors, we do the following:

- Identify stimuli that we receive. As part of the identification process, we detect and recognize familiar patterns. Most responses require us to pick out meaningful patterns of features in the stimuli presented (eg, how fast is that car traveling toward me?).
- Select a number of stimulus response alternatives and decide upon the possible options.
- Program a response based on the selection. This involves organizing and initiating a reaction.
- Produce a response at the level of the effector.

As an information processor, we have a lot of control over the stimuli we attend to and the subsequent responses we select. Those processes are influenced by a number of factors. Understanding those factors assists us in being aware of their impact on the patients we treat, and therefore we can better assist them in selecting a response that leads to improved function.

Attention and Information Processing

We all have a limited potential for attention at any given moment. We may be bombarded by stimuli and sensory input, and it is not possible to attend to all of the input we receive; however, we do not cut off the sensory input at the level of the receptors. Our nervous systems are picking up all of the sounds, sensations, visual inputs, and stimuli that surround us. The stimuli pass through some sort of attention filter, and we "decide" which ones require our response.

What factors impact the filter? Have you ever attended a noisy party? You've probably carried on conversations with friends and acquaintances while tuning out those sounds that interfered with your attention to the conversation. In fact, you were probably minimally aware of other conversations around you. If you suddenly heard your name mentioned in a conversation nearby or shouted across the room, however, you would likely switch attention to the individual(s) who voiced your name. This example demonstrates that you do not cut off stimuli at the level of your sensory receptors or you would not have heard your name in the first place.

Stimuli that are somehow meaningful to us based on our experiences and emotions make it through the filter and command our attention. You may not have noticed a particular model and make of a car until you purchased one yourself. Then suddenly, the road appears to be full of that particular vehicle. It likely was not the number of cars that changed but that the filter of your attention was adjusted by your recent car purchase. Intense stimuli also have a tendency to make it through the filter. Loud noises, bright lights, and intense sensations generally make us sit up and take notice.

We all have a limited capacity for attention, and it requires effort to direct our attention. Probably all of us have read a page or paragraph without effort and attention and when we came to the last sentence had no clue what we had just finished reading. Our capacity to attend improves with practice, and we can learn how to expend the required effort. Nevertheless, we can only attend to one task at a single point in time. We are single-channel operators with limited capacity. This is true for motor tasks as well as mental skills.

Stop and Reflect

Have you ever tried to listen to 2 people talking at the same time?

- How successfully and accurately could you recount both conversations?
- What strategies did you use to try to listen to both people simultaneously?
- If you opted to attend to one conversation versus the other, what prompted you to attend to the selected conversation?

Is multitasking possible? Can you attend to 2 tasks simultaneously? The answer is both yes and no. It is possible to perform 2 tasks simultaneously if one of the tasks does not require attention. If a task is so well learned or so simple that it can be performed automatically, it does not use up the limited capacity for attention, and the individual can perform that task while performing the more attention-requiring task. Most of us can walk and talk simultaneously, but the limited capacity we have for processing 2 tasks simultaneously is one of the arguments against permitting the use of cell phones while driving. Although driving is a well-rehearsed skill that often does not require much mental effort, unexpected shifts in traffic, velocity, and flow do require full attention, making any attention diverted to a cell phone hazardous.

Interference

There are 2 main types of interferences to attention: *capacity* and *physical*. Let's continue to use the example of cell phones to illustrate both types of interference. If you are speaking to another party using a hands-free headset while you are driving and someone makes a sudden lane change ahead of you requiring you to swerve, your conversation on the cell phone may interfere with your capacity for attention. If you are holding a cell phone and have to make a sudden swerve to avoid the vehicle that is making a sudden lane change, now you are experiencing a physical interference in addition to the capacity interference.

It is our responsibility as therapists to analyze the possible interferences patients will experience in performing important functional tasks. A patient relearning independent ambulation may experience capacity interference while walking in a crowded room. If the patient is using an assistive device and has to navigate a lot of obstacles, physical interference may also come into play.

Factors Affecting the Response Time

Before we take action, we review the response alternatives based on the stimuli and other factors. The interval between this review and the implementation of a movement is called a *response time*. A number of factors affect the length of the response time. We are going to describe some of those factors and then discuss why they are important in teaching patients new motor skills.

Hick's Law

The number of response alternatives impacts the time it takes someone to respond. Building on previous work, Hick[12] demonstrated that there is a defined relationship between response time and the number of alternative responses available. This was studied in an experiment in which the subjects had to press a variety of keys in response to a pattern of lights. The more keys that needed to be pressed, the greater amount of response time the individual required. Each time the number of response alternatives doubled (ie, they doubled the number of keys to be pressed), the response time increased by about 150 ms. We have come to know this relationship formally as *Hick's law*. In a therapeutic setting, Hick's law requires the therapist to consider the number of response alternatives being required in any task as well as the time required to process these alternatives. Hick's law can also be considered when intentionally increasing the task demands as the patient becomes more independent.

Practice and Response Time

A number of researchers, following the publication of Hick's law, investigated how accurately response time could be predicted by response alternatives. They found, of course, that a number of other variables have to be taken into consideration in order to accurately predict response times. One of the major variables to be considered was the amount of practice the individual had in assessing response alternatives and making decisions based on the detection of the pattern of stimuli. This probably already makes sense to you. Consider a beginning basketball player versus a seasoned player confronted with the same number of play options on the floor during a game. The seasoned player is more likely to rapidly detect the possible response options based on his or her experience and come to a decision more quickly than the novice player. Therapeutically, it is important to recognize that practice decreases response time and allows patients to complete tasks in a functional length of time.

Stimulus-Response Compatibility

The stimulus-response compatibility also influences the response time.[13] For example, if a subject is asked to raise his or her right hand when a light is flashed on his or her right, he or she is usually able to respond more quickly than the subject who is required to raise his or her left hand when a light flashes on the right. In the first case, the stimulus and response were spatially compatible.

Number of Movements and Response Time

The more complex the movement or the greater number of movements we need to make, the more time we typically take before responding (ie, beginning the movement or movement series). For example, consider the number of discrete movements a patient needs to perform to successfully transfer from a wheelchair to a car using a sliding board. The number of movements required impacts the amount of response time the patient needs prior to performing the task.

The Intended Final Position

When planning a complex goal-oriented movement, it is typically the final intended position that influences how we select and initiate the movement. We are more efficient and respond more quickly when we use the intended final position to influence our early posture and movement. A good example of this was described by Rosenbaum and is illustrated in Figure 6-2.[14] If the goal is for you to pick up the cup for use, you will likely adjust your initial hand position so that when you lift this cup it will be in the final intended position (ie, upright and ready to be used).

Increased Accuracy Requirement

Response time also increases as the accuracy demands of the movement increases. For example, when we throw a dart or a ball at a target while standing at a constant distance, as the target size decreases, the response time we typically need prior to initiating the throw increases. You can try this yourself. Throw a soft object trying to hit the wall in front of you, then throw the object again from the same place trying to hit a much smaller target. Therapeutically, if you were working with a patient learning to walk with crutches, consider how long it would take the patient to learn to step up onto a narrow step as opposed to a broad step.

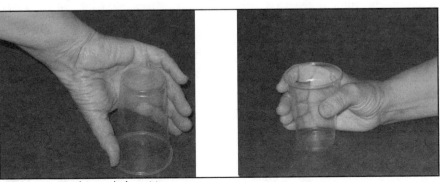

Figure 6-2. Final intended position.

Table 6-3. Humans as Information Processors: Sample Questions to Consider

- Is the individual's attention directed at the task or is there capacity or physical interference going on? If there is interference, is it possible to remove the interference?
- Based on the patient's life experiences and personal goals, is the task sufficiently meaningful to facilitate attention and effort?
- Are the stimuli being received compatible with the motor response being requested? If not, is it possible to find ways to make it more compatible?
- What are the requirements of the movement in terms of complexity and accuracy? Is it possible to decrease those demands as an initial strategy to build in early success and then progress the task?
- What is the final intended position of the movement? Would it be useful to spend more time practicing that movement? Conversely, if the final intended position is negatively impacting the required biomechanics, can the patient be made consciously aware of the deleterious effect of his or her posture selection?

Key Points to Remember

The following factors will likely increase response time:
- The greater the number of potential response alternatives required in a task
- The greater the time required to process the available response alternatives
- The greater the accuracy demands
- The greater the number of movements needed
- The more complex the movement
- The more complex the final intended position

The following factors will likely decrease response time:
- Practice
- Stimulus-response compatibility

Considering the individuals we serve as information processors helps us think about ways we can present tasks and stimuli that potentially maximize the impact of our interventions. Table 6-3 provides some sample questions we need to consider in planning our strategies for teaching and learning movement.

Conditions of Practice: Performance and Learning

The dictionary defines *practice* as "to perform or work at repeatedly so as to become proficient."[15] Practice is an essential part of learning and memory formation. It is critical that we understand how practice influences learning and proficiency and to use the best evidence when providing instructions to our patients on how to practice a skill.

Practice is essential to improving both performance and learning, and each of these effects is important to physical therapists. We want our patients to perform the skill safely, efficiently, and with spatial and temporal components consistent with functional outcomes. We also want our patients to be able to reproduce the skill whenever they need it or apply the skill to a novel task or environment when necessary. As teachers of functional movements, we need to identify practice

strategies to improve both performance and learning outcomes. We will be considering the following:

- Prepractice conditions such as motivation
- Practice schedules such as the amount of rest versus practice
- Types of practice such as part to whole and whole to part practice

It should be stated first that the absolute amount of practice time is far more important than most other practice considerations. This is referred to as the *power law of practice*.[11] Although the quality of practice is important, quality practice can never substitute for the quantity of practice. In almost all cases, the more opportunities the patient has to practice a skill, the more the patient learns. Of course, as therapists, we want to be sure that practice is being performed accurately.

We saw earlier when discussing the response time required in selecting and initiating movement that practice can alter and compensate for variables such as complexity. Important skills should be overlearned—practiced to the point that the task becomes automatic—allowing the task to be accomplished with significantly less mental effort. The individual arrives at the autonomous stage of learning, and the task can then be performed with very little cognitive monitoring.

Stop and Reflect

Think back to when you first learned to drive. Remember how much you had to think about:
- Where your hands belonged on the steering wheel
- How much pressure to apply to the brakes when you came to a stop sign
- When and how much to turn the wheel when you attempted to parallel park

Think about your driving skills now:
- Do these skills come automatically to you at this point? If so, you have overlearned these skills. What other skills have you overlearned?

Research on brain activation during the performance of learned tasks demonstrates that decreased effort is required by the cortex when the movement becomes automatic.[16] When a skill becomes overlearned, the associated brain activation patterns are more likely to be subcortical (eg, cerebellum and basal ganglia) and therefore require less cognitive processing. The value of skills being performed at this stage is that they can be performed in conjunction with other simultaneously required skills during high-level demands. Susceptibility to task interference has been minimized.

Consider the basketball player whose shot from a certain distance has been exceedingly well learned and is now almost automatic. That player has more likelihood of making the shot during an intense game because he or she can focus on the other evolving conditions on the court. A good example of this in physical therapy is working with the patient on ambulation. Ensuring that the patient has significant practice in developing the skill of ambulation in a variety of environments may increase the likelihood that he or she will be able to ambulate safely across busy the street in a timely manner.

Key Point to Remember

The absolute amount of practice time is more important than most other practice considerations.

Critical Thinking Clinical Scenario

Implications of the importance of the absolute practice time: You are treating a 62-year-old female patient with a left cerebrovascular accident and mild right hemiparesis. The patient is very motivated to regain complete functional use of her right arm so that she can go back to work as soon as possible. She does not have disability insurance and needs to work to maintain her insurance coverage and pay her bills. She works serving food in a school cafeteria and is required to lift and carry trays with both hands and serve food to children who line up at the cafeteria counter. Her insurance will only pay for 8 sessions of direct therapy.

Reflective Questions
1. Describe the movement characteristics required to lift and carry trays with both hands.

2. List some of the general strategies you will need to use to encourage this patient/client to get the amount of practice she needs in order to regain sufficient independence to return to work. Consider the settings, the people, and the tasks as you look to find ways to embed adequate practice in her daily life.

In the previous example, the therapist will need to find ways to encourage the patient to practice using the affected arm throughout the day for all tasks. That is one of the reasons that constraint-induced therapy or constraint-induced movement therapy was developed as a new treatment approach for patients who have had a stroke. The unaffected arm or the "strong"

arm is restrained for a good deal of the patient's day in order to require the individual to use the arm that was most affected by the stroke. Evidence shows that this approach has had good outcomes.[17] Consider the amount of total practice constraint-induced therapy encourages of the use of the affected arm. Although there are a number of reasons that the approach is successful from a neuroscience perspective, the influence of the total practice time is certainly a factor.

Prepractice Conditions

To learn effectively, we must be motivated to learn. This seems an obvious conclusion, but it gets more complex when we discuss what constitutes motivation and how motivation might be encouraged. One of the most obvious contributions to motivation is our perception that the task is worth learning. The task must seem important, useful, or worthwhile. If the new task is not connected to an inherent purpose that we feel is valuable, practice and rehearsal are doomed to substandard effort and a less than optimal outcome. Therefore, the therapist must understand what activities will be valued by the patient. The activities may be as demanding as a return to a sport or as fundamental as taking oneself to the bathroom independently.

Goal Setting

Motivation to put in quality practice time is usually driven by specific goals that are moderately challenging. Goals need to be precise (ie, specific in what will be accomplished) and challenging but also within reach. Kyllo and Landers[18] performed a meta-analysis of the literature in sports and exercise science. They noted that both short- and long-term goals were important to practice and performance; challenging but realistic goals improved motor learning.

Clearly, including the learner in goal setting is critical to ensuring the selected tasks will be considered worth learning. Encouragement and vague motivation such as "do your best" or "give it 100%" may be temporarily helpful and, as Schmidt[11] says, intuitively appealing, but are no substitute for specific goals. He compares it to conducting an important business meeting without an agenda. Once the goals are established, all practice can be directed toward the goal and seen as progress toward achieving the desired outcome.

Critical Thinking Clinical Scenario

A therapist is working with an individual who has had a total knee replacement. The individual tells the therapist that her goal is to be able to visit her grandchildren who live in a second-floor apartment.

Reflective Question
1. How could the therapist use this goal to encourage maximum participation in flexion and extension range of motion exercises?

Modeling and Perceptual Pretraining

In the early stages of learning at the cognitive stage, it is helpful if the learner has an overview of the task that is to be performed.[19] This assists the individual to develop what O'Sullivan[20] referred to as a *reference of correctness*. As part of developing a reference, the learner should be encouraged to associate the practice with the overall purpose and goals of the task.

Research has also demonstrated that verbal instructions are not nearly as useful as demonstrations. For example, Wulf and Shea[21] noted that demonstration or modeling may complement or even at times completely replace verbal instructions. It is often tempting for therapists to verbally overwhelm the learner with the benefit of their knowledge and experiences. Only brief and global verbal instructions are typically useful as learners can only assimilate a few directives in their first attempts at practice.

When teaching your patient to perform proprioceptive neuromuscular facilitation patterns, it would not be helpful to say, "I want you to bring your toes up toward your head and rotate your toes outward. Now raise your hip and bring your leg across the midline of your body." Your patient would be confused. Instead you might initially place the person's leg in the final intended position so he or she can get a sense of the required movement. Then you might restart the movement and say, "Toes out and up! Pull up! Go!" If you were working with someone to safely navigate stairs with crutches and bearing weight on only 1 leg, you would have to take care not to overload the patient with specific instructions while performing the task. Providing an overview and using simple commands will lead to a better outcome.

Key Points to Remember

Motivation is critical to learning. To better enhance your patient's motivation, consider:

- Setting goals that are personally relevant for your patient
- Demonstrating the task and providing a task overview
- Minimizing verbal instructions

Practice Schedules

In the next section, we will be discussing practice schedules and how they influence learning and retention (Table 6-4).

Table 6-4. Practice Schedules and How They Influence Learning and Retention

Massed versus distributed practice (ratio of practice time to rest time)	Massed practice • Massed practice occurs when the amount of practice time is greater than the amount of rest time in between trials • For example, cramming for a test the night before the exam or practicing a free-throw in basketball over and over for an hour without rest Enhances short-term recall	Distributed practice • Distributed practice occurs when the amount of rest time in between trials is greater than the amount of time for the trial • For example, studying over regular intervals the week or 2 weeks before the exam or practicing a free-throw for 10 minutes for 6 consecutive mornings Enhances overall performance and retention
Constant versus variable practice (uniform versus multiform practice)	Constant practice • Uniform practice • The learner repeats the skill in the same way each time • For example, practicing the same transfer skill under the same conditions each repetition Maximizes skill performance under specific conditions	Variable practice • Multiform practice • The conditions and type of practice vary between practice attempts • For example, practicing transfers in different rooms and between different surfaces Varying the practice requires more active learning and problem solving Enhances retention and the generalizability of the skill to novel tasks
Random versus blocked practice (practicing tasks in the same order versus practicing the tasks in an unpredictable order)	Random practice • In random practice, a number of skills are practiced in an unpredictable order; that is, practice a series of skills in differing sequences • For example, varying the order and starting position in which you practice scooting, rolling, and sitting up Enhances generalizability and retention	Blocked practice • In blocked practice, each set of skills is practiced in a "blocked" fashion; that is, practicing each set of skills until some degree of success is achieved before moving on to another skill • For example, practicing scooting, rolling, and assuming sit from supine in the same order and in the same way each time Enhances early performance

Although the absolute amount of practice is critical to success, research has demonstrated that there are optimal schedules of practice to promote performance and learning outcomes. Using practice time efficiently is an important consideration for all of us, whether you are an athlete trying to return to the field or an individual with a spinal cord injury working to re-enter the workforce. A therapist needs to consider how to set up a practice schedule that will help the patient accomplish the goals that brought him or her to therapy. For example, the type of practice that promotes optimal learning may be different than the type of practice schedule that promotes best performance. The therapist, in helping the patient plan a schedule that will encourage rehearsal of important skills, needs to be aware of the differences in likely outcomes based on the schedule.

Types of practice schedules include the following:

- Massed versus distributed practice
- Constant versus variable practice
- Random versus blocked practice

Massed Versus Distributed Practice

Massed versus distributed practice depends on the ratio of practice time to rest time (ie, time doing something unrelated to the practice).

- *Massed practice* occurs when the amount of practice time is greater than the amount of rest time in between trials.
- *Distributed practice* occurs when the amount of time in between trials is greater than the amount of time for the trial.

Students usually have no trouble differentiating between these 2 types of practice schedules when comparing massed practice as cramming for a test the night before the event versus distributed practice, which would require the student to spread the studying out over regular intervals a week or 2 weeks before the scheduled exam.

Our experiences of studying by cramming versus spreading out the content over time already highlights the different outcomes of these 2 practice schedules. When we cram the information, we may recall the content for the test but quite soon afterwards the information fades from our memory. However, information from distributed practice is more likely to be recalled several weeks later. Performance in the short term improves as a result of massed practice (that is the point of cramming, right?).

In early work, Baddely and Longman[22] investigated the differences between massed and distributed practice in postal workers. The groups were trained to use a keyboard for a total of 60 to 80 hours using different practice schedules. The group that distributed the practice time the most (1 hour once a day) at the time of retesting had retained the task and performed better than the group who had massed the practice. This principle has been verified by a great number of researchers in various contexts. Mackay et al,[23] for example, found that surgical skills were learned with better accuracy and recall when practice was distributed.

One of the reasons that massed practice is less effective for learning is the influence of fatigue on the individual practicing the task. Avoiding overfatigue should be a significant concern to therapists when considering a practice schedule for our patients. Although it is important for the individual to work hard and be maximally engaged with the practice, excess fatigue will increase the risk of injury and overuse. An additional reason for the better outcome in learning associated with distributed practice is that there is a limit to how much one can realistically learn in one session. If a person practices a task for 1 hour a day over 4 days and a second person practices the same task for 2 hours a day over 2 days, the actual practice time of the second person is likely to be less because we generally are not effective at retaining sufficient arousal and concentration to use 2 hours of practice time effectively. That means that the individual distributing the practice has actually practiced more total hours.

Key Points to Remember

- Massed practice improves performance in the short term.
- Distributed practice enhances accuracy and retention in the long term.

Constant Versus Variable Practice

Constant practice is uniform practice; the learner repeats the same skill in the same way each time. *Variable practice* by contrast is considered multiform; the conditions and type of practice vary between practice attempts. Which one is better? It depends on the desired outcome. If the goal is to be able to reproduce exactly the same movement under precisely the same condition, uniform practice works well. Think of a concert pianist who wants to be able to perform a particular piece at a concert. That person may do very well to perform that piece repeatedly in a way similar to the demands of the concert. But that is an unusual type of circumstance. Most of us, as well as our patients, need to perform the same tasks in a variety of circumstances. We need to be able to transfer our learning to novel circumstances and repeat our learned skills under a variety of conditions.

Catalano and Kleiner[24] did an experiment that demonstrated the effectiveness of variable practice on learning. They instructed subjects to press a button when a moving pattern of light arrived at a particular point. One group responded to lights moving at variable speed and another to lights that moved at a single predictable speed. When both groups were tested at a novel speed that neither group had experienced, the group that had variable practice responded with much less error than the group who had only practiced at one speed. This is just one example of the principle of being able to transfer learning best if the practice has been variable.

In a more recent example, chiropractors who practiced manipulation skills in a variety of ways in combination with visual feedback retained the skills longer and performed more accurately than chiropractors who practiced the same skill over and over without variation.[25] It appears that variable practice is easier to generalize to unique conditions. The participant is learning more than a specific task; he or she is also learning how to adapt the task to fit new circumstances.

Herbert et al[26] compared variable practice to constant practice in a group of patients with lower back pain secondary to inadequate multifidus muscle function. The patients who practiced in a variety of ways and under a variety of conditions demonstrated much better muscle recruitment that they sustained even 3 to 4 months after the training stopped. Goode et al[27] found variable practice to be much superior to repeated practice in all aspects of test performance. They hypothesized that varied practice required subjects to process the task more elaborately, which led to better learning. There is evidence that one of the best ways to build in variable practice is to ensure that learning is happening under open-task conditions—circumstances in which the participant has to adjust to unpredictable stimuli and conditions.[28]

It would be difficult to overstate the importance of the implications of this observation for the patients in therapy who are learning new movement patterns and acquiring or regaining motor skills. Most of them must perform daily tasks in a variety of open environments, and the skill is of little use to them if it cannot be performed accurately in the new environment. A patient who has transferred independently from the wheelchair to mat in a physical therapy clinic is in trouble if he or she cannot transfer independently from a chair to the bed once at home. We must take seriously the challenge of finding ways to promote variability in practice in the individuals we serve.

Key Points to Remember

- Variable practice is important to ensure learning.
- Use open-task conditions in which the participant has to adjust to unpredictable stimuli and conditions in order to build in variable practice.

Critical Thinking Clinical Scenario

You are treating a patient who has just received a new below-knee prosthesis and is learning to walk with the new prosthetic.

Reflective Questions

1. In designing a home program for this individual, what frequency and duration of practice would you recommend?

2. Consider ways to vary the practice in terms of:
   o Surfaces (texture and incline)
   o Velocity (varying speeds to cross the street in sufficient time or walk slowly in a crowd)
   o Direction (such as turning, lateral, and backward to avoid obstacles or move in small spaces)
   o Environmental background (such as noisy and crowded or empty)

Random Versus Blocked Practice

Suppose you were trying to learn how to play tennis and needed to practice serving the ball, hitting a forehand, and hitting a backhand. If you were to use *blocked practice* to learn the skill, you would practice each skill one at a time in a "blocked" fashion. So you would possibly spend several minutes doing nothing but serving the tennis ball until you achieved a modicum of success and then subsequently practiced the forehand or backhand. However, if you were to choose a *random practice* approach, you would mix it up unpredictably such that you practiced all 3 types of skills at the same time in differing sequences. Which approach is better? The answer is *it depends*.

In general, during random practice, there is contextual interference to the practice.[29] When multiple skills are practiced in a single session, the context of one skill interferes with the next when they are randomly ordered. Random practice is better than blocked practice in promoting learning. Constant training may result in better early skill acquisition and random training in better retention.[30] Tasks are better recalled and transferred to novel conditions when practiced randomly.

The caveat to this finding is in the initial phase of learning, while the individual is still learning the fundamentals of the task and is at the cognitive stage of learning. At this stage, the contextual interference may interfere with the person's ability to conceptualize the task requirements. But once some minimal task conceptualization has occurred, practicing the skills in a random order will typically lead to better long-term retention. Shumway-Cook and Woollacott[4] indicated that the factors that initially make performing a task more difficult may make learning more effective in the long run.

As discussed in earlier chapters, each individual has a unique learning style and rate. The time to switch to random practice from repeated practice is dependent on the person, and it is the therapist's responsibility to be constantly reassessing the individual's performance and retention of the skill in order to determine when to transition the practice schedule. If you were working with a patient to achieve independent bed mobility including rolling, scooting, and bridging, patient learning may be most effective if you randomly mixed the sequence of practice. However, if your patient was becoming confused with all of the varied activities, you would likely back up and include more repeated practice of a single skill.

Key Points to Remember

- Blocked practice may result in better early skill acquisition.
- Random practice is better than blocked practice in promoting learning.
- Random practice will improve transfer of tasks to novel conditions.

Type of Practice

Beyond the practice schedule and order, the type of practice should also be considered when thinking about the learning movement.

There are 3 major types of practice that must be considered in planning a motor learning session (Table 6-5):

1. Whole versus part practice
2. Discovery versus guided practice
3. Mental practice

Whole Versus Part Practice

When instructing a patient, we must consider whether to break the task down into its component parts and teach the patient to master each component prior to performing the whole task or whether it is better to practice the whole task. To break the task down into the steps or parts required to perform the task, we need to perform a task analysis. During this analysis, we identify each separate task and then the sequence of the tasks required to achieve the end result.

Critical Thinking Clinical Scenario

Task analysis: A patient is learning to transfer from a wheelchair to the mat table. Once the wheelchair is positioned at the edge of the mat table, consider all the steps and the sequence of steps required for the patient to successfully and safely move from the wheelchair to the mat table.

Reflective Questions

1. List each individual step required to complete the above skill.
2. Next, chunk or group the steps in stages that would make sense to practice as a group.

Is it better to practice each part before the whole in order to best learn the skill? Research has demonstrated that it depends on what type of task is being learned. In general, serial tasks may benefit from a task analysis and practice of component parts, whereas discrete tasks may be best practiced as a whole (even though parts may be emphasized while practicing the whole). Part-to-whole practice is beneficial if a skill is readily broken down into recognizable steps. For example, if a patient was learning how to come from supine to sitting independently,

Table 6-5. Practice Types

Practice Type	
Whole versus part	*Whole* Whole practice occurs when the task is practiced as a whole rather than practicing each component separately. *Part* Part practice occurs when a task is broken down into its component parts and the patient practices each or selected components prior to performing the whole task.
Discovery versus guided practice	*Discovery* Discovery practice uses trial and error. The patient is encouraged to try various strategies until he or she discovers one that is effective in achieving the end result. *Guided Practice* Guided practice occurs when the patient is physically guided through the task as part of the learning process.
Mental practice	Mental practice is a method by which the patient performs the task through visualization and imagination rather than physical practice.

it would be beneficial to break down the task into its smaller pieces and have the patient work on each piece. It is important, however, to put the pieces or parts back into the whole.

There is no evidence that practice of part of a quick, discrete task helps the performance and learning of the task. Generally, slow, serial tasks of long duration may benefit from part-to-whole practice. For example, if you were teaching a spouse to manage a totally dependent hoyer lift transfer of her husband from the chair to the bed, practicing parts of the activity may assist her in learning the whole task. She may want to perform the skills necessary to manage the lift as well as the placement of the sling under her husband prior to performing the entire sequence needed for a safe transfer.

It remains critical for the practice to closely resemble the inherent task. Winstein et al[31] and Seitz and Wilson,[32] working with different patient populations found little carryover to gait when working on isolated skills, such as weightshifting in standing or dorsiflexion in sitting. Brydges et al,[33] in studying complex surgical tasks, found that whole practice was always essential to optimal performance even when practicing discrete skills.

Key Points to Remember

- Discrete tasks may be best practiced as a whole.
- Serial tasks may benefit from a task analysis and practice of component parts.
- Part-to-whole practice is beneficial if a skill is readily broken down into recognizable steps.
- Slow, serial tasks of long duration may benefit from part-to-whole practice.
- Practice must closely resemble the inherent task.

Discovery Versus Guided Practice

Physical therapists are generally skilled at physically guiding our patients when they are learning or relearning a new motor skill. We have been trained at effective placement of our hands and appropriate input to achieve the desired movement. This is considered *guided learning*. The patient is physically guided through the task as part of the learning process. *Discovery learning*, on the other hand, involves trial-and-error processes. The patient is encouraged to try various strategies until he or she discovers one that is effective in achieving the end result. For example, the therapist may ask a patient with recent hemiplegia to see whether he or she can figure out how to go from supine to sitting on the edge of the bed. The patient tries a number of different strategies before discovering a method that allows him or her to sit up independently.

Which one is better? Again the answer is *it depends*. As you might have guessed, guided practice improves early performance and assists the individual in understanding the task demands.[19] Over time, however, practice under unguided conditions is critical to later retention and transfer of the skill. It is important for therapists as quickly as possible to encourage unguided practice to promote learning of the new skill.

If the patient learns to rely on guidance to complete the task, the input will end up impeding the learning of the skill. In fact, too much guidance even early on in the task may interfere with learning.[34] The individual receiving the guidance may be working too hard to remember and apply the rules, and the cognitive demands associated with that process can interfere with actually learning the task. In fact, trying to remember may interfere with trying to learn.[35] There is also research to support the principle that guidance works better for tasks that are slow rather than fast or ballistic.[11]

Key Points to Remember

- Guided practice improves early performance and assists the individual in understanding the task demands.
- Too much guidance even early in the task may interfere with learning.
- Discovery practice is critical to later retention and transfer of the skill.
- It is important for therapists to encourage unguided practice as quickly as feasible to promote retention and transfer of the new skill.

Stop and Reflect

Which of the following activities would you be most likely to use guided control to facilitate an athlete's learning/performance? Why?

- Stance position prior to serving a tennis ball
- A golf swing

Mental Practice

As therapists, we often overlook the benefits of mental practice in learning a new skill, a method used often and with much success in the training of athletes in sporting events. *Mental practice* is the method by which the individual performs the task through visualizing and imagining rather than overt physical practice. Combining both physical and mental rehearsal has been demonstrated to be productive in improving performance and learning of new motor skills. It increases the speed of learning the new task as well as the accuracy and efficiency of the task.[36] Mental practice has even been demonstrated to improve isometric muscle strength when used in conjunction with physical practice.[37]

Research suggests that mental practice is a powerful and underutilized tool. Mahmoudi and Erfanian[38] found that subjects using mental practice via motor imagery modified neuronal activity in the primary sensorimotor areas of the brain and, subsequently, the connections controlling the desired movement in the motor cortex. Electroencephalogram patterns demonstrate more efficient and accurate patterns following mental imagery of the desired movement. In subsequent work, subjects using mental imagery demonstrated changes in muscle strength and power as well as the brain waves associated with muscle activation, even without physical practice.[39] Most of the research using mental practice has been conducted with individuals without a neurological injury, but recently 10 patients with chronic stroke used mental practice in conjunction with other interventions.[40] In this group of subjects, cognitive rehearsal of activities of daily living resulted in significantly improved reaching ability with the hemiparetic arm.

Key Points to Remember

Combining both physical and mental rehearsal can:
- Improve performance and learning of new motor skills.
- Increase the speed of learning of a new task as well as the accuracy and efficiency of that task.

The Role of Feedback in Motor Learning

When an individual is learning a new task, feedback is important to develop the cognitive map of the skill and a sense of what a correct performance looks and feels like. Appropriate feedback is critical to this process. There are, however, different types of feedback, and therapists should be careful to select the appropriate feedback at the right time to enhance both performance and learning.

Types of Feedback

Intrinsic Feedback

Intrinsic or inherent feedback is input received by the individual through various aspects of the sensory system as a result of the movement itself. For example, when a child reaches too far to one side and loses balance, he or she receives immediate intrinsic feedback that the center of gravity was too far outside of his or her base of support. When someone is using discovery learning with a lot of trial and error, that person is relying on intrinsic feedback to learn the task. We continually receive intrinsic feedback from our visual, auditory, tactile, vestibular, proprioceptive, and kinesthetic senses (Table 6-6).

Stop and Reflect

Think back to a time when you were first learning a new movement task (eg, transferring a patient from a wheelchair to a bed, taking a blood pressure, performing a specific manual muscle test, etc).
- What type of feedback did you receive?
- When did you receive the feedback?
- What was helpful about the feedback and what was not?

Extrinsic Feedback

Extrinsic feedback is feedback provided in addition to the intrinsic feedback and is provided by an external source. This is also referred to as *augmented feedback* because it augments the internal sensory cues the individual receives as a result of performing the movements. When we tell the patient how he or she is doing on his or her stair-climbing task with the crutches, we are providing verbal feedback. Verbal feedback is one form of extrinsic feedback. Extrinsic feedback results in either knowledge of performance or knowledge of results:

- *Knowledge of performance* (KP): Knowledge of performance is extrinsic feedback regarding some aspect of the motor performance. For example, if the therapist says, "You are dragging your toes when you bring your right leg forward," the patient is receiving input regarding the performance of the swing phase of gait.

Table 6-6. Types of Feedback

Intrinsic Feedback	Extrinsic or Augmented Feedback	
Feedback about the movement and movement result that is inherent to the task itself. It does not rely on an external source.	Feedback from an external source	
	Knowledge of performance: Feedback about some aspect of the performance of the movement.	Knowledge of results: Feedback regarding the outcome of the movement in relationship to the goal of the movement.
Example: Your patient stubs his toe because he failed to adequately clear an obstacle in his path. The sensation provided by the toe impact is intrinsic feedback regarding the movement and movement outcome.	Example: You tell your patient, "You are putting the cane too far in front of you when you bring it forward."	Example: You tell your patient, "You have increased your strength in the muscle that straightens your knee by one muscle grade in the past week."

- *Knowledge of results* (KR): Knowledge of results is augmented feedback regarding the outcome of the movement in relationship to the goal of the movement. If the therapist says, "You gained 15 degrees of active knee extension today," the patient becomes aware of the results of all the stretching and active movement efforts he or she has expended during that session.

Intrinsic feedback is critical to error detection and learning or relearning motor movements. When a patient's intrinsic systems are injured or altered in some way, (eg, inadequate body schema awareness or an impaired visual system) learning can be severely hampered.[41]

Extrinsic or augmented feedback may also be important when learning a new motor task. For example, the learner may be able to correct errors based on the feedback provided and potentially improve a performance parameter such as accuracy, speed, or direction. Augmented feedback can also be important to reinforce a movement that has been performed correctly (eg, "That is exactly right—do it again!"). Augmented feedback and especially KR are helpful in motivating the patient. In the example of the patient being told that he or she gained 15 degrees of knee motion, that knowledge may prompt the patient to continue to put forth the required effort to make further gains.

Most therapists use feedback about the movement patterns (KP) themselves in addition to the movement outcomes (KR) to teach patients new movements. KP has been demonstrated to be successful in learning closed skills (eg, discrete tasks repeated in predictable environments, such as learning to sit up in bed), and a combination of KP and KR are best for teaching open skills such as propelling a wheelchair across a crowded room.[9] The feedback, however, should always be accurate in order to allow for appropriate correction.

Key Points to Remember

Feedback can be either intrinsic (ie, inherent) or extrinsic (ie, augmented).

- Intrinsic or inherent feedback is input received by the individual through the sensory system as a result of the movement itself.
- Extrinsic feedback is provided by an external source and is in addition to intrinsic feedback.

Feedback can result in either knowledge of performance (KP) or knowledge of results (KR).

- KP is extrinsic feedback provided on some aspect of the motor performance.
- KR is extrinsic feedback regarding the outcome of movement in relation to the intended goal of the movement.

Intrinsic feedback is critical for error detection and learning or relearning motor movements. Extrinsic feedback and especially KR are useful for motivating patients and reinforcing movements. KP has been demonstrated to be successful in learning closed skills. A combination of KP and KR is best for teaching open skills.

Timing and Frequency of Feedback

Providing augmented feedback is often helpful in assisting the patient to improve performance. The participant is better able to learn the required parameters of the movement and how he or she is performing in comparison to those parameters. But is continuous feedback a helpful strategy in physical therapy? Feedback is important, but we need to seriously consider the schedule of feedback during the progression of learning a new motor skill or task.

Too much extrinsic or augmented feedback too early in the process can overwhelm the patient.[42,43] It appears to provide excess information that patients rely on too heavily.[11] Typically, it is better to give initial instructions and then allow the person to use trial and error for several uninterrupted attempts. Following those trials, the learner is in a better position to make use of the feedback to improve performance. Picture a child learning to ride a bicycle for the first time—some general instructions for sitting on the seat, steering, and pedaling fast enough to stay upright is probably helpful. Too much detail about speed, posture, braking strategies, and turning radii would interfere with the child's ability to learn how to ride the bicycle in the initial stages of learning. More refinement can be added after the child has made several attempts. Using more KR versus KP is also generally best in improving performance and learning.[11]

Augmented feedback provided too frequently or continuously is also detrimental to learning the skill. Wulf and Schmidt[44] demonstrated that frequent feedback made the learner dependent on the external input with subsequent neglect of internal feedback. The learner does not create his or her own error detection system if he or she is relying on an external party to continuously provide feedback. In fact, too much augmented feedback may block the individual from using inherent or intrinsic feedback to correct or learn a movement task. At some point in time, the individual needs to rely on strategies learned in order to perform the task independently and apply the task in new contexts. Winstein and Schmidt[45] described this as a *fading schedule*; the amount of feedback given should decrease over the practice period. This may require the therapist to summarize or average the feedback over a succession of trials in order to enhance learning.[46,47] As the learner becomes more proficient and independent, the time between feedback sessions should progressively lengthen.

Key Points to Remember

- Too much extrinsic or augmented feedback too early in the process can overwhelm the patient.

- If you are teaching a patient a new movement skill, it is typically better to give initial instructions then allow the person to use trial-and-error for several uninterrupted attempts.

- Augmented feedback provided too frequently may make the learner dependent on the external input with subsequent neglect of internal feedback.

- The amount of feedback provided should decrease over the practice period (fading schedule).

- As feedback is decreased it is helpful to periodically summarize how the patient is performing to enhance learning.

Critical Thinking Clinical Scenario

A patient with chronic back pain is learning to maintain the appropriate alignment of the lumbar spine during all functional activities in order to minimize the risk for increased injury and more pain. The therapist is having the patient practice the position by initially providing the visual feedback of a mirror, knowledge of performance ("You need to tighten your abdominals a little more"), and knowledge of results ("You held the appropriate posture about half the time during that exercise").

Reflective Questions

1. If the therapist sees the patient 3 times per week, how might the KP and KR be gradually reduced so that the individual learns the posture and can maintain it when the therapist is not there to remind him or her?

Lifespan Differences

Motor aptitude increases in most areas for at least the first 18 years of life. In general, older children outperform younger children on most motor performance indices. It may be that younger children must also develop their capacity for processing information; they need to develop the capacity to attend, form memory, and develop the cognitive map associated with learning. Teaching a young child a motor skill often requires a different approach than teaching an adult a similar skill. Similarly, as we age, we undergo changes in cognitive and motor capacities that require some adaptations in the therapist's teaching approach. We will review some

major differences you may need to consider, though it is important to remember that each individual is unique and that it will always be up to you to determine the best way to adapt to his or her unique needs.

Younger-Aged Children

There are several important adaptations we should consider when working with younger-aged children learning new motor tasks. Motivation is a prepractice condition for all learners regardless of age, though the strategies to promote motivation are individual and may vary depending on age. Even younger children participate more readily in activities and movements they preselect versus movements that were prescribed by the instructor.[11] Up to the age of about 11 years, children do best if they are given self-referenced goals and tasks rather than goals and tasks based on social comparisons.[48] Goals should be specific for both the activity and the performance. For example, the therapist may need to say, "Let's go for a walk to the gym," suggesting the activity. Subsequently, the therapist may say, "Let's see how far you can go before you stop." Valvano[49] found that children with neurological conditions responded well to activity-related goals that were developed in collaboration with the child and the family.

Given the short attention characteristic of most young children, goals are often of short duration, and children may need reminders and reinforcement several times during a session. This is counter to the previous findings regarding the need to decrease KR and KP to enhance learning in adults and may need to be adjusted when working with a young child. The use of creative play is critical to sustain the child's motivation and engagement.

Instructions need to be adapted to the child's capability. Although children with the ability to understand language benefit from explicit verbal instruction, the directions should be short and emphasize only one or 2 key elements (eg, "Jump up as high as you can"). Generally, using visual models for instruction is an effective strategy because children rely more on visual input than adults, who tend to use a combination of visual and proprioceptive input.[4,50]

A session with a young child should include a lot of visual modeling and demonstration. Although ongoing verbal interaction with a child is critical to sustain a child's interest, it is important not to overwhelm a child with instructions. Niemeijer et al[51] found that therapists routinely gave children too many instructions and those instructions were not necessarily related to the child's performance.

Children respond to augmented feedback in similar ways as adults, which may improve performance but can have a negative impact on learning if not faded appropriately. As with instructions, verbal feedback should be provided in short and concise ways (KP: "Look at how nice and tall you are standing" or KR: "You got into your chair all by yourself today"). Encouraging the child to guess the performance outcome before giving feedback also appears to help the child focus on the necessary intrinsic feedback to develop a cognitive map (eg, "How far do you think you can throw the ball?").[9] Recent research suggests that children respond well when prompted to pay attention to internal signals and feedback while performing a motor skill.[52] So the therapist could ask the child to "feel the difference" when placed in a new position or perhaps to visually attend the limb while learning a new task.

Key Points to Remember

In teaching motor tasks to children, consider the following:

- Develop goals of short duration as a short attention span is characteristic of most young children.

- Use reminders and reinforcement frequently throughout a session (ie, you may need to adjust your feedback and not decrease the KR and KP in the same way that you would to enhance learning in adults).

- Use creative play to sustain the child's motivation and engagement.

- Use visual modeling and demonstration.

- Modify your instructions based on the child's capabilities.

- Prompt the child to attend to internal signals and feedback when performing a motor skill.

Older Adults

Motor skills also may change as we age. For example, speed and reaction times may slow down. Research on changes associated with aging has tended to focus on skills that decline with age.[11] Most people have a tendency to be more cautious and less willing to make errors as they get older.[53] This tendency can have a negative impact on the person's willingness to practice tasks that are perceived as too difficult. Older individuals,

much more than younger people, respond to negative feedback with a decline in accuracy and a decreased willingness to attempt the task.[54] Additionally, older adults are more likely than children to effectively use extrinsic rather than intrinsic feedback while learning new skills.[52] Although the comparison study contrasted feedback preferences between children and younger adults, the comparison may be even more valid for older adults with age-related changes in kinesthetic and other sensorimotor systems.

It is possible that breaking down a task into manageable components that can be successfully mastered may be especially important when working with older patients. Additionally, even healthy aging individuals have increased difficulty with motor planning and motor sequencing.[55,56] Healthy older adults demonstrated more difficulty learning multidimensional sequences of movement than middle-aged adults or younger children.[55] Most movement series have a timing component (eg, temporal requirement) and distance component (eg, spatial requirement), in addition to the motor component (eg, force requirement). The researchers found that healthy older individuals struggled to learn motor sequences when the sequences varied in all 3 dimensions. Older individuals tended to treat each element of the sequence as independent and isolated. The therapist working with older adults needs to be aware of this and embed extra practice opportunities for the acquisition of new skills. There is evidence that aging adults do have cognitive plasticity or the ability to improve as a result of practice and that improvement can even be generalized to new tasks.[57,58] Much research is still needed in this area.

Key Points to Remember

In teaching motor tasks to older adults, consider the following:

- Use positive feedback and avoid negative feedback.

- Make sure to select tasks not perceived as too hard so that the person is not afraid to try; build in success.

- Provide external cues to guide the practice sessions.

- Avoid too much variety in the practice schedule in too many simultaneous dimensions.

- Embed lots of practice into the person's daily schedule to encourage overlearning.

Critical Thinking Clinical Scenario

You are working in a sports therapy clinic that specializes in treating elite tennis players. One of the young athletes has suffered chronic pain and injury to his shoulder and elbow due to faulty mechanics while serving. In conjunction with the coach, you are working with this athlete to alter his patterns of movement during the serve in order to protect his musculoskeletal system from long-term injury and disability. The athlete is experiencing a lot of frustration with the new way of serving because he had been using the dysfunctional pattern for a number of years and is having a hard time learning a new method. Knowing that you are a motor control and learning specialist, the coach asks you for your guidance in setting up a training schedule that will maximize the motor learning for his protégé.

Reflective Questions

1. Set up a training and feedback schedule for a total of 3 weeks (specific for the serve, rather than other physical conditioning needs). Keep in mind and make decisions about the following principles/contexts:

   o What type of motor skill is a tennis serve (eg, discrete, serial, continuous)?

   o What are some prepractice conditions that may be important here?

   o Should you use a guided approach versus trial and error?

   o What type of practice would you use first: whole or part?

   o What type and schedule of augmented feedback would you recommend?

   o What type of schedule (eg, massed versus distributed practice? Constant versus variable? Block or random? A combination of these?) would you recommend?

   o What type of practice environment should this athlete practice in initially (open versus closed; be specific)?

   o What type of feedback would the athlete have that is intrinsic to the practice?

   o What type of extrinsic feedback would you provide and what type of fading schedule would you suggest?

   o How would your recommendations change as this young athlete progresses toward his goal? (Consider the stages of learning.)

Summary

Therapists are educators of skilled movement. This role requires them to not only understand the underlying processes of motor control and learning but to apply those processes in interactions with individual patients. Although the field of study is complex and expanding constantly, there are principles and concepts that we can effectively apply to teaching our patients how to learn or relearn motor skills they need in order to participate in all activities of living.

Key Points to Remember

Teaching a movement skill requires the therapist to think about how the task, environment, and patient's attributes interact to accomplish a goal.

Stages of motor learning

- There are several stages of learning a new skill, and each requires a different teaching/learning strategy:
  o Cognitive
  o Associative
  o Autonomous

Movement types

- Movements can be classified in several ways, and the desired movement type influences the teaching strategies:
  o Open versus closed
  o Discrete versus continuous
- Potential interferences and response alternatives will influence the planning and progressing of the teaching-learning session
- Sessions should focus on providing patients/clients with a lot of information about the desired end point when they are learning a new task

Practice types and practice schedules

- Goal setting, modeling, and perceptual pretraining are considered prepractice conditions that enhance motor learning
- The absolute amount of practice is the most important variable when considering practice schedules
- Massed practice leads to better performance in the short term; distributed practice leads to better learning
- Random practice is also important to learning and retention; block practice may be better during early learning of a task
- Part-to-whole practice may be useful in learning serial tasks; however, practice should always include whole practice even when part-to-whole practice strategies are included
- Trial-and-error practice enhances motor learning, although guided practice is useful during slow movements and early performance
- Mental rehearsal may improve both performance and learning of new skills

Feedback

- Intrinsic or inherent feedback is essential to detect errors and learn movements.
- Extrinsic or augmented feedback can facilitate learning, especially in the early phases of the learning process.
- Knowledge of results is generally more effective for learning, although knowledge of performance can enhance particular performance parameters
- Feedback needs to be faded over time to optimize learning and minimize feedback dependency

References

1. Brooks VB. *The Neural Basis of Motor Control*. New York, NY: Oxford University Press; 1986.
2. Bradley NS, WestCott SL. Motor control: developmental aspects of motor control in skill acquisition. In: Campbell SK, Vander Linden DW, Palisano RJ, eds. *Physical Therapy for Children*. 3rd ed. St. Louis, MO: Saunders; 2006:77-130.
3. Bernshtein N. *The Co-ordination and Regulation of Movements*. Oxford, NY: Pergamon Press; 1976.
4. Shumway-Cook A, Woollacott MH. *Motor Control: Theory and Practical Applications*. 3rd ed. Philadelphia, PA: Lippincott; 2006.
5. Mastos M, Miller K, Eliasson AC, Imms C. Goal-directed training: linking theories of treatment to clinical practice for improved functional activities in daily life. *Clin Rehabil*. 2007;21:47-55.
6. Ferguson JM, Trombly CA. The effect of added-purpose and meaningful occupation on motor learning. *Am J Occup Ther*. 1997;51:508-515.
7. Fitts P, Posner M. *Human Performance*. Belmont, CA: Brooks/Cole; 1967.
8. Luua P, Tucker DM, Stripling R. Neural mechanisms for learning actions in context. *Brain Res*. 2007;1179:89-105.
9. Gentile A. Skill acquisition: action movement, and neuromotor processes. In: Carr J, Shephard R, Gordon J, eds. *Movement Science: Foundations for Physical Therapy in Rehabilitation*. Rockville, MD: Aspen; 1987.
10. Campbell SK, Palisano RJ, Vander Linden DW. *Physical Therapy for Children*. 3rd ed. Philadelphia, PA: WB Saunders; 2006.
11. Schmidt RA, Lee TD. *Motor Control and Learning: A Behavioral Emphasis*. Champaign, IL: Human Kinetics; 2005.
12. Hick WE. On the rate of gain of information. *Q J Exp Psychol*. 1952;4:11-26.
13. Simon JR. The effects of an irrelevant directional cue on human information processing. In: Proctor RW, Reeve TG, eds. *Stimulus-Response Compatibility: An Integrated Perspective*. Amsterdam: Elsevier; 1990:31-86.
14. Rosenbaum DA. *Human Motor Control*. San Diego, CA: Academic Press; 1991.
15. Merriam Webster OnLine. Practice. Available at http://www.merriam-webster.com/dictionary/practice. Accessed August 20, 2009.
16. Puttemans V, Wenderoth N, Swinnen S. Changes in brain activation during the acquisition of a multifrequency bimanual coordination task: from the cognitive stage to advanced levels of automiticity. *J Neurosci*. 2005;25:4270-4278.
17. Leipert J, Bauder H, Wolfgang HR, Miltner WH, Taub E, Weiller C. Treatment-induced cortical reorganization after stroke in humans. *Stroke*. 2000;31:1210.
18. Kyllo LB, Landers DM. Goal setting in sport and exercise: a research synthesis to resolve the controversy. *J Sport Exerc Psychol*. 1995;17:117-137.
19. Anderson DI, Magill RA, Sekiya H, Ryan G. Support for an explanation of the guidance effect in motor skill learning. *J Mot Behav*. 2005;37:231-238.
20. O'Sullivan SB. Strategies to improve motor function. In: O'Sullivan SB, Schmitz TJ, eds. *Physical Rehabilitation*. 5th ed. Philadelphia, PA: F.A. Davis Company; 2007:472-522.
21. Wulf G, Shea CH. Principles derived from the study of simple skills do not generalize to complex skill learning. *Psychon B Rev*. 2002;9:185-211.
22. Baddely AD, Longman DJA. The influence of length and frequency of training session on the rate of learning to type. *Ergonomics*. 1978;21:627-635.
23. Mackay S, Morgan P, Datta V, Chang A, Darz A. Practice distribution in procedural skills training. *Surg Endosc*. 2002;16:957-961.
24. Catalano JF, Kleiner BM. Distant transfer and practice variability. *Percept Mot Skills*. 1984;58:851-856.
25. Enebo B, Sherwood D. Experience and practice organization in learning a simulated high-velocity low-amplitude task. *J Manipulative Physiol Ther*. 2005;28:33-43.
26. Herbert WJ, Heiss DG, Basso DM. Influence of feedback schedule in motor performance and learning of a lumbar multifidus muscle task using rehabilitative ultrasound imaging: A randomized clinical trial. *Phys Ther*. 2008;88:261-269.
27. Goode MK, Geraci L, Roediger HL III. Superiority of variable to repeated practice in transfer on anagram solution. *Psychon Bull Rev*. 2008;15:662-666.
28. Jarus T, Wughalter EH, Gianutsos JG. Effects of contextual interference and conditions of movement task on acquisition, retention, and transfer or motor skills by women. *Percept Mot Skills*. 1997;84:179-193.
29. Abrams ML, Grice JK. Effects of practice and positional variables in acquisition of a complex psychomotor skill. *Percept Mot Skills*. 1976;43:203-211.
30. Memmert D. Long-term effects of type of practice on the learning and transfer of a complex motor skill. *Percept Mot Skills*. 2006;103:912-916.
31. Winstein CJ, Gardner ER, McNeal DR, Barto PT, Nicholson DE. Standing balance training: effect on balance and locomotion in hemiparetic adults. *Arch Phys Med Rehabil*. 1989;70:755-762.
32. Seitz RH, Wilson CI. Effect of gait on motor task learning acquired in a sitting position. *Phys Ther*. 1987;67:1089-1094.
33. Brydges R, Carnahan H, Backstein D, Dubrowski A. Application of motor learning principles to complex surgical tasks: searching for the optimal practice schedule. *J Mot Behav*. 2007;39:40-48.
34. Green TD, Flowers JH. Comparison of implicit and explicit learning processes in a probabilisitic task. *Percept Mot Skills*. 2003;97:299-314.
35. Huijbers W, Pennartz CM, Cabez R, Baselaar SM. When learning and remembering compete: a functional MRI study. *PLoS Biol*. 2009;7.
36. Maring JR. Effects of mental practice on rate of skill acquisition. *Phys Ther*. 1990;70:165-172.
37. Yue G, Cole KJ. Strength increases from the motor program: comparison of training with maximal voluntary and imagined muscle contractions. *J Neurophysiol*. 1992;67:1114-1123.
38. Mahmoudi B, Erfanian A. Electro-encephalogram based brain-computer interface: improved performance by mental practice and concentration skills. *Med Biol Eng Comput*. 2006;44:959-969.
39. Fontani G, Migliorini S, Benocci R, Facchini A, Casini M, Corradesschi F. Effect of mental imagery on the development of skilled motor actions. *Percept Mot Skills*. 2007;105:803-826.
40. Page SJ, Levine P, Khoury JC. Modified constraint-induced therapy combined with mental practice: thinking through better outcomes. *Stroke*. 2009;40:551-554.
41. Peterka RJ, Loughlin PJ. Dynamic regulation of sensorimotor integration in human postural control. *J Neurophysiol*. 2004;91:410-423.
42. Boyd L, Winstein CJ. Providing explicit information disrupts implicit motor learning after basal ganglia stroke. *Learn Mem*. 2004;11:388-396.
43. Boyd L, Winstein CJ. Explicit information interferes with implicit motor learning of both continuous and discrete motor tasks after stroke. *J Neurol Phys Ther*. 2006;30:46-57.
44. Wulf G, Schmidt RA. Feedback-induced variability and the learning of generalized motor programs. *J Mot Behav*. 1994;26:348-361.
45. Winstein CJ, Schmidt RA. Reduced frequency of knowledge of results enhances motor skill learning. *J Exp Psychol Learn Mem Cogn*. 1990;16:677-691.

46. Yao WX. Average-KR schedule benefits generalized motor program learning. *Percept Mot Skills.* 2003;97:185-191.

47. Ishikura T. Average KR schedule in learning of timing: influence of length for summary knowledge of results and task complexity. *Percept Mot Skills.* 2005;101:911-924.

48. Garcia C. Gender differences in young children's interactions when learning fundamental motor skills. *Res Q Exerc Sport.* 1994;65:213-225.

49. Valvano J. Activity-focused interventions for children with neurological conditions. *Phys Occup Ther Pediatr.* 2004;24:79-107.

50. Sullivan KJ, Kantak SS, Burtner PA. Motor learning in children: feedback effects on skill acquisition. *Phys Ther.* 2008;88:720-732.

51. Niemeijer AS, Smits-Englesman BC, Reynders K, Shoemaker MM. Verbal actions of physiotherapists to enhance motor learning in children with DCD. *Hum Mov Sci.* 2003;22:567-581.

52. Emanuel M, Jarus T, Bart O. Effect of focus of attention and age on motor acquisition, retention, and transfer: a randomized trial. *Phys Ther.* 2008;88:251-260.

53. Welford AT. Between bodily changes and performance: some possible reasons for slowing with age. *Exp Aging Res.* 1984;10:73-88.

54. Wild-Wall N, Willemssen R, Falkenstein M. Feed-back related processes during a time-production task in young and older adults. *Clin Neurophysiol.* 2008;120:407-413.

55. Boyd LA, Vidoni ED, Siengsukon CE. Multidimensional motor sequence learning is impaired in older but not younger or middle-aged adults. *Phys Ther.* 2008;88:351-362.

56. Shea CH, Park JH, Braden HW. Age-related effects in sequential motor learning. *Phys Ther.* 2006;84:478-488.

57. Bherer L, Kramer AF, Peterson MS, Colcombe S, Erickson K, Becic E. Transfer effects in task-set cost and dual-task training in older and younger adults: further evidence for cognitive plasticity in attentional control in late adulthood. *Exp Aging Res.* 2008;34:188-219.

58. Smith CD, Walton A, Loveland AD, Umberger GH, Kryscio RJ, Gash DM. Memories that last in old age: motor skill learning and memory preservation. *Neurobiol Aging.* 2005;26:883-890.

SECTION III
FROM CLASSROOM TO CLINIC AND BEYOND

Communities of Practice
Learning and Professional Identity
Development in the Clinical Setting

Chapter Objectives

After reading this chapter, you will be prepared to:

- Differentiate between learning in the classroom and learning in the clinical setting.

- Recognize the complexity of teaching and learning in the clinical setting.

- Relate the concepts of apprenticeship learning and communities of practice to learning in physical therapy practice.

- Recognize the challenges students face while learning in the clinical setting.

- Differentiate between personal meaning making and shared meaning making.

- Appreciate the importance of dialogue in the negotiation of shared meaning.

- Apply the concepts of communities of practice to designing effective teaching and learning experiences in the clinical setting.

Stop and Reflect

- In what ways does learning in the clinic differ from learning in the classroom?

- In what ways does teaching in the clinic differ from teaching in the classroom?

As we know from previous chapters, teaching and learning in the classroom is much more complex than simply lecturing to an audience and hoping that they will absorb the content. Similarly, teaching and learning in the clinic is much more complex than simply matching a student and clinical instructor and having them work together with patients. Teaching and learning in the clinic are so complex because there is an expectation that the learner will develop a unique professional identity, which is much more than just accumulating knowledge and skills, assimilating core values, or even simply applying their knowledge and skills to patient care. In this chapter, we provide you with a framework to help you recognize the complexity of the clinical teaching environment so you can design effective teaching and learning situations within the clinical setting.

The development of professional behaviors and the affective domain become even more critical as students begin to interact with patients and other professionals. Professional behaviors, including communication and interpersonal skills, are emphasized because these are often the most challenging to teach and the most challenging to learn. The concepts we present can be generalized to all aspects of learning (psychomotor and cognitive) in the clinical environment. Much of the information in this chapter is a synthesis of research and personal interviews with more than 50 students and clinicians, as well as written critical incidents from close to 350 additional students.[1,2] Throughout the chapter, you will see direct quotes from students and clinicians that illustrate and reinforce the concepts being discussed. The quotes provide insight into the perspectives of both students and clinicians, and illustrate how they developed their own professional identity, which is integral to becoming a competent health care professional.

Plack M, Driscoll M. *Teaching and Learning in Physical Therapy: From Classroom to Clinic* (pp 159-176).
© 2011 SLACK Incorporated

Stop and Reflect

In 1999, Hayes et al[3] completed a study entitled "Behaviors that cause clinical instructors to question the clinical competence of physical therapist students." Issues related to which of the following domains of learning do you think most often caused clinical instructors to initially question the safety, efficacy, and overall abilities of student physical therapists?

- Psychomotor skills
- Cognitive skills
- Affective skills

Professionalism in Health Care

Though we know that it is critical for professionals to develop a level of expertise in their cognitive and psychomotor skills, we also know that this is not enough. If you think back to Chapter 4 on developing presentations, you will remember that learning occurs in 3 domains (cognitive, psychomotor, and affective). You will also remember that Dettmer[4] advocates the addition of a fourth domain, the social domain. To develop high-quality, competent, caring practitioners who have assimilated the core values of the profession, we need to facilitate development in all domains of learning.

In the "Stop and Reflect" above, if you selected "affective behaviors," you would be correct. It is truly our affective behaviors and social skills that enable us to interact effectively with patients.[5] In any health care profession, the patient must be at the heart of all that we do. Without developing the values, attitudes, and beliefs that enable us to communicate and interact professionally and effectively with our patients, clients, and other health care providers, our own professional competence may be called into question. This is particularly true when we are interacting with lay people, who may have limited knowledge of health care in general, specifically physical therapy.[3,6-8]

Stop and Reflect

Patients place a great deal of trust in their health care providers and often assume that they are prepared to practice because they hold a license.[7]

1. What are your thoughts on the statement above?

2. How do patients with limited knowledge of health care judge whether their providers are good or not?

3. Have you ever worked with a health care provider who had a poor bedside manner? What did that make you think about that person's overall competence and skill? Did it make you feel confident in your choice of providers? If you had a choice, would you return to that provider for follow-up care?

Beliefs, attitudes, values, norms, and standards are the noncognitive behaviors that comprise the affective domain. In the eyes of some patients, these skills may be even more important than some of the more technical skills because they often assume that because you have a license you must be a competent practitioner. How do they really judge whether you are good or not? They may very well make this judgment based solely on how you interact with them (ie, on your bedside manner).[7] We live in a society of consumerism, and patients are now much savvier and more consumer-oriented than individuals from previous generations. They know that there are plenty of very smart and very skilled clinicians available, so why would they work with someone who does not appear to respect or value them as individuals? Very often, it is the behaviors in the affective or social domains—your interpersonal skills—that will set you apart from other clinicians and place you "a notch above." Professional practice is not complete without the ability to demonstrate the attitudes, values, and beliefs established by our profession.

The *Code of Ethics*, the *Standards of Practice*, and the *Core Values*[9,10] of the physical therapy profession provide us with a set of expectations of professional abilities and behaviors. For some of us, these behaviors come easily; they are intuitive. Altruism, care and compassion, accountability, and social responsibility are values that perhaps we grew up with and simply take for granted. For others, these behaviors are not so simple and straightforward; they do not come so naturally. In fact, research has shown that these behaviors, though critical, have been problematic not only in physical therapy but throughout the medical community.[11-17] It has also been shown that problems with these behaviors raise "red flags" for clinical instructors. When a clinical instructor observes students having difficulty with professional behaviors, they often begin to question the safety and efficacy of their overall performance.[3,15]

Stop and Reflect

Pause for a minute and think about the 7 Core Values* of the physical therapy profession: accountability, altruism, care and compassion, excellence, integrity, professional duty, social responsibility

- What does each one of these values mean to you?
- How would you define each of these values?
- How might your definitions differ from someone from another generation? From another culture?
- How might you reconcile those differences?

*If you are not familiar with the Core Values of the physical therapy profession, they can be found on the American Physical Therapy Association Web site at http://www.apta.org.

Why has the development of professional behaviors been such a challenge in the health professions? Attitudes, values, and beliefs are abstract and complex concepts. They are more complex than what is written in the American Physical Therapy Association (APTA) *Code of Ethics, Standards of Practice*, or *Core Values* documents. These behaviors are not technical skills, so they cannot necessarily be taught or measured objectively. Addressing issues of unprofessional behaviors or poor interpersonal skills can also feel very personal and uncomfortable at times. Though we do have a set of standards and expectations in the profession, these standards are reinterpreted with subtle differences in each setting. For example, as a young physical therapist, I worked in 2 very different organizations. One organization was a well-known rehabilitation setting, and the other was a well-known pediatric school setting. Expectations in each facility were quite different; behaviors and activities acceptable in the less formal pediatric setting would likely not be acceptable in the other more formal rehabilitation setting. In addition, after reading Chapter 2, we recognize that these attitudes, beliefs, and values are quite interconnected with our own past histories, cultures, and generational experiences, making them ingrained and at times unconscious. Each clinical setting or community has its own history and culture, which adds to the expectations of professionalism.

Critical Thinking Clinical Scenarios

- A student routinely arrives late to clinic (ie, anywhere from 5 minutes before his first patient is to be seen to 10 minutes after the session has begun). He always has an excuse but never seems to have a strategy to improve his performance.

- A student was observed reviewing a chart on a patient that was not on his caseload. When asked, he commented that he had overheard another therapist speaking about this patient's illness and he was just curious and wanted to learn more. He did not recognize that his behavior violated the rules of confidentiality.

- A clinical instructor came to her student to tell her that she needs to see a patient immediately because the patient was scheduled for a procedure later in the afternoon. The student responded that she will come, but this is the only break she had so she needed to finish her lunch first.

Reflective Questions

1. What is going on in each of these situations? Consider the perspectives of the student, clinical instructor, and patient.

2. Limitations in which of the core values are demonstrated by each of the scenarios above?

3. To address these limitations, what goals might the clinical instructor develop for the student to make the expectations more explicit?

How are appropriate professional behaviors learned and how do we teach them? Very often, it is simply assumed that by the time you come to a professional program you should already have the attitudes, values, and beliefs needed to be a professional, or otherwise you will learn them when you get to the clinic.[3,11,18,19] As with any other skill, these abstract attitudes and behaviors must be practiced, and an openness and willingness to both provide and accept feedback is essential. We know, and research has shown, that academic faculty and clinical instructors hesitate to provide adequate feedback on affective behaviors because they often consider it too personal.[3,11,14,20] As instructors, whether in the classroom or the clinic, we often emphasize the cognitive and psychomotor domains of learning and minimize the importance of learning in the affective domain. This may be because cognitive and psychomotor domains can be evaluated more easily and more objectively, whereas the affective domain requires substantially more subjectivity in evaluation. If you think back to Chapter 2, this is exactly what Schön[21] referred to when he suggested that professional programs focus too much on "technical rationalism" almost to the exclusion of professional development. This is why it is so critical, as noted in Chapter 4, to develop the skill of creating objectives that incorporate all domains of learning.

Professional behaviors in the affective domain are not so easily defined, taught, or evaluated. We also know that although passing the licensing exam gives us a certain degree of credibility, it does not guarantee that we have acquired the professional behaviors needed to become a fully functioning and competent therapist.[22] We first learn about these behaviors in the abstract setting of the classroom, and then we apply and continually refine them in our day-to-day clinical experiences. John Dewey[23] suggested that just because we have had these experiences does not guarantee that we will learn from them. This is particularly true now in our rapidly changing, fast-paced, health care environments where students are expected to arrive in the clinic well prepared to work collaboratively, not be a burden on their clinical instructor, and perhaps even add to the productivity of the department. We typically expect that the students will "hit the ground running" as they enter the clinical setting.

Theoretical Perspectives on Learning in the Clinical Setting

As you will remember from previous chapters, learning is grounded in experience, and it is only through the application and interpretation of knowledge that education occurs.[23] Kolb believed that learning is a cyclic "process whereby concepts are derived from and continuously modified by experience."[24] In Chapter 1, we learned that the cycle of learning starts with our concrete experiences and moves through reflection and observation, abstract conceptualization, active experimentation, and finally back to concrete experiences. It is this cycle that helps us transform abstract academic theories into practical clinical application.[25] This is particularly relevant in physical therapy and the other health care professions because we not only need to develop the knowledge, skills, and behaviors essential for practice, but we must be able to apply them in the practice setting as well. Clinical internships and other clinical education experiences are what provide the real-life or contextual, social, and interactive experiences that help us translate some of the abstract theories learned in the classroom to actual clinical practice.

Stop and Reflect

- How did you learn what the appropriate personal space is when interacting with other people? How does it feel when someone stands too close to you when conversing?

- How did you learn how you were supposed to act in the classroom in first grade?

- How did you learn about your parents' value system regarding work, service, and education?

In thinking about the "Stop and Reflect" questions, you may have indicated that you learned through observation or by listening to and engaging in conversations with your parents and others. Some theorists suggest that our goals, values, and interests are developed tacitly; we learn them essentially through osmosis. Because professional behaviors are so complex, they cannot simply be taught through explicit instruction in an academic setting. These behaviors must be experienced and learned on the job, through demonstration, practice, and indirect instruction.[26] We know that theorists like Schön[21] and Mezirow[27] believe that through the use of the reflective process we can make what we have learned tacitly more explicit, and therefore more fully recognized and understood. Not only do students need to learn and assimilate the core values of the profession but they also must learn the sociocultural

expectations of each new setting.[28] Whereas Bandura[29] proposed that much of this acculturation process occurs through observation within the social context, Lave and Wenger[22] and Wenger[30] suggested that it takes much more than simple observation and imitation; rather, to make sense of the sociocultural expectations of each new clinical environment, active engagement in practice is critical.

This is a real paradigm shift in our thinking about how we learn. We now recognize that learning, particularly in the physical therapy practice, is not simply an accumulation of facts or the processing of information, but more importantly it is how we apply what we have learned in a given context.[22,30,31] Problem-based learning, patient simulations, and the use of cases to simulate real-world problems are examples of classroom strategies we use to create real-life situations from which we learn to problem-solve. In contrast, clinical practice requires us to actually function within a much more complex clinical environment. As authentic as we can try to make a classroom scenario, it is still quite different from what occurs in real-world situations. Often, in simulations, we are given the problem and asked to come up with a solution, but in real-world practice, we often do not even know what problem to address. In simulations, it is the instructor's responsibility to create the problem, and our role as students is simply to solve it. In real-world practice, we own the problem, the instructor does not. It is our patient who presents with a problem, and it is our responsibility to first define the problem and then develop the strategies we might use to address that problem within the context of the unique clinical scenario.

Stop and Reflect

- How does *learning about* physical therapy differ from *learning to become* a physical therapist?

- How does the phrase *learning to talk, not learning from talk*, relate to physical therapy education?

- What are the implications of these statements to teaching and learning in physical therapy practice?

Though the differences noted earlier are substantial, perhaps the most significant difference in learning in the clinical setting versus the classroom setting is that learning takes place in a community of practice. Learning is no longer solely focused on gaining knowledge and skills or problem solving; rather, of equal importance is how we function effectively within the community. When you are in the clinical setting, you are no longer learning *about* physical therapy; rather, you are learning to *become* a physical therapist.

If we think about physical therapy, we can see that it is inherently a social practice, and therefore learning is inherently a social process. Learning in physical therapy, or in any community of practice, is not simply the acquisition of skills and knowledge but rather the development of an identity and a sense of belonging within that community. Wenger[30] suggested that within a community, this process is both reciprocal and evolutionary—not only does the newcomer learn from those already in practice, but those in practice learn from the newcomer. Newcomers often add different perspectives that may actually result in changes within the community (ie, an evolution). Students learn from and add to the community as much as the community learns from and adds to the development of the student. For example, because students are required to frequently search through literature and utilize current evidence to support their work in the classroom, they bring these skills to the clinic. Simultaneously, clinicians bring years of experience to bear on how that literature and evidence is used in a given real-world context.

Communities of Practice

Unlike the classroom, learning in the clinical setting is improvisational or extemporaneous and is driven by the unpredictable real-life problems that we encounter on a day-to-day basis. These problems are embedded in the complex social and physical environment within which we practice. Perspectives on how this impacts teaching and learning have evolved over time. As noted earlier, numerous educational theorists have explored the importance of different factors in the teaching-learning situation. Because of their efforts, effective instructional strategies in professional education today include social interactions, context, and active participation in practice.[21-24,30,32,33]

Active participation in practice is what helps students and novice clinicians learn how experienced practitioners act and interact throughout the day, how they interact as professionals, and how they communicate with patients and other health care providers.[30] It helps shape how they think, what they do, and how they make sense of their experiences. Actively engaging in practice involves negotiating ways of being and interacting with one another within the community. It is through this negotiation process that students ultimately learn what it truly takes to belong and to become fully participating members of the profession.[30] Each new experience reshapes how we understand practice. This continuous renegotiation of the meaning of our day-to-day experiences results in our own professional identity development. Shepard and Jensen[34] described this transmission of shared meanings as an acculturation process and suggested that it is

the means by which students become socialized into the physical therapy profession. This renegotiation process holds true for newcomers as well as for those who have been in practice for some time and forms the basis for lifelong learning in the profession.

Key Points to Remember

Active participation in the community of practice of the clinical setting enables students to do the following:

- Develop their own identities as professionals.
- Turn their theoretical knowledge into practical knowledge.
- Further validate their understanding of the norms, standards, and ethics of the profession at large.
- Learn how experienced practitioners act and interact throughout the day and how they communicate both within the community of practice as well outside of the community.
- Learn what it truly takes to belong to and become fully participating members of a profession.

Critical Thinking Clinical Scenario

As a physical therapist, my first job was at a very large, prestigious, metropolitan rehabilitation center. This was a traditional hospital environment that included formal meetings, presentations, and formal rounds with families, physicians, and other health care providers. We wore uniforms with blue pants, white tops, and name tags. Patients were identified by surnames, as were supervisors. Appointment times were structured, and patients waited for you in the waiting room. We worked with patients one-on-one in a quiet setting with minimal distraction. My second job was at a school for children with developmental disabilities. It was a much less formal environment, with drawings on the walls and frequent impromptu meetings. We wore pants (some even jeans) and colorful shirts. Families were in the gym at all times, working with some therapists and waiting for others. There was always lots of chatter and lots of activity including laughing, joking, and playing in the gym.

Reflective Questions

1. How did the expectations of professional behavior differ in each setting?
2. How do you think I reacted on my first day of my second job? How do you think my colleagues in the pediatric facility reacted to me on that day?
3. How do you think I learned what was expected of me in each setting?
4. What kind of influence do you think my colleagues and these environments had on my development as a young clinician, and vice versa?
5. How might my acculturation have been different if I had started at the pediatric facility and moved to the rehabilitation facility?

Legitimate Peripheral Participation: Making Your Way Into the Community

Based on the previous scenario, you can begin to recognize the complexity of becoming a physical therapist in a specific clinical setting. Even experienced clinicians need to learn what the expectations of the community are and adjust accordingly. How can we help newcomers make that transition more easily, whether from classroom to clinic or clinic to clinic?

In physical therapy, we learn from experienced practitioners much like an apprentice learns from a master craftsman. Lave and Wenger[22] studied apprenticeship learning in a variety of settings. They broadened the traditional concept of apprenticeships to include communities in which increasing levels of participation lead to identity development, much like in physical therapy and most other health care professions.[30] The goal of their work was to find the common threads that facilitated and inhibited learning in social practice. Common to all of these apprenticeships, as with physical therapy internships, is the concept of legitimate peripheral participation.

Legitimate peripheral participation is a framework for understanding how newcomers learn by engaging with members of the community in progressively more complex and inclusive ways. In physical therapy, students start by simply observing, asking questions, and performing a component of patient management under close supervision. As they demonstrate increased competence, they gain credibility in the eyes of the clinical instructor, who then allows them to perform more complex skills with greater independence. Over time and with additional experiences, the novice clinician gains full membership into the community as a practicing clinician with responsibility for a total patient caseload. Throughout this transition from student to novice clinician, the learner is interacting with many individuals throughout the community of practice in the clinical setting. It is this progressively more complex engagement with other members of the community of practice that allows newcomers to continually enhance and modify their skills and interactions. Even for me as an experienced clinician, yet as a new member of the pediatric community, I had to go through a similar process of learning about the culture of this new environment, and it reshaped the way I practiced and interacted with all members of the community, including my patients.

Stop and Reflect

Think back over a time when you started a new job, joined a new club or social group, or experienced your first clinical immersion or internship.

- How did you figure out what was expected of you?
- How did you figure out the social norms of the community where you were (ie, how you were expected to act, dress, communicate, etc)?
- What helped your learning?
- Did you ever feel like you really belonged? If so, at what point did you really feel like you belonged? How did that happen? If not, why not?
- What most helped you develop a sense of belonging? Or what hindered you from developing a sense of belonging?
- In what ways did you influence how things were done in your new setting?

In physical therapy, all students experience a period of adjustment in each new clinical setting, and they begin their learning on the periphery. They are given the opportunity to observe and to participate in practice activities that carry minimal risk or cost for error, and they share minimal responsibility for the total outcome. This is what Lave and Wenger called "way in."[22] Students and newcomers need time to orient themselves and recognize the culture of their new environment, and it is important that we, as experienced clinicians, provide them with insight into the expectations of the community before we can expect them to contribute in a meaningful way. Regardless of the time frame involved, all newcomers need time to experience this gradual integration into the community.

As they gain competence and credibility, the "way in" period is followed by a practice period where students and newcomers become increasingly more engaged in the total process. They are given more responsibility, begin to take ownership of the activities of the group, and become integral members of the community of practice. Engagement in practice expands, and the complexity of their role and responsibility becomes increasingly more sophisticated. In this way, students and newcomers continually enhance and modify their skills and interactions as they begin to develop a sense of belonging within the community itself. Throughout this practice period, students as active participants go beyond imitation of behaviors to begin to construct their own professional identities. The ultimate goal of legitimate peripheral participation is the development of an identity and sense of belonging within the community of practice of physical therapy.

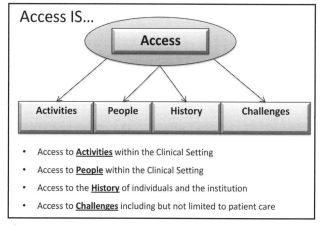

Access IS...

- Access to **Activities** within the Clinical Setting
- Access to **People** within the Clinical Setting
- Access to the **History** of individuals and the institution
- Access to **Challenges** including but not limited to patient care

Figure 7-1. Access.

Apprenticeship Learning in Physical Therapy Education

Having explored apprenticeship learning from a theoretical perspective, this next section will provide you with insight into physical therapy students' and clinicians' perceptions of how learning takes place in the clinical setting. Using real-life examples from students and novice clinicians, we will provide you with tools to use in enhancing the educational experiences of students and newcomers in your clinical setting. If you are a student, understanding how learning occurs in the clinical setting can better prepare you to be proactive in your educational and professional development. As noted earlier, direct quotes will be used to illustrate how students and clinical instructors believed they developed their own professional identities through their clinical education experiences. Underscoring the complexity of moving from the classroom to the clinic, one student commented:

> [There is a] big difference between being in the classroom … and being in the physical therapy setting. Everything sounds good and easy in the book, but it's not always that way. … You learn a thousand times more in a week than you learn in a semester in the classroom by just being in the facility and interacting with people as opposed to just sitting there and listening to the teacher talk about the way it should be.

Access as an Essential Ingredient to Learning in Physical Therapy Practice

Once you enter the clinical setting, your first challenge is to determine how to fit in, which includes figuring out the accepted culture and norms of behavior.[30] Though we have written standards in the physical therapy profession,[9,10] as you saw in an earlier scenario, the norms for behavior and practice may be different in each clinical setting. As Wenger[30] suggested, written standards must be renegotiated in each practice setting. This makes it particularly challenging for newcomers. Clinics can range from those that are very relaxed, with minimal rules, where clinicians are open to all types of professional and social discussions, to those that are more structured, with more rigid rules, where discussions are centered solely on patient care and issues of professional practice. Behaviors acceptable in one setting are not always acceptable in another setting, and expectations of one setting may differ from another. It is not surprising that the student quoted previously valued her learning in the clinical setting so much, because it is only through access to the clinical environment and engagement with clinicians that you can begin to make sense of these different expectations. One of the things that I learned from the students and clinicians I interviewed was that access means much more than simply placing a student in the clinic to observe physical therapy practice; it means giving them access to various activities, people, history, and challenges (Figure 7-1).

Stop and Reflect

Consider the quote above in which the student distinguishes between learning in the classroom and learning in the clinic.

- What is your reaction to that quote?

- How accurate is that quote for you?

- Why do you think the student feels that she learned more in 1 week in the clinic than an entire semester in the classroom?

Table 7-1. Access to Activities

Activity	Exemplary Quotes
Rounds	"The situation that had the most impact on me was the first time I sat in on rounds during my clinical affiliation. All these individuals seemed to interact with each other in a certain way … no matter how strongly a person felt about a patient and their ability to increase their functional abilities everything was handled very professionally. When it was my turn to report, I wanted to seem just as professional. I learned a lot by watching others do what I thought was the correct way to interact with other professionals." "Rounds are a huge thing. It was amazing just to sit there, not the pressure of participating, but just watching how someone reports; how there can be an argument, a conflict, people saying different things, yet it all being professional. So I think that is a great way to learn communication and interpersonal skills."
Lunch	"Lunch breaks helped. I could discuss freely what had happened in the clinic, without feeling [like] it was infringing upon my grade, or that I was being watched. It was very relaxing; it was [a] very comfortable setting to learn in." "Most of the students go out and they go sit in the cafeteria. They sit amongst themselves, and they try to bond with each other. She'd actually come in and listen to us talking. People really felt like she'd been here for months and she [the student] became part of the staff after a while." One student even commented: "I felt the distance. No one else sat and ate lunch together. I would sit by myself. I didn't feel comfortable, so I just went on my own." Later in the interview, she described the impact that this type of interaction had on her, saying it made her feel more distanced and less apt to engage in conversation or to ask questions throughout the day. Though most felt that lunch was an important time to sit together, the reverse was also heard by students and clinicians in both summative focus groups. "Sometimes I need that downtime. Lunch is a time for me to regroup and not feel like I am on or teaching all the time."

Stop and Reflect

Think back to a time when you just started a new clinical internship or a new job.

- What types of activities did you learn the most from?

- What people most helped your learning?

- What challenges did you face that you learned the most from?

- Looking back, what would you have liked to know before going into that particular setting?

Access to Activities

As a student or newcomer in any new situation, you begin to engage in all aspects of the environment and like you are part of the team. In physical therapy, you learn during formal activities such as rounds and meetings, as well as during informal or social activities, such as lunch. Being involved in informal gatherings may actually increase your comfort level with those around you and enable you to interact more fully, engage in dialogue, and ask questions, which can help you validate the sense you are making of your own experiences. Without this sense of comfort and belonging, it can sometimes begin to feel like you are an outsider. As an outsider, you probably would not fully engage, which would ultimately hinder your own learning and acculturation process. As stated earlier, in physical therapy, learning is a social practice, so having access to engage with other members of the profession is essential to the learning process.[2] Table 7-1 provides examples of what newcomers (students and new graduates) and clinicians told us about the importance of having access to engage in a variety of activities typical of the clinical setting.

Access to People

Being in the clinic can help you as a student and newcomer become more aware of how physical therapists communicate and interact on a day-to-day basis. You observe clinicians interacting with different patients, different family members, and different health care professionals. You observe therapists manage conflicts and very sensitive issues, which can provide a model for you to follow as you begin to identify the norms of the community. Though we all learn about these behaviors in school, it is not until you actually encounter them in the clinic that you often make sense of what you have learned. You begin to realize that what you have learned in school can be applied in a variety of ways in the clinic, sometimes in ways you might not have ever considered while in the classroom. In essence, it is by observing and working with other physical therapists that you can begin to link theory to real-world practice.[35] While in the clinic, you may observe both professional and unprofessional interactions. By being exposed to these differences, you begin to determine which behaviors you want to emulate and which ones you do not. This will ultimately help you shape your own professional identities. Table 7-2 provides examples of what some newcomers (students

Table 7-2. Access to People

People	Exemplary Quotes
Positive and negative role models	"I learned a lot from different people. One physical therapist I work with is outgoing, a funny, witty type of person. I also worked with the other side of the spectrum—very professional. He didn't make small chatter. They both had different approaches, and they both worked." "I worked for 2 brothers who were PTs. One brother was very professional at all times. He had great interpersonal skills: very attentive, good listener, knowledgeable. Brother #2 was the very opposite. The biggest problem seemed to be his interpersonal skills. Before I worked for the 'brothers,' I never really thought about professionalism. After working with them, I saw how important it is not to JUST HAVE good hands-on skills."
Patients	One student said, "Give the difficult and medium and easy patients. That definitely helps their experience because if you give them only easy patients, they are going to come out of the clinical thinking 'oh it's easy,' and they will have too much confidence. Then, when they become a real physical therapist, they are going to have a problem [treating] patients."

PT indicates physical therapist.

and new graduates) and clinicians have said about how having access to different people while in the clinical setting helped their learning and development.

Stop and Reflect

Think back to your experiences in the clinic either as a volunteer, a student, or a professional.

Complete the following sentences:

- "The worst display of unprofessional behavior I have ever observed was …"

- "I hope when I become a therapist I never …"

- "The most memorable display of professional behavior I have ever observed was …"

- "I hope when I am a therapist, people will look to me because I …"

Access to Shared History

Shared history is also an important concept in the development of professionals.[30] Having access to the history or background of people in the clinic can help you make sense of what you are observing. It can also help you understand the uniqueness of each individual and how he or she fits into the community. For example, one student on her clinical internship commented on how one of the clinicians, unlike most clinicians in that setting, took a great deal of time with every patient. The student was quite impressed and began to model that behavior. It was only after the student spoke with her clinical instructor that she realized that this behavior was not the norm and perhaps should not be emulated. In fact, the therapist she observed was quite slow and the way she managed her patients was really not acceptable to either the patients themselves or to the clinic director. Without this "history of the community" or "insider information," newcomers might imitate behaviors they observe, which actually might not be fully accepted by all of the members in the community.

Students also found it particularly helpful when their clinical instructors shared their own journeys toward professional development. One clinical instructor described what it took for her to develop expertise in pediatric physical therapy when she worked with students. She explained that students often fail to recognize that development of expertise truly takes time and practice and that it is not an expectation of entry-level practice. When clinical instructors share what they were like as novices, how they too made errors, and what it really took for them to develop competence, confidence, and ultimately expertise, they help students and novices modulate and clarify their own expectations and assumptions. Shared history enables them to envision themselves as future physical therapists and can provide them with a path to follow in attaining their goals.[35] Table 7-3 provides some examples of what some newcomers (students and new graduates) and clinicians told us about the importance of access to history in the clinical environment.

Stop and Reflect

Think of a time when you may have benefited from having access to history of an environment or situation before you entered that environment (perhaps you "put your foot in your mouth" or felt very awkward because you were not aware of the culture or expectations of the setting).

Table 7-3. Access to History

History	Exemplary Quotes
Development of expertise	"I just make it clear—I have been here for a long time. I wasn't expected to do any of this when I first began. I try not to make the students' assumptions real. I get a sense that they're saying, 'Were you put into this situation from day one or did you work towards that?' So I let them know—so and so has 25 years of experience; this one has 15 years of experience; someone else has 2 years of experience. There are big differences, and we all have different responsibilities, but it took us some time to get to where we are. We did not know everything when we first started."
Insider's view of the department	"I felt at times many of the staff members ranging from my CI to the supervisor were very moody. I would come in and say 'Hi' when I arrived in the morning and hardly received a response. When I spoke to other staff members in OT/PT/ST/RT, etc, they reassured me that I should not take it personally, that they had felt the same. It has changed my perspective for when I am a future CI. I have become more sensitive to the student and their transitions."
Insider's view of the patient's behavior	"I didn't know what happened. I just came out of the room, I smiled and the patient said, 'Why are you laughing at me, get out of my face!' I was shocked. Then the therapist took me aside and said, 'Don't feel bad, she does it to the other therapist, too.' I felt really bad, at that moment, but I realized it was not directed at me and that I had to just stop and let her get over that emotion."

CI indicates clinical instructor; OT, occupational therapy; PT, physical therapy; ST, speech therapy; RT, recreational therapy.

Access to Challenges

Our role as educators is to challenge students, and it is through these challenges that students learn. In the clinical setting, students face at least 3 major challenges that provide excellent learning opportunities: (1) learning activities explicitly designed by the clinical instructor to challenge the student and facilitate learning, (2) novel or unfamiliar situations, and (3) situations in which students must manage their own attributes and those of their clinical instructor, patients, and the environment, as well.

Good clinical instructors routinely design challenges that facilitate student learning (eg, problem-solving activities, independent treatment sessions, on-the-spot questions, role plays, mock evaluations, and case scenarios). Masterful clinical instructors design activities to facilitate learning as well as take advantage of those "teachable moments"–they take every opportunity to turn clinical experiences into learning opportunities. Table 7-4 provides examples of how newcomers (students and new graduates) and clinicians described some of the challenges, explicitly designed by clinical instructors, that helped them apply and refine their knowledge and skills.

Learning opportunities are easily recognized by skilled clinicians; however, these are not the only challenges students face. Students and novice clinicians often face challenges that are long forgotten and taken for granted by the experienced clinician. For example, when students walk in the door for the first time, not only do they have to meet many new people, but they must rather quickly decipher the norms and expectations of the entire community. Moreover, given that clinical education is time limited and is an evaluative process, students must learn very quickly to comply with these expectations. As new learners gain credibility and are given greater responsibility and independence, they are challenged to become more authoritative, to delegate responsibilities, and to problem-solve independently.

Most of the time, these challenges are beneficial; however, some students have shared that they felt like they were always being put on-the-spot or given too much independence too soon. In fact, some students commented how at times it felt more like they were being tested constantly for grading purposes, rather than challenged for learning purposes. Some find this quite stressful. If you remember back to the chapter on the brain, you will realize that some stress can facilitate learning and retention, but if the stress is perceived as being excessive, it may actually interfere with and become a barrier to learning. As instructors, it is important for us to recognize these stressors and potential barriers and provide appropriate supports to optimize learning. Table 7-4 provides examples of what newcomers (students and new graduates) and clinicians described as some of the novel situations they found particularly challenging.

Not only are students and novice clinicians challenged by all of the new activities they are experiencing, but they must learn to modify their approach to meet the needs of each patient and are expected to interact effectively with other members of the community as well. To function fully within the community, they have to manage their own personal characteristics (eg, shyness, insecurity) and adapt to the unique characteristics of each member of the community (clinical instructor, patient, and environment). Table 7-4 provides examples of some of the characteristics newcomers (students and new graduates) and clinicians found particularly challenging about themselves, their clinical instructors, their patients, and even the environment.

Table 7-4. Access to Challenges

Challenges	Examples	Exemplary Quotes
Activities designed by the clinical instructor	Asking questions	"He was constantly bombarding me. I told him how I didn't think I did well answering questions head-on like that, but he just kept it up. By the end, I was more comfortable with it, and I would say things I didn't even remember that I knew." "My supervisor thought a good way to teach me was to question me in front of the patient. That was a bad approach because if I was wrong, it would look bad and that particular patient would have no confidence in me." "She would give me case scenarios and quiz me. Sometimes it was frustrating because I'm like, 'Does she think I'm dumb?' But at the end, I realized why she was doing it."
	Figure it out	"Instead of just going and telling you what to do, my CI waited until I figured out how to work with this child on my own. It took me about 3 treatment sessions, but she wanted me to figure it out on my own instead of telling me what to do." "I'm not going to tell my students to 'go home and figure out how you can do it better' because it's virtually impossible; you don't know how to do it better; you are already doing the best that you can. There is no way to do it better in your mind, because you are trying already so hard."
Novel situations	Fitting in	"Getting the feel of what type of people are around and how should I react to these people? Are they going to write me up? How do I have to act? Who's important, who's not? Who are the people I can kid around with? You see, there is a pecking order, and a lot of times you realize very quickly who's listening to who and who is reporting back to who."
	Taking charge and delegating	"She was a bit shy, and it took her a little while to talk to patients in a way that was authoritative." "I can do it myself, I can set up the patient. I wanted to do it with the patient. I wanted to do everything with the patient. It is your first time, and you really want to get more hands on, but there is this time management thing—you've got so many patients to see and you just have to be able to delegate to the aides. Sometimes you realize you have to let it go so that way you can treat other patients that need your skills, which is kind of hard for me."
Personal characteristics	Need to be liked	"I always want people to like me so I'm nice. Then, at the end of the session, I realize that we haven't really done anything, and I realized that I have to be firmer and not worry so much as to win their sympathy as to win their respect."
	Being too personal	"At times, I hesitate to ask a question because I'm thinking, 'is that too personal?' Even though the question might be very important, I hesitate to ask, concerned, 'Am I stepping over the line?' I felt as though it was kind of private. Maybe because I don't want people to step over the line with me, to ask me questions that I don't want to answer."
	Culture and English as a second language	"Sometimes, they say things I don't understand and I don't know how to respond. But if I would just stop, I would feel like they think that I don't want to talk to them or they think that I am stupid or I don't know how to say things. In some situations, they talk about something I don't even know about because it happened before I came to the US, some TV show let's say. I have no idea what they are talking about, and it's hard for me to tell them. I feel kind of weird and don't know how to respond."
Clinical instructor characteristics	Overly demanding	"I come in 30 minutes early. As soon as she sees me, she says, 'We're going to go now and start doing chart reviews.' She never stopped to ask if I was in early for a specific reason. During lunch break, she would say, 'You better grab something fast. Why not bring your food because by the time you go into the cafeteria you could do 2 notes.' At one point, I told her my doctor wanted me to go for a stress test because I was having chest pain and she said, 'When you finish, come back to work.' I said I might not be finished until 2 or 3. She said, 'It doesn't matter even if you finish at 3 or 4, still come.'"
	Inconsistent	"He gave me mixed messages. Sometimes he was my best friend, and other times he was this superior being. I was very confused. I was afraid to tell him anything. One minute he would say I've already shown you that and then later he would show me like nothing happened. It was a little like trying to follow a ping pong ball. I never quite knew how to act."
Patient characteristics	Culture	"We have a variety of patients from everywhere, and I have a difficult time when someone doesn't speak English. It's difficult to get your comments across. For example, this couple from the Middle East, the wife was the patient but you had to speak only to the husband. It was very uncomfortable. It was very difficult because the husband would not let us approach the woman, so it was really an issue of culture, that you had to be respectful of that person's culture."

(continued)

Table 7-4. Access to Challenges (continued)

Challenges	Examples	Exemplary Quotes
Patient characteristics (continued)	Diagnoses	"Expressive aphasia patients, it's difficult to understand what they are saying at first. I would just nod my head, 'Ok, oh yeah,' but I don't really know what they are talking about. I don't want them to be disappointed by my lack of understanding, so I would pretend I understood what they were saying. It ends up not so good because from the way that I respond, he knows that I don't understand. That gets into a weird situation because now I am like lying, if I'm pretending, he is going to think, 'Am I going to be able to trust you again?' because now you are pretending you understand." "I was dealing with a cognitively impaired population. I knew what to expect and was prepared in terms of my treatment strategies, but the communication aspect was challenging. I felt 'helpless.' I took for granted the ease most patients understand your directions but with this population, you have to be more creative. This helped me realize how our interpersonal skills are critical in all different patient populations. I realized how you have to be able to relate to a whole range of patients."
Environmental characteristics	The clinical setting	"One place was much more professional. Really straight and narrow. There wasn't a lot of extra chit-chat. At another facility, there was talk going on about the weekend. It was much more acceptable to talk to my CI about things other than therapy. Then I went to my peds affiliation, and there were no rules—they'd talk about anything and everything. So it was totally different."
	The role of the student	"You have to know your place—you're a student and a student has a certain role, certain guidelines they should follow. You should be what you would be normally, respectful and polite, but even more so. Especially with some clinical instructors because they can be unfair and look for anything to take points off. So I'm always on my tippy toes. Students have a pretty bad job they've got to learn, work hard, watch for 8 weeks, and be this perfect person. Or, they don't have to, and then they might not pass."

CI indicates clinical instructor.

Critical Thinking Clinical Scenario

Take some time to review and reflect on the quotes provided in Table 7-4.

Reflective Questions

1. Which of those quotes resonates most with you? Why?

2. Did you find any of the challenges surprising? If so, which one(s)? Why?

3. Considering your own personality traits:
   o How might your own personal traits add to the challenge of being new to a clinical setting?
   o What strategies might you use to help manage your own challenging traits?

4. What strategies might you consider:
   o In trying to fit in on the first day of your internship?
   o During your first independent treatment session?

5. What strategies might you consider if you were faced with:
   o An overly demanding clinical instructor?
   o A clinical instructor who has inconsistent behaviors or expectations?
   o A patient who does not speak English?
   o A patient who does not adhere to the recommendations?
   o A patient with a challenging diagnosis?
   o A setting (eg, acute care, rehabilitation center) that you find particularly challenging?

Moving Beyond Individual Learning to Developing Shared Meaning in the Clinical Setting

Giving students access to the clinical environment through clinical education provides them with access to people, activities, history, and a variety of challenges essential to their own learning and professional development. However, just having access does not guarantee they will learn. Once they start their immersion or internship, they must begin to make sense (ie, personal meaning) of what is happening around them so that they can learn from their experiences. We each have our own learning styles or preferences; however, we know that to be effective teachers and learners we must use all of the different learning styles. The same is true in the clinical setting. In the clinic, we use a variety of learning strategies, which may be very different from the strategies we use in the classroom. Students, newcomers, and clinicians noted that to truly make sense of their surroundings they used the following learning strategies:

- Engagement (ie, doing)
- Reflection (ie, thinking)
- Observation (ie, watching)
- Dialogue (ie, talking)

Table 7-5. Personal Meaning-Making Strategies

Personal Meaning-Making Strategies	Exemplary Quotes
Learning by doing (engagement; eg, patient treatment, rounds, lunch)	"I learn the most from my patients. They tell me how I'm doing and how I should react, like, if I'm trying to tell them something and they don't understand it, I have to make changes. I have to change the way I'm communicating so they can understand it, so I think a lot of it is from my patients."
Learning by reflecting (eg, role plays, case scenarios, and mock evaluations)	"While working in a hospital, I kind of rushed through a treatment. I really didn't communicate with the [patient] nor did she really communicate with me. At the end, I realized that I didn't know anything about the patient besides her diagnosis. I realized that despite my hard work, it is important to communicate, to learn more about a patient as an individual."
Learning by observing or watching	"I really learned a lot about communication from my CI. I observed how she interacted with the patients in the hospital setting, specifically how at the end of the treatment she made sure they could reach their phone, had their remote, etc. Prior to this, I wouldn't have even thought of doing these things. The patients responded very positively, and it enabled me to interact with patients as 'people' and not just 'patients.'" "By observing how each person relates, you get a sense of what's appropriate. Paying attention to the chemistry in your environment you see where you fit in."
Learning through dialogue (eg, gaining feedback, asking questions, being asked questions, and clarifying expectations)	"I had a lot of time to discuss things with my CI. It was helpful because maybe I would go back 3 steps—maybe I took a wrong turn in my thinking 3 steps backwards. And so we would talk about it. I got to learn everything. I wanted to show him all my faults, let's fix things at the ground level."

CI indicates clinical instructor.

Table 7-5 provides quotes shared by students and novice clinicians illustrating how each of these different learning strategies was used in the clinical setting. Figure 7-2 provides a schematic of these learning strategies.

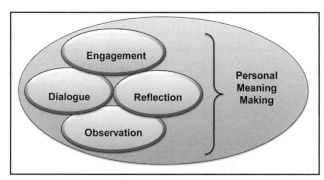

Figure 7-2. Personal meaning-making strategies.

Stop and Reflect

Think back to Chapter 2. Compare the learnng strategies described by the students and novice clinicians in Figure 7-2 to the learning styles described by Kolb.[24]

Students and clinicians alike told us that they learned by engaging in practice, observing others in practice, taking time to reflect, and engaging in a dialogue about what they were observing and learning.

Dialogue is the one strategy that is not explicitly a component of Kolb's[24] learning styles, yet it is critical to learning in the clinical setting. Dialogue is what allows us to link our own personal thoughts and experiences, and what we learned from those experiences, to that of others. As Figure 7-2 demonstrates, these strategies help us individually make sense of our experiences in the clinic. To validate our own learning, we need to develop a shared understanding of our experiences. We also need to be sure that the meaning we make, or how we understand our experiences, is consistent with the clinical community and its members. We need to be sure that what we are thinking is accurate. Recall the scenario of the student earlier who observed a therapist spending a great deal of time with each patient and began to emulate this behavior. What made sense in her mind was that the therapist was taking a long time and therefore must have been very thorough and because a great deal of time was spent with the patient, this must have been patient-centered care. It was only through dialogue with her clinical instructor that she realized that this therapist was spending an inordinate amount of time with patients, which was not always beneficial to the clinic or the patient. Through dialogue, she was able to clarify what she was thinking and correct the inaccurate assumptions she was making. In fact, rather than being thorough, she learned that the therapist was quite inefficient; rather than being patient centered, the therapist gave little thought to the time that patients were wasting while they waited for her.

It may make more sense if we put this in the context of an earlier chapter in which we discussed the concepts of intention and impact. It is possible that you and your clinical instructor may observe the same treatment session and walk away thinking 2 different things. For example, as the director of a physical therapy program, I remember a student coming to me to tell me that her clinical instructor was "awful." When I asked what made her so awful, the student explained that she had no idea how to evaluate a patient, she rarely did more than 1 or 2 special tests, and never fully evaluated any patient. In reality, her clinical instructor was an expert clinician, who had both excellent history-taking skills and keen observation skills. The expertise that the clinician had developed enabled her to make critical decisions without completing unnecessary tests. The problem was that the student was unaware of the clinical decisions her clinical instructor was making throughout the session. Had the student been aware of her clinical instructor's clinical decision-making process, she may have come to a very different conclusion about her clinical instructor's skills. The student observed, engaged in practice, and even reflected; however, what she did not do was take time to dialogue about what she was learning with her clinical instructor.

We continually make sense of our own experiences but we must move beyond personal meaning making to ensure that our thinking is accurate. To do so, we must actively seek and engage in dialogue with others. By asking questions, we can better understand how and why decisions are made. By sharing our thoughts, we can help students and others validate their thought processes and confirm the accuracy of the conclusions they are drawing. Of course, the reverse is also true. Students must work to make their thought process as explicit as possible as well. Wenger[30] referred to this as negotiation of shared meaning (Figure 7-3).

If you look back over the individual learning strategies described above, dialogue was the one strategy that appears to be inconsistent with Kolb's[24] model of learning. This is in part due to the fact that Kolb emphasized learning within the individual and did not account for learning within a social practice. When placed within a community of practice, dialogue becomes a mechanism through which reflection can occur not only within an individual but between and among individuals. Dialogue is the one mechanism that can help make what is tacit explicit. Without this dialogue, individuals can make personal meaning of an experience but cannot develop a shared meaning or understanding of experiences or expectations.

Implicit in any discussion of dialogue as a strategy for learning is the assumption that both parties have at least adequate communication skills. At the very least, we assume that people use respectful language, listen without interruption, and paraphrase or use periodic summaries to let one another know their message has been heard and understood. Additionally, the guideline presented in Chapter 2 for asking effective questions can enhance the dialogue process. Development of effective therapeutic communication is beyond the scope of this chapter; however, there are many available comprehensive texts and resources that address this issue.[36]

Figure 7-3 provides a schematic of the negotiation of *shared meaning*, or the process of moving from personal meaning making to shared meaning making through dialogue, which is essential to learning in the clinical setting. Table 7-6 provides quotes illustrating the concepts of learning through dialogue and the negotiation of shared meaning.

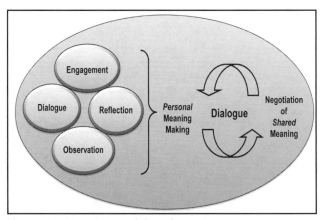

Figure 7-3. Negotiation of shared meaning.

Table 7-6. Negotiation of Shared Meaning: Learning Through Dialogue

"My CI sat me down the first day and said what she expected of me, what we were working towards. It put me at ease. I knew this is what I have to work towards and this is where I fit in."
"My student would be doing things, and I'd see she wasn't getting anywhere and would just keep trying and trying. I said to the student, tell me about what's going on—instead of just saying, 'I'm good' and then just trying something else, I could see she was struggling but it made me think she thought what she was doing was perfect, and I knew there was something really wrong with it. So I finally had to say to her, 'Tell me what you're thinking or when you're struggling, just tell me. This is not what you want to be happening.' Then I could say, so, what do you see is wrong? What's the problem? What are you having difficulty with?"
"I learned the most when I had the time to discuss things with my CI. Even if I feel like I was completely wrong, it was helpful that I said things like that because maybe I took a wrong turn in my thinking 3 steps backwards. And so we would talk about these things, and I got to understand things better. I wanted to show him all my faults so we could fix things at the ground level."

CI indicates clinical instructor.

In the clinical setting, some students are reluctant to engage in dialogue, ask questions, or discuss their concerns with their clinical instructors at times because they know they are being graded and do not want their clinical instructor to think they do not know something. This is problematic because without the dialogue, shared meaning cannot develop. For example, one student described how she often avoided dialogue for fear of conflict. She shared how when she was growing up she had many negative interactions with her father. Because of her immature ability to engage in effective dialogue with her father, these interactions often resulted in conflict and discomfort. This pattern of behavior stayed with her, and her fear of conflict made her avoid raising concerns, asking questions, or clarifying expectations throughout her internship. This hindered the dialogue and ultimately the shared understanding she developed with her clinical instructor. As a result, this student never fully met her clinical instructor's expectations, and the clinical instructor never fully understood the cause of this student's apparent noncompliance. The clinical instructor and student each developed personal meaning of the situation. The clinical instructor viewed the student as a noncompliant student who did not listen to what was expected and was not interested in learning. The student viewed the clinical instructor as being inconsistent in her expectations and was concerned that a conflict would ensue if she asked any questions. In this situation, dialogue did not occur, and, as a result, a shared understanding of the situation never developed.

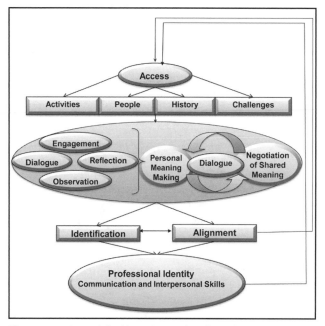

Figure 7-4. A model of learning in the clinical setting.

Though many theorists agree that experience is the basis for learning, their focus has been more on the individual and less on the interaction between the newcomer and the community.[21,23,24,35,37,38] Conversely, although Wenger[30] views learning as a social practice, his model of learning within a community of practice fails to fully capture the individual strategies that are used. Learning in the clinical setting is a complex process that requires us to look at the intersection between individual and social learning theories. It combines access to the community of physical therapy practice and all of its challenges (see Figure 7-1) with learning strategies for the development of both personal meaning making and shared meaning making through the negotiation of meaning (see Figures 7-2 and 7-3). Figure 7-4 depicts a process of learning in the clinical setting that incorporates both personal and shared meaning in the development of a professional identity (see Figure 7-4).

Key Points to Remember

Dialogue:

- Connects individual learning and develops shared meaning within the community of practice.

- Enables us to explore our roles within the community, make meaning from our experiences, validate what we see and do in practice, and develop a sense of belonging.

- Allows us to explore the development and the history of individuals, the community, and the profession.

Shared meaning provides us with clarification and validation, enables us to make informed decisions about which behaviors we want to emulate, and serves to enhance our professional identity development.

Stop and Reflect

Consider the scenario in which the student and clinical instructor did not develop shared meaning through dialogue.

- What might the student have done to facilitate the dialogue?

- What might the clinical instructor have done to facilitate the dialogue?

Identification, Alignment, and Professional Identity as Outcomes of Clinical Education

Becoming a PT is more than simply applying knowledge amassed in school.[30] It is a negotiation of ways of being and interacting within the community. This not only includes being recognized as a member of the professional community (ie, being identified as a PT) but developing a sense of belonging within the community and with other members of the larger community of physical therapy professionals (ie, identifying with other members of the profession). This requires both the process of identification, as well as that of alignment.

As we develop a shared understanding of the community of practice, we begin to identify those characteristics (eg, care, compassion, empathy, honesty) that we would like to emulate. We also identify important skills, attitudes, and values essential to being an excellent physical therapist. As we develop this internal image of what we want to become, we begin to identify ourselves with other practitioners and begin to identify ourselves as a physical therapist to others in society (identification). Simultaneously, we begin to conform to the expectations of the profession, including the *Core Values, Code of Ethics,* and *Standards of Practice* of the profession, as well as the goals, values, and expectations of our patients and the local clinical community (alignment). Both identification and alignment are essential components of our professional identify development.[30] Table 7-7 provides quotes illustrating how the concepts of identification and alignment are outcomes of the learning process in the physical therapy clinical setting.

Critical Thinking Clinical Scenario

Congratulations! You have all graduated and have been practicing for about a year. Your supervisor comes to you and says you have been assigned your first student and she will be starting next month. Even though she is only a first-year student, you are very nervous.

Reflective Questions

1. Based on the concepts presented in this chapter, what will you be sure to address during orientation? What strategies and activities will you put in place to maximize the potential for learning for this student?

2. Be sure to consider:
   - Access
   - Challenges
   - Learning strategies/styles
   - Dialogue and the negotiation of shared meaning

Table 7-7. Learning Outcomes

Learning Outcomes	Exemplary Quotes
Identification (eg, characteristics, skills, roles, values and responsibilities)	"One day, this 77-year-old Italian man started crying. My CI stopped what he was doing and spoke softly. [He] put his hand on the resident and showed this man compassion and sympathy without feeling sorry for him. I could not believe that this was part of the job of a PT, maybe because for the past year I have been focused on the academics. For the rest of my affil, I noticed how my CI spoke to people (patients) with such respect and compassion, and I feel like he was a mentor." "On my first affiliation, I was working with a patient who had an ACL repair. One day as she was exercising, she started crying and telling me about some problems in her personal life. At that point, I realized that as a physical therapist my role is not just to instruct patients on their exercises, but to be an active listener. In the future, I know that a priority should be on treating the patient as a whole." "A lot of the therapists would go to rounds so that they could learn about the patients. That was very professional. It was really nice to see therapists take their time out to learn everything they can about their patients. I want to do that as a therapist." "It was just amazing to sit there at rounds, watching how there can be an argument, a conflict, people saying different things, yet it all be [sic] professional."
Alignment	"You just have to take the time to really know exactly where they're coming from and try to really understand what this person's going through—asking questions and really listening." "At first, you kind of mold to the facility and try to figure out and then slowly you try to change things that you don't like. However, the world isn't perfect. In school and everywhere else, they are teaching that if you don't like something, approach the person and explain it, but in the real world it doesn't work that way. If your supervisors are not open to suggestion, they can really make you miserable so you do have to mold." "One new graduate shared numerous examples of how he disagreed with his supervisor and at one point commented to a co-worker, 'Just because that's the way he is, doesn't mean we should just accept it.' He had difficulty complying with the expectations of the facility and after several months called this researcher to inform her that he had resigned from that facility."

CI indicates clinical instructor; ACL, anterior cruciate ligament.

Summary

This chapter is based on the lived experiences of a number of students and new graduates, and it provides us with a model of how learning takes place within the physical therapy community of practice. Participants' stories showed how clinicians acted as role models and provided access for newcomers. They described how access goes beyond simply being in the clinical environment to treat patients. Access to activities, people, history, and challenges helps students and new graduates develop a sense of belonging and a sense of becoming physical therapists. Participants described the learning strategies they used and how active engagement and dialogue with experienced clinicians were critical to their development. Their stories also showed how shared meaning, consistent with that of their supervisors and others within the clinical setting, could only be developed through dialogue. Finally, they provided examples of how they were able to assimilate the attitudes, values, and beliefs of the profession while developing professional communication and interpersonal skills, which formed the basis of their own professional identities.

This model has significant implications for designing effective clinical education experiences as well as for developing effective orientation and mentoring processes for new graduates. Providing access is insufficient without encouraging dialogue with experienced members of the community to develop shared meaning and make learning explicit. Dialogue allows community members to negotiate meaning that is consistent with the expectations of the clinical setting. Dialogue not only makes the community's expectations explicit but provides the newcomer with an opportunity to share new ideas and add to the ongoing evolution of the community. In this way, lifelong learning can be facilitated in all members of the community of physical therapy practice.

Key Points to Remember

Learning requires access to the clinical setting.

- Access does not simply mean being in the clinical environment to treat patients.
- Access includes the following:
  - Access to people
  - Access to history
  - Access to activities
  - Access to challenges

Learning in the clinical setting requires a variety of strategies, including the following:

- Engagement in practice
- Observation
- Reflection
- Dialogue

Learning in the clinical setting requires more than just personal meaning making.

- Learning requires the negotiation of shared meaning.
- Personal meaning making does not necessarily mean shared meaning.
- Dialogue is critical to the development of shared meaning.

Learning in the clinical setting requires both identification and alignment.

- Newcomers must begin to identify with and be identified as a member of the community of practice.
- Identification as a new member of the community of practice will require the newcomer to align his or her values, beliefs, and behaviors with those of the community.

References

1. Plack MM. *Learning Communication and Interpersonal Skills Essential for Physical Therapy Practice: A Study of Emergent Clinicians.* New York, NY: Teachers College, Columbia University; 2003.

2. Plack MM. Developing communication, interpersonal skills and a professional identity within the physical therapy community of practice. *J Phys Ther Educ.* 2006;20:37-46.

3. Hayes K, Huber G, Rogers J, Sanders B. Behaviors that cause clinical instructors to question the clinical competence of physical therapist students. *Phys Ther.* 1999;79:653-671.

4. Dettmer P. New Bloom's in established fields: four domains of learning and doing. *Roeper Rev.* 2006;28:70-78.

5. Chambers DW. Professional development. *J Am Coll Dent.* 1999;66:43-47.

6. May WW, Morgan BJ, Lemke JC, Karst GM, Stone HL. Model for ability-based assessment in physical therapy education. *J Phys Ther Educ.* 1995;9:3-6.

7. Haddad S, Fournier P, Machouf N, Yatara F. What does quality mean to lay people? Community perceptions of primary health care services in Guinea. *Soc Sci Med.* 1998;47:381-394.

8. May W, Stroker G. Critical thinking and self-assessment: the key to developing professional behavior. Paper presented at: National Clinical Education Conference; March 23, 2001; San Francisco, Calif.

9. Guide to physical therapist practice. *Phys Ther.* 2001;81:1-768.

10. *Professionalism in Physical Therapy: Core Values.* Alexandria, VA: American Physical Therapy Association; 2004.

11. Hojat M, Borenstein BD, Veloski JJ. Cognitive and noncognitive factors in predicting the clinical performance of medical school graduates. *J Med Educ.* 1988;63:323-325.

12. Fidler GS. Developing a repertoire of professional behaviors. *Am J Occup Ther.* 1996;50:583-587.

13. Benatar SR. The meaning of professionalism in medicine. *S Afr Med J.* 1997;87:427-431.

14. Cross V, Hicks C. What do clinical educators look for in physiotherapy students? *Physiotherapy.* 1997;83:249-259.

15. Hayward LM, Noonan AC, Shain D. Qualitative case study of physical therapist students' attitudes motivations and affective behaviors. *J Allied Health.* 1999;28:155-164.

16. Mostrom E. Professionalism in physical therapy: a reflection on ways of being in physical therapy education. *J Phys Ther Educ.* 2004;18:23.

17. Papadakis MA, Hodgson CS, Teherani A, Kohatsu ND. Unprofessional behavior in medical school is associated with subsequent disciplinary action by state medical board. *Acad Med.* 2004;79:244-249.

18. Altmaier EM, McGuinness G, Wood P, Ross RR, Bartley J, Smith W. Defining successful performance among pediatric residents. *Pediatrics.* 1990;85:139-143.

19. Duke M. Clinical evaluation–difficulties experienced by sessional clinical teachers of nursing: a qualitative study. *J Adv Nurs.* 1996;23:408-414.

20. Carey JR, Ness KK. Erosion of professional behaviors in physical therapist students. *J Phys Ther Educ.* 2001;15:20-22.

21. Schön DA. *Educating the Reflective Practitioner.* San Francisco, CA: Jossey-Bass Publishers; 1987.

22. Lave J, Wenger E. *Situated Learning: Legitimate Peripheral Participation.* Cambridge, UK: Cambridge University Press; 1991.

23. Dewey J. *Experience and Education.* New York, NY: Simon & Schuster; 1938.

24. Kolb D. *Experiential Learning: Experience as the Source of Learning and Development.* Englewood Cliffs, NJ: Prentice-Hall; 1984.

25. Korthagen FA, Kessels JP. Linking theory and practice: changing the pedagogy of teacher education. *Educ Res.* 1999;28:4-17.

26. Tennant MP, Pogson P. *Learning and Change in the Adult Years: A Developmental Perspective.* San Francisco, CA: Jossey-Bass Publishers; 1995.

27. J Mezirow. *Fostering Critical Reflection in Adulthood: A Guide to Transformative and Emancipatory Learning.* San Francisco, CA: Jossey-Bass Publishers; 1990.

28. Schein EH. *Organizational Culture and Leadership.* San Francisco, CA: Jossey-Bass; 1992.

29. Bandura A. *Social Foundations of Thought and Action: A Social Cognitive Theory.* Englewood, NJ: Prentice-Hall; 1986.

30. Wenger E. *Communities of Practice: Learning, Meaning and Identity.* Cambridge, UK: Cambridge University Press; 1998.

31. Barab SA, Duffy TM. From practice fields to communities of practice. In: Jonassen DH, Land SM, eds. *Theoretical Foundations of Learning Environments.* Mahwah, NJ: Lawrence Erlbaum Associates; 2000:25-56.

32. Brown JS, Collins A, Duguid P. Situated cognition and the culture of learning. *Educ Res.* 1989;18:32-42.

33. Jarvis P. *Paradoxes of Learning: On Becoming an Individual in Society.* San Francisco, CA: Jossey-Bass Publishers; 1992.

34. Shepard KF, Jensen GM, eds. *Handbook of Teaching for Physical Therapists.* Boston, MA: Butterworth-Heinemann; 1997.

35. Boud D, Keogh R, Walker D. *Reflection: Turning Experience Into Learning.* New York, NY: Kogan Page/Nichols Publishing; 1985.

36. Davis CM. *Patient Practitioner Interaction: An Experiential Manual for Developing the Art of Health Care.* 4th ed. Thorofare, NJ: SLACK Incorporated; 2006.

37. Jarvis P. *Adult and Continuing Education: Theory and Practice.* 2nd ed. London: Routledge; 1995.

38. Jarvis P, Holford J, Griffin C. *The Theory and Practice of Learning.* London: Kogan Page; 1998.

The Learning Triad
Strategies for Optimizing Supports and Minimizing Barriers to Facilitate Learning in the Clinical Setting

Chapter Objectives

After reading this chapter, you will be prepared to:

- Compare and contrast learning in the classroom and clinic settings.

- Apply the concept of the learning triad that emerges in the clinical setting to developing effective teaching and learning strategies.

- Analyze the potential barriers to learning in the clinical setting.

- Analyze the potential supports to learning in the clinical setting.

- Apply the concept of mentorship within a community of practice to design effective learning experiences for students and new clinicians.

- Use a comprehensive and systematic approach to optimize learning in the clinical setting.

As we discovered in the previous chapter, learning in physical therapy requires total immersion in the physical therapy community of practice.[1] This is true in other health professions as well.[2] Though classroom learning is critical to our success, for many of us, the abstract concepts learned in the classroom do not begin to make sense until we apply them in practice. Gaining access to and engaging in practice with professionals enables us to begin to develop a shared understanding of our role as practitioners.[3,4] However, simply gaining access to observe practice is not enough.[1,2] Observation is important in the learning process, but in the health professions it is equally if not more important to gain personal experience and be actively engaged in all aspects of practice. Through active participation, we learn how experienced practitioners act, interact, and ultimately learn what it truly takes to become a fully participating member of the profession.[3,4] Active participation allows for dialogue, which enables us to negotiate meaning and develop a shared understanding of the values, beliefs, behaviors, and expectations of professional practice.[1] Dialogue and engagement are social processes that are essential to learning and professional development in the health professions, and they begin with the sponsorship of a mentor. In physical therapy, that mentor is the clinical instructor.

Stop and Reflect

You are at the end of your first year in physical therapy school, and next week you will be starting your first full-time clinical experience. You are excited and nervous.

Think for a minute:

- What are you excited about? What are you nervous about?

- Who do you anticipate learning the most from in the clinical setting?

- Where will you turn if you run into a problem or situation you cannot seem to solve?

- What if that situation involves your clinical instructor?

In this chapter, we present the concept of a learning triad, which includes the learner, the instructor, and the clinical community. We examine the role of mentorship within the physical therapy community of practice and how mentorship moves beyond the one-to-one relationship of the student and clinical

Plack M, Driscoll M. *Teaching and Learning in Physical Therapy:
From Classroom to Clinic* (pp 177-196).
© 2011 SLACK Incorporated

instructor to include the entire learning triad. We examine the role of the student, the clinical instructor, and the rest of the clinical community in supporting learning. Of course, the director of clinical education and all faculty members within the academic program are essential in supporting student learning, whether it be in the classroom or the clinic; however, this chapter focuses on the clinical environment specifically. We will also explore how the same components that support learning in the clinical environment can potentially hinder learning as well. Finally, we present a framework for learning that optimizes the supports and minimizes the barriers or hindrances to learning in the clinical setting.

As in the previous chapter, you will see direct quotes from students and clinicians that illustrate, reinforce, and provide additional opportunities to apply the concepts discussed. These quotes provide evidence of how learning in the physical therapy clinical environment is similar to, yet different from, a more traditional mentorship or apprenticeship model of learning.

Mentorship: The Master and the Apprentice

Wenger[3] and Lave and Wenger[4] discussed apprenticeship learning within a community of practice. They studied apprenticeship learning in a variety of professions; however, little mention was made of the actual relationship between the "master" and the "apprentice" or the teacher and the learner. They described this relationship as ranging from almost nonexistent to a well-defined and explicit relationship, without which the apprentice would not have had access to the community. Spouse[2,5,6] specifically studied nursing students and noted that support from clinicians in the mentorship role significantly increased the student's adjustment to the clinical environment and ultimately enhanced learning. Similarly in physical therapy, the clinical instructor becomes a significant teacher and mentor in the life of students and novice clinicians.[7,8]

Stop and Reflect

Think about someone who has been a mentor to you in your life. Perhaps you have had more than one mentor, or perhaps you have been a mentor to someone else.

- What was your relationship like with this person(s)?
- How did this relationship(s) come about?
- How long did this mentorship relationship(s) last?
- What role did your mentor(s) play in your life? Or, if you were a mentor, what role did you play in the life of your protégé?

The term *mentor* comes from Homer's *Odyssey* in which Mentor was a trusted friend of Odysseus to whom he entrusted his son, Telemachus. Mentor was a teacher, guide, friend, adviser, protector, and even surrogate father to Telemachus at times.[9-12] This mythological story depicts the essence of a traditional mentorship—an older, wiser, more experienced person influencing and guiding a younger, less experienced individual or protégé through life's transitions. Has this been your experience, either as a mentor or as a protégé? Terms such as *sponsor, role model, coach, supervisor, preceptor, advisor, gatekeeper, guide, counselor,* and *friend* have been used synonymously with the term *mentor.*[2,9,11-13]

Stop and Reflect

- Of the term(s) used in the text above (eg, counselor, guide, friend, etc), which term(s) best describe your mentor(s)? If none, what term would you use to describe your mentor's role in your life?
- If you had more than one mentor, did they come at different times in your life? Did they have different functions in your life?
- In what ways did your mentor(s) help you develop? Or, if you were a mentor, in what ways did you help your mentor grow and develop?

Just as the term *mentor* is a complex one that means different things to different people, the role of the mentor is also quite complex. If you take even a few minutes to compare your mentorship experiences with those of some of your peers, you are likely to find that your experiences may have some similarities but they may have been quite different as well. Mentors can play many different roles and provide many different functions in the life of a protégé. In his text entitled *Mentor,* Daloz[9] described 3 distinct functions of a mentor: support, challenge, and vision.

Daloz[9] defined *support* as the affirmation and validation of the protégé's experiences. Kram[13] more explicitly delineated the mentor's role as having 2 distinct support functions, career and psychosocial functions, although certainly there is overlap between the 2 of them.

1. Career functions are those functions that help orient a protégé and advance the protégé's career, such as providing sponsorship, visibility, exposure to challenging assignments, and coaching. Career functions also include protecting protégés from situations for which they are not yet prepared.

2. Psychosocial functions are "those aspects of the relationship that enhance a [protégé's] sense of

competence, identity, and effectiveness in a professional role,"[13] such as providing acceptance, confirmation, counseling, friendship, and being a role model.

Kram[13] noted that career functions are generally the result of the longevity, position, and influence of the mentor within the organization, whereas the psychosocial functions are the result of the interpersonal relationship or bond that forms between the mentor and protégé.

Stop and Reflect

Think back on your mentor(s).

- In what ways were their roles consistent with what Kram and Daloz described?

- In what ways were their roles inconsistent with what Kram and Daloz described?

In physical therapy, both career and psychosocial functions are critical for newcomers to any clinical practice. When we first enter the clinical environment as students, we look to our clinical instructor (mentor) for emotional support, as well as for guidance in the areas of career and psychosocial functioning. In an acute-care setting, student physical therapists may work directly with seriously ill patients for the first time. They may even experience the death of a patient to whom they have come to know and value. The clinical instructor becomes a role model for how to experience strong emotional reactions, even sadness and a sense of loss, while continuing to provide care and treatment for other patients on that day's schedule. Whether it is during lunch or at an interdepartmental meeting, the function of the mentor is to facilitate learning for the protégé through social engagement in the community of practice.[2] It is often through this mentorship relationship that clinicians share their professional values, beliefs, and behaviors, often tacitly, in the midst of being actively engaged in everyday activities.[14]

Some authors also suggest that mentors have a "political function" and "power perspective" as well.[15,16] This may be particularly critical in a physical therapy setting where newcomers are expected to quickly recognize and adapt to the expectations of the community. First impressions are important, and we must quickly figure out what we can and cannot do, how we should and should not act, and with whom we should and should not interact—we must learn to navigate the subtleties of each community of practice. For example, in a hospital setting, the physical therapist is part of a multidisciplinary team. Students must very quickly learn who is in charge at the nursing station or what questions to pose to the social worker versus the nurse or the physician. In an outpatient setting, it can be equally important to recognize who has the power to even influence basic aspects of practice management such as scheduling and patient assignment. It is often the mentor who helps the newcomer learn to effectively negotiate through the community's political and social structures as he or she moves toward becoming an active participant in that community.[15-18] Spouse[2] believes that it is this early mentoring relationship that allows students to feel comfortable in an unfamiliar environment and enables them to move beyond the one-to-one mentoring relationship to engage with others in the community of practice besides the clinical instructor.

Stop and Reflect

Think back to a time when you were a newcomer to a particular environment. Consider your first day of physical therapy school.

- How did you figure out what was expected of you?

- Who helped you figure that out?

- What did that person(s) do to help you?

- How does that compare with our previous discussion of the role of the mentor?

Think back also on some of the challenges you faced during your first semester of physical therapy school or your first clinical internship.

- How did you overcome each of those challenges?

- What did you learn by overcoming those challenges?

As noted, the role of the mentor is not only to support the protégé but also to challenge the protégé because it is through those challenges that we learn. Mentors challenge us by providing experiences that result in a tension or a gap between what we know and what we do not know. To resolve this tension or bridge this gap, learning must occur.[5,9]

From the previous chapter, you know that challenges, like supports, can take many forms. You also know that clinical instructors use different strategies to challenge students, such as providing novel tasks, facilitating reflection, discussing problems, questioning hypotheses and solutions, exploring new ideas and alternative perspectives, experimenting with new approaches, and setting high standards.[1,19] We also know that students are faced with many more challenges in the clinical setting than those explicitly designed by the clinical instructor. Being exposed to novel situations and having to manage the different attributes of the student, clinical instructor, and community (including the patient and environment) can be quite a challenge.[1] Though challenging, these strategies and activities are critical to our learning, and our clinical instructor can help us master these challenges through coaching,[20] role modeling,[18,21] scaffolding our learning,[5] and facilitating our engagement in practice.[2-4,22]

Daloz[9] and Zachary[10] noted that the third role of the mentor is to provide vision for the protégé. Mentors bring a great deal of experience to any given situation and as a result can provide us with a sense of what our own careers might look like some day and can share with us how they achieved success, which can give us a sense of how we might work to reach that vision. Effective mentors are our role models and are role models for the profession. In his theory on social learning, Bandura[21] discussed the importance of role models and how true mentors embody the role of a professional to provide us with a vision to achieve. True role models also provide a path for us to follow as we strive to achieve that vision; they help us understand what it takes to achieve competence and expertise in our profession. Wenger,[3] on the other hand, argued that it is more important for newcomers to be exposed to a wide variety of career paths so that we can each begin to negotiate our own way in developing a professional identity. As students, we have many mentors, and each may have taken a different path to success. By being exposed to a variety of clinicians with varying levels and types of success, we can begin to define who it is we want to be and how we want to be viewed as professionals. In the previous chapter, this was defined as providing the learner with access to history.

Key Points to Remember

The role of the mentor is to provide:
- Support
- Challenge
- Vision

A mentor helps the protégé to navigate the sociopolitical landscape of a new environment and provides both career and psychosocial functions.

Mentorship in Physical Therapy Education

Stop and Reflect

- In what ways do you think the role of a clinical instructor is similar to that of a mentor as described above? What functions are the same?
- In what ways do you think the role of a clinical instructor is different from that of a mentor as described above? What functions are different?

The Role of the Clinical Instructor in Mentoring Students

When we enter the clinical setting as physical therapy students, typically we are assigned to a clinical instructor for the purpose of orientation and socialization and to help us make sense of and apply our theoretical knowledge. The role of the clinical instructor in physical therapy education is similar to, yet somewhat different from, that described by Daloz[9] and Kram.[13] Responsibilities of the clinical instructor include planning for and orienting the student, developing objectives, designing and implementing learning experiences, identifying problems, providing feedback, and completing formative and summative evaluation.[23] The role of the clinical instructor as assessor or evaluator, is not traditionally viewed as a function of a mentor, although assessment is critical to the mentor's ability to provide appropriate challenges and supports and to identify potential barriers to learning. The clinical internship is a component of the professional curriculum, and although clinical instructors may not award grades, they do provide input on student performance, which ultimately impacts the overall grade awarded. Assessment for the purpose of grading raises an issue of power in physical therapy education that may, in some cases, change the dynamics of a traditional mentoring relationship. On the other hand, the clinical instructor-student relationship may lay a foundation for future mentoring experiences.

The Learning Triad: Moving Beyond the Clinical Instructor

Physical therapy clinical education today is most often provided in a one-to-one mentoring model consisting of a student-clinical instructor dyad. Some would describe this as a formal mentoring relationship even though it is relatively short lived and focuses primarily on career functions and on-the-job training.[11,13] In physical therapy clinical education, this mentoring relationship takes place within a community of practice. So although Daloz[9] suggested that it is the mentor who provides the vision, challenges, and supports, recent research shows that vision, challenges, supports, and barriers can emerge from many aspects of the clinical setting.[1,19,24] Our learning and development in the clinical setting are really the result of our interactions with many different individuals. These interactions result in a complex learning triad consisting of the student, the clinical instructor, and the entire health care community (eg, patients, families, other therapists, doctors, nurses, other health care workers, other students, etc) (Figure 8-1).

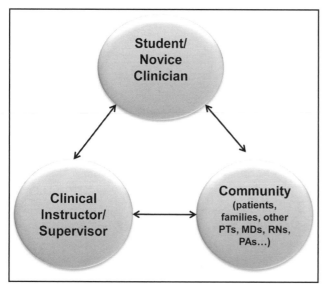

Figure 8-1. The learning triad.

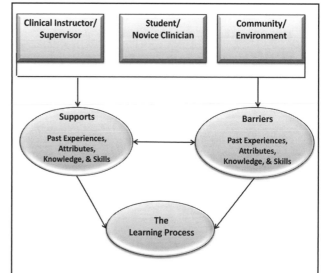

Figure 8-2. Barriers to and supports for the learning process.

Potential Barriers and Supports to Learning in the Clinical Setting

We already described the importance of having access to different challenges in the learning environment, and we defined challenges as those activities, experiences, or ordeals that we are faced with while in the clinical setting, which we need to overcome or master as we learn. In contrast, *barriers* are factors that hinder our learning, make it more difficult for us to overcome or master these challenges, or constrain or restrict us from fully participating in the community of practice. Our research highlighted how we each bring our own personal history and experiences with us to any learning situation, as do the members of the already established community of practice. Interactions that occur within the learning triad have the potential to facilitate as well as hinder our learning because both supports and barriers can emanate from each component of this triad (Figure 8-2). Each member of the learning triad presents with his or her own unique set of attributes, knowledge, and skills, so each learning situation is a unique confluence of factors that can support, and at times impede, learning.

Barriers

Boud and Walker[25] noted that personal assumptions; negative past experiences; expectations; inadequate preparation; lack of time; a hostile, unreceptive, or threatening environment; and the like can present barriers to learning. Many of the students and practicing clinicians we spoke with agreed and shared examples from their own experiences. They discussed how their

own past experiences and attributes sometimes negatively influenced the learning situation and described how their own lack of confidence, fear, shyness, language limitations, or cultural differences sometimes hindered their learning (Table 8-1).

You may remember, from the last chapter, the student who shared a prime example of how her presuppositions and negative past experiences became barriers to her own learning. She tried to avoid conflict with her father at all costs because of his explosive nature. Stories she shared about her interactions with her clinical instructor showed that she continued to avoid conflict in a similar manner in the clinical setting as well. As a result, she avoided asking questions of her clinical instructor and limited the dialogue that occurred. Without dialogue, assumptions were made, both by the student and her clinical instructor, which further limited learning. Shared meaning is central to the learning process, and without dialogue shared meaning cannot develop.[1,3]

Several interviewees described how their own lack of confidence, fear of being wrong or making a mistake, prevented them from asking questions or sharing their thoughts. More often than not, they shared how they decided not to disagree or ask questions because they were afraid to look bad in front of their clinical instructors. This not only limited the dialogue that took place but the potential for learning. On the contrary, one student commented on how he much preferred to let his clinical instructor see his weaknesses. He found that by doing so the clinical instructor could help him correct his thinking, and this often resulted in rich discussions that enhanced his learning. In a recent study, a few of the students and novice clinicians described how the reverse—excessive confidence—could be a barrier to their learning as well. Overly confident individuals

Table 8-1. Potential Barriers to Learning Resulting From Learner Characteristics

Students and novice clinicians both experienced that personal characteristics can act as potential barriers to their own learning; these characteristics include **a lack of confidence, excessive confidence, language or cultural differences, defensiveness, inability to accept constructive criticism, or a lack of respect.**
Illustrative quotes: "Every time I go into these clinics, I feel very nervous and insecure. If I were more secure, I would probably communicate more openly." "Students are always worried that they're going to do the wrong thing. Their biggest fear when they get to clinic is that they are not going to know what to do. It's a new working environment, much different than actual school. So the student is always worried that they are going to screw up, especially the first few weeks—Am I going to give this person the wrong answer, is he going to think I'm dumb, is he going to fail me?—They are always worried, it takes them a few weeks to get adjusted to making mistakes and saying, 'It's okay, I'll think about it harder.'" "Your pride and your confidence can really hinder you from establishing a relationship because if you are over confident and you are over proud, you cannot ask for help, and without asking for help, you just going to be stuck where you are; you're never going to grow, and you're never going to learn." "At times, I feel as though I can't get the words out. You want to say it but, the words just ain't coming. Sometimes I know the perfect way to respond in Chinese, but no one here understands what I want to say so you're trying to find a similar response in English but there's not really a response that's similar enough to relate the meaning you want to express." "Not truly being open to criticism. When there's a difficulty accepting criticism, it starts to build a wall, and that wall expands across the whole department. You could tell from the sound of their voice, sometimes body language—they're defensive and stand-offish." "As Americans, we have so much freedom to speak. Sometimes with our CIs, we cross the line; we speak our mind, and we're completely disrespectful. Instead of complying with what they know and who they are, it has to be taught to some students that because the CIs have more experience than we do, even though they might be younger, we have to respect it as students and not question. A lot of people are not used to that. We're all used to being these outstanding personalities, but it really hinders our success in situation[s] like this. Students are given so many rights and so few responsibilities, and they really lose respect. And they carry this to the clinic when a lot of CIs came from different countries and that's unacceptable behavior."

CI indicates clinical instructor.

tend not to ask for confirmation or clarification, making the assumption that they are correct, again limiting the potential for open dialogue and the development of shared meaning.[19]

The attributes of the students can pose potential barriers to learning, and certain attributes of the clinical instructors and supervisors can be equally problematic. It can be challenging to work with a clinical instructor who has a limited knowledge or skill base, but the same can be said for students who lack knowledge or skill as well (Tables 8-2 and 8-3). What students found to be more of a hindrance to their learning was working with clinical instructors who were inconsistent, overly demanding, condescending, uncaring, or disrespectful. Some students found themselves in clinical settings where the community itself was not receptive or responsive to their needs. They also expressed how working with clinical instructors who lacked skill in providing clear expectations, feedback, and supervision was problematic at times. Even the pace and evaluative nature of the environment can be a potential barrier to learning for some in the clinical setting. Table 8-4 provides some quotes that exemplify potential barriers to learning resulting from the characteristics of the clinical instructor.

Several students and novice clinicians described their experiences with disrespectful clinicians. They described the sense of embarrassment they felt after being reprimanded in front of others and how these reprimands often came without any attempt to actively listen or understand their thinking. The resulting embarrassment closed down communication and made it difficult for them to face other professionals with any sense of credibility. Sometimes this fear of embarrassment followed them to their next internship and is a reminder of how negative past experiences can influence future actions. Once communication was closed down, the negotiation process could not progress, and shared meaning was never developed. Furthermore, having lost credibility, access to additional challenges and activities may very well be limited, further impeding the entire learning process.[1]

A number of students described a power differential and how they chose not to risk disagreement or share differences of opinion because they were afraid of receiving a lower grade. This power differential significantly limited their freedom to ask questions and ultimately engage in effective dialogue. To truly engage in dialogue, it is important that each person has the ability to contribute by asking questions, agreeing, disagreeing, or challenging what is being said. It is also important that both participants in any dialogue are open to truly hearing what the other is saying.[26] A power differential, where one participant feels more empowered than the

Table 8-2. Potential Barriers to Learning Resulting From Clinician Characteristics

The personal characteristics of clinical instructors and supervisors can act as potential barriers to student learning; these characteristics include **inconsistency, an overly-demanding and uncaring nature, disrespect, intimidation, unreceptiveness, or unresponsiveness.**

Illustrative quotes:

"She would say, 'You should know what that is' or 'Go look it up.' It just got to the point where I was afraid to ask her a question so the communication just really closed down."

"I never passed the stage of, 'I don't measure up.' There was always anxiety and tension. Every time she spoke to me, I froze and that's really not conducive to learning."

"A person that projects this superiority makes you feel that it doesn't matter what you do, you will never be as smart as I am. My previous CI was like that. Even though she was only 3 years out of college, she made a big deal of how important she is and how superior she is and how I won't even come close."

"My CI put me down in front of the patient. It made me feel stupid and inadequate; it made the patient lose all trust in me. I will never do that to anyone, particularly a student."

"I didn't feel like she was approachable, she always went in her office and shut the door. She was like 'Please don't come in' so I never was able to ask her question. If we were doing rounds, she was watching me like a hawk. It was very uncomfortable. I could have learned much more from her but I didn't know how to get if from her. I couldn't get anything out of her. I was scared to death of her."

"I had to deal with a CI that made me feel inept and was not open and receptive. Communication was virtually impossible and was made worse by the fact that I was forced to remain quiet even if I disapproved of her methods or her techniques. I was not allowed to justify my rationales for treatment. Since she would rather 'I did as she did,' I was forced to remain a silent recipient because my future depended on her midterm and final evaluation of my performance."

CI indicates clinical instructor.

Table 8-3. Potential Barriers to Learning Resulting From a Lack of Knowledge

Students and novice clinicians noted that having **a limited knowledge base** or being in an **unfamiliar situation** was a potential barrier.

Illustrative quote:

"It is a totally new environment, totally new people, and you're just very hesitant about what you are going to say and do. You are afraid of what you will say. You're afraid of how you'll react and that in a sense hinders what you are as a person."

Table 8-4. Potential Barriers to Learning Resulting From the Clinical Instructor's Lack of Skill

Some students and novice clinicians encountered **clinical instructors with limited teaching and supervisory skills.** Their comments suggest that how, when, and how much feedback and independence their clinical instructors provided were potential barriers.

Illustrative quotes:

"You have a million things running through your head. You don't really concentrate on the patient you are with. You're back-playing the beginning of the day—freaking out about your mistakes. It showers you with this anxiety. You can't think you're so stressed. It's just horrible. You don't care so much about the patients, I just concentrated on avoiding mistakes. I didn't learn anything."

"A lot of CIs just assume, 'Okay, let's just throw them in there and see how they do.' How are you supposed to know you're supposed to do something or be a certain way if someone doesn't tell you as a student?"

CI indicates clinical instructor.

other, can limit effective dialogue. At times, this power differential was exacerbated by clinical instructors who were overly judgmental, authoritative, condescending, or overly demanding. All of this led to limited communication. Without this communication, both access and negotiation of shared meaning were impeded.[1]

Communication is integral to effective teaching and learning. Communication is a collaborative process that requires openness on the part of both the student and clinical instructor. It is also a skill that needs to be developed and refined. Just as students have responsibility to seek and receive feedback on their communication skills, it is equally important that the clinical instructor share this responsibility in providing feedback and in seeking feedback on their own skills.

Critical Thinking Clinical Scenario

You just started your second full-time internship and you are preparing for orientation with your new clinical instructor. In your last setting, you felt very uncomfortable and were afraid to speak up. Your clinical instructor tended not to give you any feedback until the end of the week or would comment directly in front of patients.

Reflective Questions

1. What strategies would you discuss with your new clinical instructor that would help minimize the chances that you would be faced with some of the issues described above?

2. What suggestions would you give your clinical instructor regarding how and when you find feedback most effective?

The clinical environment itself can be stressful for newcomers, in part because of its novelty.[1] Ideally, it is important for clinical education experiences to occur in environments that support learning.[27] Some of the students and clinicians we spoke with described how they perceived that this was not always the case and that their stress was exacerbated by a community that lacked empathy, was too busy, or was unwelcoming; this is consistent with what Boud and Walker[25] described as a hostile environment. This, too, has the potential to limit learning. A number of the individuals described how being in such an environment left each of them feeling like an outsider. It did not empower them to develop a sense of belonging, which is critical to professional identity development.[3] An unwelcoming environment can limit your ability to gain access and fully engage in all of the activities of the community, again hindering the learning process.

To optimize learning in the clinical setting, it is critical that students and clinicians alike be actively engaged in the teaching and learning process. If the student or the clinicians or the community is not receptive to engaging in this process, learning can be hindered.[19] Learning in an established community of practice such as the clinic requires a true give-and-take from both the newcomer and those within the community. As noted in the previous chapter, Wenger[3] described this as production and reproduction. Experienced clinicians who have been in a certain environment for some time are invested in maintaining the established expectations and traditions of the community and passing them on to newcomers (ie, reproduction); simultaneously, newcomers bring new information and ideas to the community that can result in changes and add to the evolution of the community (ie, production). Newcomers need to feel valued, respected, and listened to for what they bring to the community; likewise, experienced clinicians need to feel valued for the experience and wisdom they bring to practice.

Being valued and respected may mean different things to different people.[19] Compliance and reproduction (ie, the concept of following the traditions and established expectations of the community) generally are accepted by most students in the clinical setting. This is evidenced by comments such as "You need to comply," "You need to make your clinical instructor happy," or "Your role as a student is to absorb all you can." For new graduates, being valued and respected often meant that their ideas and suggestions were considered by members of the community. One new graduate shared how disempowered he felt when his supervisor never listened to any of his suggestions. He felt like he was not accepted or respected, and this prevented him from developing a sense of belonging within that community. He ultimately left that position to accept one where he felt that he could be valued for what he brought to the community. In this situation, a lack of receptivity posed such a barrier that neither the graduate nor the community could move through the negotiation process successfully.

Characteristics of the clinical environment itself can also pose potential impediments to learning (see Table 8-5). Some of the students and new graduates we spoke with described the environment as being too fast paced for learning, although the reverse was also noted to be problematic. For students, the grading process was an additional threat and potential barrier to learning. Some described their internship experiences like "taking a test every day." Table 8-5 provides some quotes that exemplify how the characteristics of the environment and community can potentially hinder learning.

Critical Thinking Clinical Scenario

The director of clinical education (DCE) is meeting with a student who is in the middle of her second internship. The clinical instructor asked for the meeting because she was concerned that the student was not taking initiative in working with patients, was not completing the homework assignments as requested, and seemed to be lacking both in knowledge and skill. In speaking with the student, the DCE realized that the student had a negative experience with her first clinical instructor, who provided very little feedback. Whenever the student tried to take initiative or offer suggestions, her first clinical instructor was very critical. As a result, she was afraid to try anything new or even to start patient care without first asking permission. She indicated that she did all of her assignments but did not want to bother the clinical instructor in the morning because she knew she was very busy. The student also indicated that the environment is very fast paced, and she has little time to communicate with her clinical instructor about what she does and does not know.

Reflective Questions

1. What potential barriers are represented in this scenario? Consider the student, the clinical instructor, and the community.

2. As the DCE, what advice might you give to the student and to the clinical instructor?

Table 8-5. Potential Barriers to Learning Resulting From Community or Environmental Characteristics

Below are characteristics of the clinical environment or community that students and novice clinicians experienced as having the potential to impede their abilities to interact, communicate, and ultimately learn; these characteristics most notably included **a lack of receptivity (ie, an unwelcoming disposition), a lack of responsiveness, grading, pace, and competition.**

Illustrative quotes:

"It was like, 'Ok, good she's [the student] here, I'm taking off.' They would take off days, call in sick, come in late. And I was like, wait a minute, 'How is this a typical work situation?' I felt I wasn't getting the full feel for things. It was just, 'Oh, good here's the student, she'll pick up the slack.'"

"All the PTs go out to lunch, and no one invited the students. Students eat in their corner, and the therapists go wherever. If you are the only student in the place, that's really hard. No one says, 'Oh, you want to come along? We are going to eat lunch.' It's a weird feeling."

"My second day at my affiliation, I sat down, and the one therapist said to me, 'Ok, you can leave now. We are having a meeting now. Students aren't welcome; you have to go.' It made me feel very uncomfortable, and I feel it very definitely set the stage for later on or throughout the rest of the clinic because they definitely made me feel uncomfortable."

"I felt very reluctant to say anything because I was a student, and when you're in those kinds of settings, being graded by them, you can't really do anything or say anything, because I have to be graded. I said to myself, 'Just bite your tongue don't say anything. If you rock the boat too much, you might not do as well.' So I sat back and said nothing."

"Pass and fail, that's your major concern when you come in. If you are stuck in this phase, 'Oh, I might fail,' you don't really care about learning, you're just desperate for passing."

"In my first clinical experience, we saw so many patients a day I just felt that was the worst learning experience for me. There wasn't enough time with each patient. There wasn't enough time to communicate. It was really hard for me to discuss anything with my CI; he didn't have time to talk."

"It just wasn't a busy office, so I was there at one point, and we would see 7 patients for the day. There were 3 of us students, so I did a lot of sitting around as opposed to treating patients, so it wasn't a good learning experience."

"It became competitive between the 2 students, and that actually hindered the student that was doing poorly in particular. It became a vicious cycle; the more you compete with somebody and compare yourself, the more pressure that put on her and she fell further behind and got more frustrated. It wasn't a healthy relationship."

PT indicates physical therapist; CI, clinical instructor.

Key Points to Remember

- Potential barriers to learning can emanate from all aspects of the learning triad.
- Knowledge, skill, and characteristics of the student, clinical instructor, and community all can present potential barriers to learning in the clinical environment.
- Personal assumptions, unclear or false expectations, past negative experiences, and inadequate preparation (ie, lack of knowledge or skills) all can potentially impede learning.
- Student characteristics that have the potential to be problematic include a lack of confidence, overconfidence, lack of motivation, or lack of willingness to admit error.
- CI characteristics that have the potential to be problematic include being condescending, authoritative, or overly demanding.
- Community characteristics that have the potential to be problematic include being unwelcoming, unreceptive, or uncaring.
- The environment itself can be a potential impediment to learning if it is too fast paced or even too slow paced.
- These are considered potential barriers to learning because what may be a barrier to one may not be a barrier to another (eg, fast-paced environment).

Supports

Just as barriers can emerge from all 3 components of the learning triad, so too can supports. Past work and clinical experiences helped prepare some students to engage in activities in the clinical setting. Particular characteristics of students, novice clinicians, clinical instructors, supervisors, the community, and the environment can also support learning. Being familiar with the environment and the patient population and being paired with clinical instructors who are knowledgeable and skillful in providing clear expectations, feedback, and supervision can certainly facilitate the learning process.[19]

Stop and Reflect

What characteristics (cognitive, psychomotor, and affective) would you ascribe to a good clinical instructor?

Emery[28] described the characteristics of an effective clinical instructor, which included effective:

- Communication skills (eg, sharing information, providing feedback, actively listening, and encouraging dialogue)

- Interpersonal skills (eg, creating a comfortable environment, empathetic and supportive of students)

- Professional skills (eg, practicing competently, systematic in problem solving)

- Teaching skills (eg, allowing for progressive student independence while also providing constructive criticism).

Kelly[27] added the importance of making time for students as well as having a work environment that is supportive of clinical education. Daloz[9] suggested that a key function of the mentor is to provide support to the protégé, and Kram[13] suggested that support from the mentor went beyond coaching and sponsoring (ie, career functions) to include the psychosocial functions of acceptance, confirmation, and friendship. In a complex system like the community of practice of the clinical setting, providing support is not limited solely to the mentor.[19] Just as with the potential barriers to learning, the potential supports to learning can emerge from past experiences, attributes, knowledge, and skills of the entire learning triad (ie, the newcomer, the mentor, and the community; see Figure 8-2). Exemplary quotes illustrating each of the concepts we will be describing can be found in Tables 8-6 to 8-11.

When a mentor or clinical instructor possesses effective skills in providing supervision and feedback and is consistent and clear in establishing expectations, newcomers feel supported in their learning.[19,27,28] Having clear expectations establishes the norms of the community and facilitates the newcomer's understanding of those norms, while at the same time, providing consistent and effective supervision and feedback can help ensure the accuracy of the learning. Effective supervision includes providing newcomers with access to engage with other clinicians and role models, thus making them mentors to the process as well[19] (see Tables 8-6 and 8-7).

Table 8-6. Potential Supports to Learning Resulting From the Skills of the Supervisor

Students and clinicians experienced skillful clinical instructors and supervisors that facilitated their learning. The skills these clinicians possessed included **their ability to provide clear expectations, effective supervision, and constructive feedback.**

Illustrative quotes:

"My CI sat me down the first day and said what she expected of me. It put me such at ease, and I knew right away that it was okay. This is where I fit in."

"Clearly determined objectives at the start of the affiliation made it less stressful since I knew what was expected of me and what to work for from the beginning."

"Supportive supervision is what M. was doing. She would observe what I was doing; she would teach me how I could do it better; give me feedback, not just staring over my shoulder simply pointing out your every mistake."

"Giving me more responsibility definitely helped me. It made me feel a little bit more confident, and that opened me up even more. I was able to bring more questions to the table because I had different experiences so that helped."

"At least once a week, we would talk about how things were going. Throughout that week, I would also get feedback. But, this was definitely a time when we could sit down. He [was] always in the room to listen and comment. He gave constant feedback; he didn't leave it for the end of the week."

"If there is a problem, we'd sit down; we'd talk about it. Ongoing communication works best, rather than waiting for a specific time at the end of the week. If there is a situation on Monday, I'm not going to wait until Friday to discuss it, I'm going to correct it immediately and be ready to move on."

"She would not say, 'Oh you did a great job' no matter what I tried to do until the CCCE (supervisor) asked her, 'How will the student know anything? How will the student have self confidence if you don't tell the student, You did this good?' If you had a patient you're not telling this patient, 'Oh very good oh keep trying.' How would the patient know that they are making progress?"

"She took me in a private place away from everybody, and nobody was able to hear what she was saying. She was calm, made each point clear, gave me particular examples, gave me a solution, and didn't say go and figure it out, that's probably the best thing."

"At the end of the day, she would discuss everything with me. She would give me positive feedback, and she would give me negative. She would say this is what you need to work on, this is where you are now; you are doing so great."

"During my first clinical, I was very nervous about what my CI would say in front of a patient if I was doing something incorrectly. It was important to me that the patient had confidence in my skills. She recognized this and discussed my concerns with me before starting treatments. Together, we developed a system in which I was very comfortable receiving feedback in front of the patient. She would make eye contact with me and give me a questioning look. I would then pause and discuss what I was doing and adjust accordingly. It felt very collegial and decreased my stress level to almost nothing."

CI indicates clinical instructor.

Table 8-7. Potential Supports to Learning Resulting From Characteristics of the Clinical Instructor

Students and novice clinicians cited that certain characteristics that clinical instructors possessed were beneficial to the teaching-learning situation, which included being **approachable, adaptable, intuitive, caring, constructive, respectful, open, and honest.**

Illustrative quotes:

"This is the advice I would have for new CIs: be very easy to approach; don't be a nitpicker; give them some leeway; let them have room for mistakes; don't jump on their case when they do make mistakes."

"One of the things that we try to do is make people feel comfortable so they have less apprehension about approaching their clinical instructor or any of the physical therapists at work."

"You can't be too controlling. You really do have to be flexible to that person's particular needs. You can't treat every student the same. You have to be adaptable to their particular needs. And make them feel as though this is a good learning experience."

"My biggest challenge is to ask for help, so, for me to ask for help I better be stuck there. This CI, she would offer me help by herself without my having to ask. Whenever she saw me stuck, she would say, 'Oh, you need help? Do you want me to show you?' She was not too proud to ask me if I needed help because she saw that I was not asking for help. Unlike my previous CI, she didn't say, 'Oh, you are not asking for help. You are a terrible person.'"

"The experience I had which helped me was the 2 therapists I worked with gave me a lot of positive feedback about my work. They would bring up specific things I did and praise me for it. This encouraged me to work harder as well as feel more comfortable in the work environment. With my newfound confidence, I was better able to interact with patients and faculty."

"I let them develop their skills and their confidence. I don't cut them off; I let them say whatever they need to say and if they don't say it right, then I would interject at the end. I never make them feel bad in front of the patient. I know that once you belittle somebody in front of somebody else when you're trying to establish yourself, it's the worst knock you can give somebody; it just makes you feel stupid."

"I had this patient who took me aside and told me that I was very hesitant and nervous. She said, 'Can sense it.' And she told me I should just get over it and be more relaxed. Then, towards the end of my clinical, she was still there, and she said, 'I'm so proud of you; you made a great improvement.' That is when I realized that my communication skills improved."

CI indicates clinical instructor.

Creating a supportive learning environment requires more than the skills of a single individual. Emery,[28] Kram,[13] and Kelly[27] described the characteristics of a good mentor and clinical instructor. In addition to skills in teaching and supervision, the mentor must possess effective interpersonal skills. It is important to remember that the characteristics of the community also can contribute to the development of a supportive learning environment.[19] Responsiveness, care, respect, and empathy from both the clinical instructor and from the community can all result in a comfortable, supportive learning environment, which reduces stress and opens the lines of communication necessary for students to ask questions, admit error, and begin to negotiate meaning (see Table 8-8).

The characteristics of the student also play a critical role in the learning situation (see Tables 8-9 and 8-10). Past personal and work experiences (ie, fast-paced jobs and familiarity resulting from previous clinical experiences) can make the learning situation more manageable for students. Equally important is that students who are more self-directed, adaptable, and confident are empowered to more fully engage in practice, dialogue, and in the negotiation process. Other important traits include motivation, persistence, and receptivity. It is clear that when the student, the mentor, and the community all are knowledgeable, skilled, and receptive to learning, more information is shared and discussed; newcomers are made to feel comfortable and welcomed, and ultimately they are provided with more access to people activities and history, all of which we now know are critical to learning in the clinical environment[1] (see Table 8-11).

Critical Thinking Clinical Scenario

Refer back to the scenario in which the Director of Clinical Education is meeting with a student who is in the middle of her second internship. Consider that prior to coming to physical therapy school, she had a responsible position in corporate finance. Academically, she is a good student and well connected with her peers. The facility where she is interning has a large staff of physical therapists, physical therapist assistants, and currently has 2 other students on site. She is excited to be in this outpatient facility because she sees herself ultimately working in a similar facility in the future.

Reflective Questions

1. What potential supports are represented in this scenario? Consider the student, clinical instructor, and community.

2. Did the advice you gave incorporate use of all of the potential supports available?

Table 8-8. Potential Supports Resulting From Environmental and Community Characteristics

Students and clinicians cited certain environmental and community characteristics as being beneficial to the teaching learning situation, which included being **welcoming, open, and receptive to students.**

Illustrative quotes:

"The staff members at each facility were very warm and accepting. They were able to understand that, as a student, I did not have much clinical experience."

"What made it easy was the people around. At my clinical setting, they were very open, very friendly, and that helped. They were good at communicating, which helped me get over my uncomfortableness in the beginning."

"The patient knew I was a student. I was learning, and she was okay with that. She was intrigued by what I knew and was open to suggestion and understood where I was coming from, and the interaction was very beneficial and made me feel good as far as a student, knowing that you got that kind of response."

"The patients weren't asking questions to test her; they were asking her because they were interested in her as their practitioner and that helped her more than me complimenting her. It was really the reinforcement from the patient that really did it."

"One of my patients wrote a very nice note to the 'floor' about me. I never treated her just like another patient, her well being mattered to me, and it really showed in my actions with her, but I was just doing my job. However, her ability to acknowledge it and to take action by writing a nice letter made me feel great. I'll never forget her."

"The patient population here is pretty friendly. People here chat all day. It's a pretty friendly environment. Everybody here would help each other out. Unlike at my last place where everybody was just very busy, they don't really help you as much. Here, in a sense, it is kind of like a family."

"There was plenty of time to sit down with my CI and discuss things and to sit down with the patient at the same time. I could learn a lot of his techniques, and he could see how I was doing. Time really was a plus. Time to actually sit down and talk to other therapists was very helpful."

CI indicates clinical instructor.

Table 8-9. Potential Supports to Learning Resulting From Past Experiences

Students and novice clinicians reported that **personal past experiences** (ie, personal, work, and/or clinical) helped to prepare them to interact and communicate on a professional level.

Illustrative quotes:

"I used to teach skiing. I taught for about 5 years so I became very comfortable with just my interpersonal skills on that basis 'cause I had interactions from different people from all over the countries, all different backgrounds, and you really get to know all different types of people."

"This may sound silly, but the fast-paced stuff, being a waitress helped me a lot. I remember being at the private practice, and we had 6 rooms, so it was almost like 6 tables. You ordered this, she ordered that. Having to keep it in my head helped me a lot. Also interaction with people. I'm a shy person, but being a waitress, I wasn't shy. So being a therapist, I'm not shy."

"Definitely working as an aide for a couple of years, I got to see a lot. I knew a lot about PT before I even had my first affiliation. For a lot of people, just being in the environment is overwhelming, so I was accustomed to the PT environment already. I was accustomed to the interaction between therapists and knowing what that's like as much as I could without being that person."

"You acquire your interpersonal skills throughout life. You pick up on others' actions, how your peers act and how they conduct themselves. I cannot recall a specific incident. It's more of a cumulative effect you see how people are treated and act, and you think that's how I should act or shouldn't or I'd like to be treated like that or not treated like that. It's those personal experiences which help mold your skills."

PT indicates physical therapist.

Table 8-10. Potential Supports to Learning Resulting From Learner Characteristics

Students and clinicians both reported that certain characteristics of the learner were beneficial to the teaching-learning situation; these characteristics include **adaptability, self-directedness, motivation, receptiveness, responsiveness, caring, empathy, respect, and confidence.**

Illustrative quotes:

"Her easygoing nature, ability to be flexible, ability to accept constructive feedback without being defensive, her social skills."

"She's just somebody who's really been able to kind of come in and assimilate with everybody. She just goes with the flow, and she's flexible."

"She had great initiative. I never had to tell her. She'd see patients waiting, and she would automatically know they're our patients. She was just so prepared for the day; not every student does that. For her, it was just very automatic. The initiative was just there."

"She was quiet, a little quieter than most students but she had initiative. So in terms of fitting in with the therapists, there was an acceptance. She was doing the things that you asked; taking an active role in their clinical education. That automatically let's you take that person in as part of the group. She fit in very well."

"Some students get very frustrated. She didn't; she stayed with it, which is exactly the way I would handle it. She wanted to come up with the answer; it was very motivating to her. Her personality was like, 'I'm going to figure this out; I'm not going to give up.'"

"She observed, and she took in everything. She knew her weaknesses, and she knew her strengths. If I gave her criticism, she would never say, 'But.' A lot of students would give a defensive answer; she would totally say, fine, thank you, and she would go on. She always learned from her mistakes."

"'I'm a new graduate. I know I have a lot to learn from everyone, and I'm willing to learn.' She gave that feeling that I'm open to your input. And that was really important."

"She's so confident. I am so amazed because as a student I wasn't like that at all. It took me a few years to gain that confidence to be able to just walk over to anybody and introduce myself. I've never seen that in a student before. It opened a lot of doors for her. She got a lot of experience, she learned a lot. Surgeons were drawing pictures for her. She walked over to an orthopedic surgeon asked about a new kind of surgery, and the guy just threw off his scrubs and explained everything to her."

"Even if I feel like I was completely wrong, I said it anyway, because maybe I would have to go back 3 steps, maybe I took a wrong turn in my thinking—so we would talk about it. I wouldn't keep my mouth shut just so I would not sound stupid. I let him know how stupid I am. I wanted to show him all my faults so we could fix things at the ground level, so I did let him know how stupid I was."

"He was confident in who he was and that's the thing that most helped him. That was atypical."

"She would come in at lunch and listen to us talking. We knew her, and she knew everybody. She was comfortable talking to other therapists and so she became part of the staff after a while."

Table 8-11. Potential Supports to Learning Resulting From Knowledgeable Students, Clinical Instructors, and Patients

Besides past experiences and attributes, students and novice clinicians cited knowledge as being a support to their ability to communicate and interact on a professional level. This knowledge included **familiarity with the patient population, familiarity with the setting and the individuals within that setting, as well as having knowledgeable supervisors and patients.** They commented on how their communication flowed more smoothly when they had the didactic knowledge to support what they were saying.

Illustrative quotes:

"I feel so much more comfortable providing information when I have something I know so much about."

"If I'm talking about a condition or pathology of which I have a good understanding, it tends to flow better. It tends to be more accurate. Whereas if you ask me something I don't know, I may just be limited in what I can say."

"I am just much more relaxed with the diagnosis I am more familiar with … so when I approach a patient I am more relaxed and can communicate better."

"My CI was really helpful; she was just there every step of the way, explaining things. It is very supportive when they are there and explain it to you, because not every patient is the same."

"A great CI is someone who is knowledgeable in what they are doing and who is willing to share that knowledge with you."

"It was the background knowledge of the patient that helped because one of the patients never had the problem, so it was kind of hard to explain it to her, while this other patient had a similar problem, and it was so much easier to explain to her because she was already familiar with it. It is definitely the patient's knowledge."

CI indicates clinical instructor.

Key Points to Remember

- Supports can emerge from the knowledge, skills, and attributes of all 3 components of the learning triad: the student, clinical instructor, and community/environment.
- Past personal, work, and clinical experiences along with familiarity with the environment and the patient population help prepare students to engage in activities in the clinical setting.
- The personal characteristics of students, novice clinicians, clinical instructors, supervisors, the community, and the environment can support learning.
  - Students: Self-directed, adaptable, confident, motivated, persistent, and receptive
  - Clinical instructors and the community: Open, welcoming, responsive, respectful, caring, and empathetic
- Knowledge and skills (eg, being paired with clinical instructors who are knowledgeable and skillful in providing clear expectations, feedback, and supervision) can facilitate the learning process.

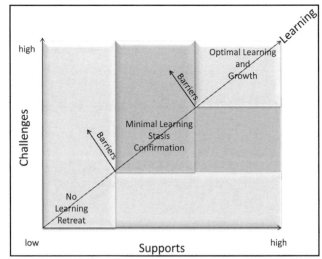

Figure 8-3. Challenges, supports, and barriers.

Barriers and Supports as Uniquely Defined

Though some commonalities may exist, barriers and supports are uniquely defined by the individual within a given context. Two students named Eva and Jackie discussed similarly demanding and critical clinical instructors. Eva described how this negatively affected her learning and stated that she ultimately learned very little from that setting; whereas, Jackie viewed it as a challenge to be mastered. Jackie commented that although she felt that her clinical instructor was trying to punish her by giving her an excessive workload, she took it as a challenge and learned a great deal from her experience. By the end of her internship, Jackie was glad that her clinical instructor had been so demanding because she felt she had developed a true sense of what it will be like to be a physical therapist functioning independently and responsibly.

Similarly, 2 other students described their experiences with clinical instructors who gave them a great deal of independence very early on in their clinical internship. Jan noted how the independence really made her take charge and helped her to learn how to communicate with patients, staff, doctors, and other therapists within the community. On the other hand, Kayla saw this independence as "throwing [her] to the lions" without any preparation. She viewed this as a barrier to her overall learning.

We have found that what one student may consider a challenge to be mastered, another may consider a barrier to learning, and yet another student may consider it

a support to learning. There is an interplay among the challenges, supports, and potential barriers that new clinicians face in the clinical setting, and this interplay is integral to the learning process that occurs in the community of practice.[19]

Knefelkamp et al[29] and Daloz[9] discussed the impact of challenge and support on the developmental process, suggesting that if as a student you are:

- Highly challenged and highly supported, you will learn and grow
- Highly challenged and minimally supported, you will retreat
- Minimally challenged and highly supported, your knowledge will simply be confirmed
- Minimally challenged and unsupported, your knowledge will remain static

In addition to challenges and supports, potential barriers to learning must be considered in this matrix as well.[19] Learning results from the mastery of challenges and optimal learning occurs when a novice is highly challenged and highly supported.[9,29] As we have already seen, barriers may exist that impede learning, and they may be present anywhere along the learning continuum (Figure 8-3). For example, a student may be faced with examining a patient for the first time (ie, high challenge) by a clinical instructor who is willing to coach her through the examination process (ie, high support). On the surface, this appears to be an optimal learning situation; however, the student may lack confidence and be so fearful of making a mistake that her own personal attributes present a barrier to her learning. In this case, the student may need more support than anticipated by the clinical instructor. Engaging the student in dialogue to develop a shared understanding of her concerns, along with strategies to facilitate her learning, may optimize this learning situation.

Barriers can emerge at any point in the clinical internship, and given the evaluative nature of the internship, ongoing dialogue is essential to ensure that learning is continually optimized. Optimizing supports and minimizing barriers will enable students and novice clinicians to master the challenges they face. It is important that we, as learners or teachers, take time to identify potential barriers to learning and seek supports to optimize learning and growth.

In our research, many of the scenarios shared by the interviewees fell neatly into the categories described by Knefelkamp et al[29] and Daloz,[9] where the students were simultaneously supported and challenged to grow and learn. Others illustrated how some newcomers seemed to grow and learn despite the limited support they received from their mentors in the clinical setting. In a community of practice, supports come from the individual and the community as well as the clinical instructor. In the previous scenario about Jackie, who had an overly demanding clinical instructor, though she did not necessarily feel supported by her clinical instructor, other clinicians within the community provided the support she needed by offering to speak with the clinical instructor or to help her with her patient load. Jackie was a self-confident individual, which provided an additional support and helped optimize her learning situation. Finally, Jackie viewed her situation as a challenge to be mastered, rather than an actual barrier to her learning. Her personal attributes, coupled with the support she received from the community, enabled her to overcome the excessive demands placed on her by her clinical instructor, and as a result she thrived (Figure 8-4).

faced. Not receiving support from their clinical instructors or supervisors, these individuals also relied heavily on the other 2 components of the learning triad.

To optimize learning as described by Knefelkamp et al[29] and Daloz,[9] students need to be simultaneously supported and challenged. Most often in the clinical setting, students receive an excellent balance of challenge and support. As noted in the previous example, there are times when students thrive in the clinical setting despite limited support from the clinical instructor or despite the excessive challenges. There are 2 primary reasons for this apparent discrepancy. First, in the community of practice, supports from other community members can compensate for an overly challenging clinical instructor or supervisor. Though a student who has not developed a good rapport with her clinical instructor may not necessarily feel supported by her clinical instructor, she may have developed an excellent rapport with other members of the clinical or academic community. The support received from those other members may very well be sufficient to optimize the learning experience for that student. Secondly, supports can also emerge from the attributes of the students themselves. A student may be working with a demanding clinical instructor who continually puts the student on the spot. Self-confidence on its own may provide just the right amount of support needed to overcome any potential barriers in this given learning situation. A student may be highly challenged and receive little to no support from his or her mentor but may still be able to view this potential barrier as a challenge to be mastered. This individual will learn and grow despite the challenges or barriers that he or she may face.

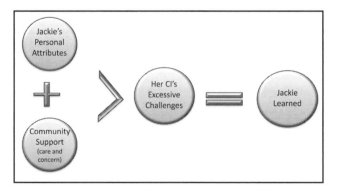

Figure 8-4. Jackie's learning triad.

Other students have found themselves in environments that they did not find very challenging, but because they were self-directed in their own learning, they were able to find activities to challenge themselves, which optimized their own learning. These individuals learned and grew despite the challenges or barriers they

<u>**Stop and Reflect**</u>

You are a clinical instructor and you are working with a student on her third internship.

- Knowing what you now know about the adult learner and the novice to expert continuum, what assumptions might you hold about the role of the student and the role of the clinical instructor in this scenario?

- How will you know if she is feeling sufficiently challenged or overwhelmed?

- What types of reflective questions might you ask the student to facilitate dialogue and determine how to best challenge and support the student while minimizing barriers to learning?

- In Chapter 4, you learned about classroom assessment techniques (CATs) and how you might modify some of these CATs to be used in the clinical setting. Refer back to these CATs, and reflect on which one(s) you might use to help you assess your student's progress.

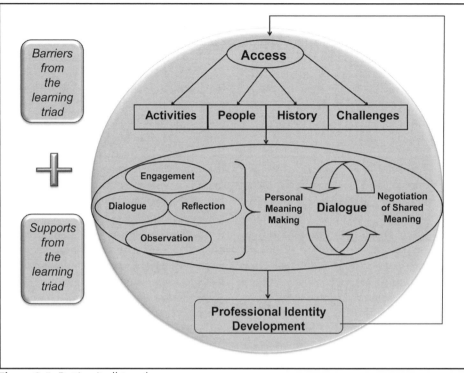

Figure 8-5. Putting it all together.

Critical Thinking Clinical Scenario

Fiona is a third-year student in an entry-level doctor of physical therapy program. She is on her final clinical internship and has done fine in her 2 previous internships. Fiona is also the mother of a 4-year-old and 2-year-old triplets. Before coming to the clinic in the morning, she is responsible for getting all of the children ready, and she brings them to day care on her way to the clinic. She gets to the clinic 30 to 45 minutes early so that she can breathe a bit and place a focus on her learning. Barbara is a new clinical instructor, and Fiona is her first student. She is anxious to do a good job and to make sure that Fiona has a good experience. She gets to work about 30 minutes early as well. As soon as Barbara arrives, she says to Fiona, "Let's go, so we can start reading the charts in the ICU." At lunch time, she asks Fiona, "Why don't you tell me what you want for lunch. I will go get it for you so you can just stay right here and work on your notes." This bothers Fiona, and she says, "I don't even know what is downstairs so how can I tell her what I want?" After a few days, Barbara says, "You know, you should just bring your lunch. It would save you time." Again, Fiona is bothered because she knows that she eats only ethnic food at home, and she does not want to bring it in because some people might not like the smell of it heating in the kitchen microwave. This goes on for some time, and the other therapists notice Barbara really working Fiona hard. A few of the therapists actually came up to Fiona and asked her, "Would you like me to speak with Barbara for you?" Fiona simply said, "No thank you." Fiona was determined to do her best and to show Barbara her skills. She was determined to "rise to the occasion and meet this challenge head on." One day, Fiona started to experience some chest pains. She called her doctor, who said she wanted to see Fiona the very next day. Fiona told Barbara what happened and that she would need to go for a stress test. Barbara said, "That is fine, but be sure to come back when you are done." Fiona said, "I might not be finished until about 3 or 4." Barbara said, "That is fine, come when you are done." These are some examples of how the clinical experience went with Barbara and Fiona. In the end, Fiona excelled, and Barbara told her how pleased she was with her performance. When it was all over, Fiona had a long talk with Barbara and suggested that she never treat a student like that again. Barbara listened, said she was sorry, and commented that the reason she was so tough on Fiona was because that is how her CI treated her when she was a student.

Reflective Questions

1. What challenges did the student in this scenario face?
2. What supports did Fiona draw on to make this a successful learning experience?
3. What other supports were needed?
4. Where and from whom could Fiona have gotten the supports she needed?
5. Where and from whom could Barbara have gotten the supports she needed?
6. What strategies would you use if you were faced with this situation?

> ### Key Points to Remember
>
> - Challenges, supports, and barriers emerge from all aspects of the learning triad.
> - Maximizing challenges and supports while minimizing the barriers will optimize learning.
> - To optimize learning, students and clinicians alike should look to their own personal attributes, knowledge, and skills, as well as those of the other members of the learning triad.
> - Learning in the clinical setting is a collaborative process requiring the student, clinical instructor, and community to be proactive in identifying challenges, supports, and potential strategies to overcome any barriers to learning.
> - Ongoing dialogue is essential to effective teaching and learning in the clinical setting.

Putting It All Together— How Students and Novice Clinicians Learn in the Clinic: A Confluence of Factors

Learning in the clinical environment is a complex process. As we have discussed, instructors and students alike must consider multiple factors in designing and preparing for effective teaching and learning experiences (See Figure 8-5 for a pictorial display of how learning takes place within the clinical setting).

Whether you are a new student, an experienced student, or a new graduate, before entering the clinical environment, you must have achieved a certain level of competence. This competence in physical therapy typically means academic success.[30] It is this academic success that provides you with the initial credibility needed to be accepted in the clinical environment as a legitimate peripheral participant.[4,31] Credibility allows you into the environment, but it is the access that is achieved once you are in the clinical setting that optimizes your learning.

As a student, you are assigned to a clinical instructor to act as your mentor. Your clinical instructor is the conduit through which you gain initial access. This traditional dyadic relationship becomes a triadic one in which the entire community is involved in the teaching-learning process. Access provides you with the opportunity to engage in practice with other community members, to observe, and to interact with a variety of people and role models, including patients and therapists as they move through their daily routine. Engagement is more than observing and interacting; it is acting, belonging, and becoming an actual member of the community, albeit rather limited at first.

Engagement provides you with a sense of belonging and a sense of becoming—an idea of what it takes to be a physical therapist.

Though the mentor is your initial conduit to this engagement, it is your involvement with the entire community that provides you with a full vision of what professionalism and skill look like within this community of practice. As Wenger[3] suggested, having access to several members of the community allows you to view the range of possibilities that exist within the profession. Engagement with the mentor and other community members also provides you with a bridge to help connect past, present, and future. By sharing their history, their expertise, and how they developed from novice to expert, you can begin to make sense of where you currently fit in, where you would like to ultimately see yourself as a professional, and how you can get there.

Access includes exposure to and involvement with the full array of challenges that therapists face in the clinical setting. For students, unlike novice clinicians, this also includes the challenges that the mentor designs to assess and enhance learning. It is important for all members of the community to recognize that these challenges exist and that students and newcomers may need to be supported in their endeavor to master the challenges they face.

Through your engagement in the daily routines of your mentor and the community, you begin your process of trying to reconcile your abstract knowledge with its practical application; that is, you try to make sense of the clinical environment. Literature suggests that learners display learning preferences; what is evident in the clinical setting is that you utilize a variety of learning strategies to make personal meaning of your engagement within that particular community.

More important perhaps is the need to incorporate dialogue into all learning situations. You may attempt to make sense of the environment; however, it is only through discussion with your clinical instructor or another member of the community that your thoughts can be confirmed and validated, or refuted and clarified. It is only through this dialogic process that you can begin to fully identify, understand, and assimilate the meaning of the attitudes, values, and norms of the community and the profession. Because people vary greatly in their ability to communicate effectively, it is essential for students and mentors alike to practice the skills of assertive communication, role play potentially difficult conversations ahead of time, and ask for feedback from one another periodically.

As you make sense of your experiences through engagement in practice and the dialogic process, you begin to identify behavioral expectations. These behavioral expectations include, but are not limited to, communication, interpersonal skills, and professionalism. You begin to identify the political and social nuances of various practice settings as you determine your current and future roles. You begin to sort out those attitudes, values, and beliefs that you will ultimately choose to emulate and those that you will not. In identifying yourself with the community and its members, you begin to align yourself with the implicit and explicit expectations of that community. You assimilate certain community traditions and behaviors, and at the same time work to enhance the community with what you as an individual bring to the table.

By identifying the implicit and explicit expectations of the community and coming into alignment with those expectations, you begin to identify with community members and at the same time begin to be identified as a member of the community. These processes of identification and alignment further enhance your credibility, and the cycle begins again. With each cycle, you are given greater access and greater responsibility, which leads to your role as a full-fledged physical therapist and member of the broader professional community. Professional development is an ongoing process. With each new experience, previous knowledge and understanding is renegotiated and its meaning reconfirmed or new meaning created. As you move through the processes of identification and alignment, you continually enhance your own professional identity. As your professional identity grows, so too does your credibility—continuing the cycle of professional growth and development.

Given the triadic relationship that is established within the physical therapy community of practice, challenges, barriers, and supports can emerge from any component of this triad and can impact any point throughout the process (ie, facilitate or impede your professional identity development). Challenges, barriers, or supports emerging from one component of the triad can be mitigated or exacerbated by those that might emerge from another component of the triad. These cannot be deconstructed and viewed in isolation; rather, each must be viewed as a component of the whole in order to establish an effective triadic learning relationship.

Summary

Learning in a professional setting is a complex interaction between the individual, the mentor (clinical instructor/supervisor), and the community. It begins with gaining access to the community and all of its challenges and requires both personal meaning making and the negotiation of shared meaning through dialogue. This process moves far beyond the development of knowledge and skills to include the identification and assimilation of the norms, values, and beliefs that underlie professional practice. Challenges, supports, and barriers are individually defined and emerge from all components of the triadic relationship of newcomer, mentor, and community (See Figure 8-5 for a pictorial display of how learning takes place within the clinical setting).

Stop and Reflect

Take some time to reflect on the major concepts presented in this and the last chapter. What recommendations do you have for the following individuals that may help to minimize barriers to learning and optimize the supports to learning in the clinical setting?

- Academic educators
- Students and new clinicians
- Clinicians, clinical instructors, and supervisors
- Academic and clinical coordinators of clinical education

Key Points to Remember

The process of learning in the clinical environment includes the following:

- Learning requires a triadic, not a dyadic relationship, which includes the following:
  - Learner (the student, novice clinician, or newcomer)
  - Clinical instructor or supervisor
  - The community (including the patient, family, and other members of the clinical community)
- Challenges, supports, and potential barriers to learning may emerge from all aspects of the learning triad.
- Challenges and supports need to be balanced for optimal learning to occur.
- Dialogue is critical to the development of shared meaning.

Clinical education truly is a collaborative process. The student must be proactive in seeking out challenges and supports as well as potential strategies to overcome any barriers to their learning.

Pearls of Wisdom

Exemplary quotes on advice for new clinical instructors from students and novice clinicians:

- "Explain what is expected."
- "Never give any kind of criticism in front of a patient … it can be … very demeaning."
- "Talk about it. Bring it to the student's attention; it's something that [they] have to work on as much as their manual skills, sometimes even more. Give them regular feedback on their communication skills, and comment on how they communicate with patients. It's important."
- "I would tell them right up front that part of your training is going to be communication and interpersonal skills. Lay down some guidelines, and stress that it's important."
- "The clinical setting should be more aware of communication skills. A lot of times, it's so academic. Here's your treatment skill, how do you treat … but they forget about interpersonal skills."
- "Listen and give frequent feedback, ongoing feedback."
- "Be patient.
- "Create an environment where the student will immediately feel comfortable; always be open, helpful, and respectful."
- "They are going to make mistakes; let them. Just because it's not what you would do doesn't mean it's wrong."
- "Don't put yourself on a pedestal, there is no gain from intimidating a student."
- "Make them feel comfortable, like you want to help them, not like you're out to get them. Be open minded, and always give feedback."
- "Don't be judgmental."
- "Be receptive, and give the student a chance to express themselves."
- "Feedback is essential."
- "Give the student both positive feedback and negative feedback."

References

1. Plack MM. Developing communication, interpersonal skills and a professional identity within the physical therapy community of practice. *J Phys Ther Educ.* 2006;20:37-46.
2. Spouse J. Bridging theory and practice in the supervisory relationship: a sociocultural perspective. *Issues Innov Nurs Educ.* 2001;33:512-522.
3. Wenger E. *Communities of Practice: Learning, Meaning and Identity.* Cambridge, UK: Cambridge University Press; 1998.
4. Lave J, Wenger E. *Situated Learning: Legitimate Peripheral Participation.* Cambridge, UK: Cambridge University Press; 1991.
5. Spouse J. Scaffolding student learning in clinical practice. *Nurs Educ Today.* 1998;18:259-266.
6. Spouse J. The effective mentor: a model for student-centered learning in clinical practice. *NT Res.* 1996;1:120-134.
7. Shepard KF, Jensen GM, eds. *Handbook of Teaching for Physical Therapists.* 2nd ed. Boston, MA: Butterworth-Heinemann; 2002.
8. Gandy JS. *Train the Trainer Clinical Instructor Credentialing Course.* Alexandria, VA: 2002.
9. Daloz LA. *Mentor: Guiding the Journey of Adult Learners.* San Francisco, CA: Jossey-Bass Publishers; 1999.
10. Zachary LJ. *The Mentor's Guide: Facilitating Effective Learning Relationships.* San Francisco, CA: Jossey-Bass; 2000.
11. Murray M. *Beyond the Myths and Magic of Mentoring: How to Facilitate an Effective Mentoring Process.* San Francisco, CA: Jossey-Bass; 2001.
12. Gandy JS. *Mentoring. Orthopaedic Practice.* 1993;5:6-9.
13. Kram KE. *Mentoring at Work: Developmental Relationships in Organizational Life.* Lanham, MD: University Press of America; 1988.
14. Swap W, Leonard D, Shields M, Abrams L. Using mentoring and storytelling to transfer knowledge in the workplace. *J Manage Inform Syst.* 2001;18:95-114.
15. Ragins BR. Diversified mentoring relationships in organizations: a power perspective. *Acad Manage Rev.* 1997;22:482-521.
16. Benabou C, Benabou R. Establishing a formal mentoring program for organizational success. *Nat Prod Rev.* 1999;18:7-14.
17. Wilson JA, Elman NS. Organizational benefits of mentoring. *Acad Manage Exec.* 1990;4:88-96.
18. O'Reilly D. The mentoring of employees: is your organization taking advantage of this professional development tool? *Ohio CPA J.* 2001;60:51-54.
19. Plack MM. The learning triad: potential barriers and supports to learning in the physical therapy clinical environment. *J Phys Ther Educ.* 2008;22:7-18.
20. Schön DA. *Educating the Reflective Practitioner.* San Francisco, CA: Jossey-Bass Publishers; 1987.
21. Bandura A. *Social Foundations of Thought and Action: A Social Cognitive Theory.* Englewood, NJ: Prentice-Hall; 1986.
22. Brown JS, Collins A, Duguid P. Situated cognition and the culture of learning. *Educ Res.* 1989;18:32-42.
23. *Physical Therapy Clinical Instructor Educator Credentialing Manual.* Alexandria, VA: American Physical Therapy Association; 1997.
24. Plack MM. *Learning Communication and Interpersonal Skills Essential for Physical Therapy Practice: A Study of Emergent Clinicians.* New York, NY: Teachers College, Columbia University; 2003.
25. Boud D, Walker D. Barriers to reflection on experience. In: Boud D, Cohen R, Walker D, eds. *Using Experience for Learning.* Bristol, PA: The Society for Research Into Higher Education and Open University Press; 1993:73-87.
26. J Mezirow & Associates. *Fostering Critical Reflection in Adulthood: A Guide to Transformative and Emancipatory Learning.* San Francisco, CA: Jossey-Bass Publishers; 1990.
27. Kelly S. The exemplary clinical instructor: a qualitative case study. *J Phys Ther Educ.* 2007;21:63-69.
28. Emery MJ. Effectiveness of the clinical instructor: students' perspective. *Phys Ther.* 1984;64:1079-1083.
29. Knefelkamp L, Widick C, Parker C, eds. *Applying New Developmental Findings.* San Francisco, CA: Jossey-Bass; 1978.
30. Gherardi S, Nicolini D, Odella F. Towards a social understanding of how people learn in organizations. *Manage Learn.* 1998;29:273-297.
31. Spouse J. Learning to nurse through legitimate peripheral participation. *Nurs Educ Today.* 1998;18:345-351.

Patient Education
Facilitating Behavior Change

Chapter Objectives

After reading this chapter, you will be prepared to:

- Appreciate the role of the physical therapist in patient education and in facilitating behavior change.

- Assess your patient's readiness to change.

- Identify potential barriers to adherence.

- Assess your patient's health beliefs and explanatory model.

- Design effective patient education.

- Create effective patient education materials.

- Use a 5-step model of behavior counseling to facilitate and maintain behavior change.

- Select an appropriate approach to patient education based on your patient's health beliefs, explanatory model, learning style, literacy level, and readiness to change.

As described in the introduction to this text, health care providers teach every day; it is integral to what we do. Thus far, we have discussed teaching in the context of the classroom, in the context of professional and community presentations, and in the context of how students learn in the clinical setting. However, perhaps the most important aspect of our role as teachers or educators is teaching our patients and their families. Although our goal in all teaching-learning situations is to help our learners learn, in the context of patient care, learning becomes even more critical. Our goal is to ensure that our patients are fully educated about their dysfunction so they can make informed choices, be effective advocates for themselves and others, become valuable partners in the therapeutic process, and remain actively engaged in their own health and wellness.

In this chapter, we examine the complexities of patient education. We describe the importance of education from a number of perspectives and explore the many factors that need to be considered in designing effective learning experiences for your patients. Before you can begin any educational sessions with your patients, it is important to assess their readiness to learn, both physically and emotionally. To do so, we link back to adult learning principles and motivation theory. We then describe the importance of placing your patients at the center of the decision-making process and how you can negotiate shared meaning using explanatory models.

After developing goals that meet your patients' needs, we discuss strategies and processes to facilitate behavior change by understanding your patients' health beliefs. We explore the stages of change and suggest different strategies for teaching and learning to help move your patient along the continuum of behavior change. We examine some of the factors (including comorbid conditions) that may facilitate or hinder adherence and present the communities of practice framework to help identify supports that may facilitate adherence in your patients. Because literacy is quite prevalent in the United States, we also provide you with strategies to assess your patient's literacy level and mechanisms to design educational materials that will be optimally accessible to your patients. Finally, we provide you with a mechanism to facilitate long-term maintenance of behavior change in your patients using behavioral counseling strategies. Throughout, we use

Plack M, Driscoll M. *Teaching and Learning in Physical Therapy: From Classroom to Clinic* (pp 197-224).
© 2011 SLACK Incorporated

a communities of practice framework to problem solve strategies to support your patients and optimize their success in the rehabilitation and wellness process.

lifestyles, and the like. By now, you also know that educating your patients is much more than simply telling them what they should or should not do.

Patient Education: What Is It?

The *Guide to Physical Therapist Practice 2nd ed*[3] describes 5 elements of patient management that lead to optimal outcomes: *examination, evaluation, diagnosis, prognosis,* and *intervention. Intervention* is defined as "purposeful and skilled interaction of the physical therapist with the patient/client and, if appropriate, with other individuals involved in the care of the patient/client, using various physical therapy procedures and techniques to produce changes in the condition that is consistent with the diagnosis and prognosis." The *Guide* further differentiates 3 types of intervention: (1) procedural interventions; (2) coordination, communication, and documentation; and (3) patient-related instruction. Patient instruction is described as "the process of informing, educating, or training patients, families, significant others, and caregivers, [which] is intended to promote and optimize physical therapy services. Instruction may be related to the following:

- The current condition
- Specific impairments, functional limitations, or disabilities
- Plan of care
- The need for enhanced performance
- Transition to a different role or setting
- The need for health, wellness, or fitness programs

Stop and Reflect

Think back to a time when you either participated in or observed a physical therapy session.
1. Was patient education part of that session?
2. If so, what strategies did the therapist use in educating the patient?
3. Was it effective? How do you know?
4. Knowing what you now know about teaching strategies and learning styles, would you consider using different strategies? If so, which ones and why?

Physical therapists are responsible for patient-related instruction across all settings for all patients."

Patient education is much more than instructing patients on exercises and therapeutic interventions; it includes education about illness, resources, healthy

Patient Education: Why Is It Important?

Patient education is clearly an integral part of what we do as physical therapists. Patient education is what extends the therapy session beyond the 30 to 45 minutes that you might spend with your patient and can help to optimize patient outcomes. Patient education is necessary to promote adherence to exercise programs, facilitate changes in behaviors, and help cultivate healthy lifestyles.

Standards from the Joint Commission require all accredited inpatient facilities to have a multidisciplinary program of patient and family education.[4-6] Joint Commission's educational criteria mandate that patient education be grounded in sound educational principles and based on the patient's needs and readiness to learn. Education should be ongoing, systematic, interactive, and individualized to the patient's learning preferences and educational level. The Joint Commission's standards mandate facilities to have policies and procedures that delineate good patient-centered educational practices, including the following:

- *Assessing* patient/family needs
- Considering *individual differences*
- Having a *written plan* that addresses the needs of the patient
- Providing relevant *information and skills*
- Using a *variety of educational tools*
- *Actively engaging* the patient and caregiver in the process
- *Evaluating* the learning achieved

Stop and Reflect

Compare the Joint Commision's mandates for effective patient instruction to the elements of systematic effective instruction noted in a previous chapter. How are they similar? How are they different?
- Needs assessment
- Individual filters
- Objectives
- Content
- Content boosters
- Active learning strategies
- Formative and summative assessment

Not only does the Joint Commission mandate the use of good pedagogical practices, the Commission goes further to mandate that patient education include information about diagnosis, treatment, safe use of medications, drug interactions and reactions, nutrition counseling, diet, oral health, rehabilitation needs and techniques to maximize independence, pain and pain management, community resources, and postdischarge treatment.[4]

The American Hospital Association's *Patient Bill of Rights*, more recently replaced by the *Patient Care Partnership: Understanding Rights and Responsibilities*, also notes that it is the patient's responsibility to be a partner in the decision-making process. For it to be an effective partnership, patients must be informed about treatment and expected outcomes, including risks and benefits, sources of follow-up care, and training in self-help.[4-6] Medicare also requires patient education to be a part of the documented plan of care,[4,6] as does the Commission on Accreditation of Rehabilitation Facilities.[7]

In physical therapy specifically, the *Guide to Physical Therapist Practice*, which sets the standard for good practice in physical therapy, includes patient-related instruction as an integral component of the patient management model.[3] The *Normative Model for Physical Therapist Education* also provides the following sample objectives as expected outcomes of all entry-level physical therapist education curricula: "Demonstrate and document effective patient/client education" and "Employ patient/client-specific instructional strategies."[8] To ensure that this happens, the Commission on Accreditation of Physical Therapist Education (CAPTE) accreditation criteria[9] included criterion CC-5.26 in its 2006 *Evaluative Criteria for Accreditation of Education Programs for the Preparation of Physical Therapists*, which reads, "Effectively educate others using culturally appropriate teaching methods that are commensurate with the needs of the learner." Based on these standards and guidelines, it is clear that patient education is a valued activity in health care.

Finally, and perhaps most important, given the changes in health care today, patients have a limited number of therapy sessions available to them. The ultimate goal in health care is to empower and motivate patients to manage their own health. Patient education provides a mechanism for therapists to optimize patient adherence and extend necessary interventions beyond the limited time available in therapy. The more informed our patients are about their own health and how to manage their illnesses, the more prepared they are to become effective partners in making health care decisions, follow through on home exercise programs, and adhere to best practices in health and wellness.

Patient Education: What Do You Need to Consider in Preparing to Teach?

Traditionally, patient education has consisted of telling the patient what you expect, demonstrating it, and then having him or her do it (ie, tell, show, do). From there, health practitioners simply expected patients to follow their instructions and recommendations. By now, you are well aware that teaching is much more complex than show and tell. Educators must assess their learners' needs and develop effective strategies that meet those needs.

In physical therapy, we assess our patients from the biopsychosocial perspective (ie, we consider not only biology but also environmental [physical, social, and psychological], lifestyle, and behavioral factors). From there, we develop effective intervention strategies to meet the needs of our patients and clients. Just as we select interventions based on solid rationale and the best evidence, it is similarly important that we select patient education strategies based on solid rationale and the best evidence. Having a solid rationale for selecting the appropriate teaching strategy requires you to know the educational theories available upon which to build your strategies. A complete exploration of educational theory is beyond the scope of this text; therefore, we will focus on 2 major educational theories commonly used in patient education: *behaviorism* and *constructivism*.

Behaviorism is among the more traditional theories in education. Proponents of the behaviorist approach to learning focus on observable human behaviors and seek to shape those behaviors by reinforcing effective behaviors while extinguishing ineffective behaviors.[10,11] Behavioral theorists believe that learning occurs through stimulus, response, and conditioning activities. The role of the teacher is to create an environment that facilitates behavior change. Behavioral theorists break down the learning task into its component parts (ie, small steps). Each small step is then reinforced using positive reinforcement to facilitate learning or behavior change. Adherents to the behaviorist approach rely primarily on drill, practice, and reinforcement.

Using this approach, the therapist or educator develops specific measureable and behavioral objectives based on each component of the task and focuses on attainment of each goal. The therapist provides clear instructions and frequent feedback and positively reinforces performance. For example, you are teaching your patient, Mrs. G, to get out of her wheelchair and use her cane to walk. Mrs. G has weakness in her left upper extremity (LUE) and left lower extremity (LLE). A task analysis might reveal the following steps involved in transferring from a wheelchair to standing:

- Lock your brakes.
- Unbuckle your seat belt.
- Place the cane on your right side—slightly in front and to the side of the right armrest.
- Move your buttocks forward toward the front of the chair seat.
- Position your feet flat on the floor with your right foot slightly behind your left foot.
- Place your right hand on the armrest of the wheelchair.
- Lean your body forward and push up with your right arm and leg, letting your left arm and leg help as much as possible.
- Grab your cane with your right hand and stand fully upright.
- Maintain your balance before you start walking.[12]

You will then work with Mrs. G to determine which of these steps is most challenging for her. You might have her practice just that component of the transfer until she can perform it safely, efficiently, and effectively. At that point, you might chunk the tasks together so that there are fewer steps for Mrs. G to remember. Finally, you would be sure to put it together as a whole. This approach is consistent with the part-to-whole strategy previously discussed in the chapter on teaching and learning motor tasks. The behaviorist approach is especially effective for discrete tasks with patients who prefer a sequential and detailed plan for learning or who require a very structured environment (eg, a patient who has sustained a traumatic brain injury).[11,13,14]

Constructivism, on the other hand, is an approach to learning whereby learners actively make sense of their experiences based on their own values, beliefs, knowledge, skills, and prior learning.[15] Constructivists believe that all tasks are context-dependent and each task should be viewed as a whole. Proponents of the constructivist approach believe that tasks should not be broken down into discrete components to be mastered individually by the learner; rather, the learner must actively engage in problem solving (ie, how best to accomplish the task within the context of how and when the learner actually needs to perform that task). Constructivists do not view the teacher as the expert or authority but rather as a facilitator. Instruction is learner focused rather than teacher directed. The role of the teacher is to facilitate the learner's own problem-solving ability.[16]

The constructivist approach to teaching and learning comes from Dewey's work in learning from experience. Educators draw on the patients' own experiences and let them solve problems in ways that work best for them. In using this approach, you would engage your patient in authentic activities in realistic settings. Your role as the therapist is to set up an environment that is safe for experimentation and risk-taking. As the therapist, you would not tell your patient what to do but rather support your patient by creating a safe environment in which to try different strategies and ultimately to figure out which strategy works best for that particular patient.

For example, rather than breaking down the task of transferring from a wheelchair to standing into its component parts, you might instead prepare the room for your patient by placing the wheelchair in a safe spot away from the crowded gym and then stand by for safety purposes. You might then have your patient strategize on how she would approach the task of getting up from the wheelchair. This would allow your patient to draw on some of her own past experiences in determining how best to complete the task. Clearly, this approach requires that the patient is able to participate cognitively and physically in the problem-solving process. If this is not the case (eg, if the patient has significant sensory or cognitive limitations), the patient educator may use the more structured, behaviorist approach.

As a patient educator, it is important for you to understand the various theoretical approaches available so that you can select the approach that is most congruent with the given situation as well as with your patient's learning preference. Just as it is important for you to have solid rationale for the types of assessments or treatment interventions you select, it is equally important for you to have a clear rationale for the educational approach you select with your patient. In selecting the appropriate educational approach, it is important to consider the following:

- Your patient's cognitive, sensory, emotional, and physical capabilities
- Your patient's experience, beliefs, knowledge, skill, learning style
- The task itself
- The environment

Stop and Reflect

Think back over some of the patient education sessions you have observed.

- Did the therapist use a a behaviorist approach, a constructivist approach, or some combination?
- Have you observed the same therapist using different approaches to meet the needs of different learners and different tasks?
- Compare 2 different sessions and consider:
  - The patient
  - The task
  - The environment

Patient Education: Is Your Patient Ready to Learn?

In an earlier "Stop and Reflect" exercise, you were asked to compare and contrast the Joint Commission's educational criteria to the concepts of systematic effective instruction presented earlier in this book. If you did this exercise, you would have noticed that the one component of systematic effective instruction that was missing in the Joint Commission's criteria is the *motivational hook*. As we saw earlier, the motivational hook is what grabs the audience's attention, and it is important to recognize what is grabbing your patient's attention during any given education session. If your patient is in pain, his focus may be on his pain and he may not be ready to learn. If your patient is fearful of falling, her attention may be on her potential fall and not on what you are trying to teach her. If your patient does not believe that the exercises you are teaching him will help, you may not have his full attention.

For your educational session to be effective, your patient must be both ready and willing (ie, motivated) to participate. In an earlier chapter, we discussed how adults generally bring with them a readiness to learn. However, we also know that each person is an individual with different life stressors and different personal motivators.[17] *Readiness* means that your patient is both emotionally and physically able to participate in the teaching and learning situation. *Motivation* means that your patient has some drive to act.[17] If your patient is not ready or willing, you will have to adjust your strategies to ensure that the educational session occurs at a time when your patient is more available to participate. This concept of physical and emotional readiness takes on even greater importance in physical therapy where active engagement is essential and where we often work with patients with neurological, cognitive, psychological, and/or communication disorders. A more detailed discussion of educational strategies for use with special populations will appear later in this chapter.

Having the drive, willingness, or motivation to participate on a basic level includes both intrinsic and extrinsic motivation.[17] You may have a patient who is intrinsically motivated because he finds the activity personally valuable, interesting, and perhaps enjoyable. On the other hand, you may have a patient who is extrinsically motivated, doing his exercises solely to please his spouse or therapist. You may also have a patient who is not motivated to participate at all. Our goal is to help our patients develop an intrinsic motivation to optimize their learning, retention, and follow-through. Though we cannot intrinsically motivate our patients, we can provide certain social and environmental conditions in the teaching-learning situation that may facilitate a level of intrinsic motivation. Ryan and Deci[17] suggested 3 major factors that may help our patients develop intrinsic motivation. Patients are more likely to be intrinsically motivated if they feel a sense of the following:

- *Connectedness*, which can come from a sense of being trusted, respected, and cared for by the therapist.
- *Self-efficacy*, or a feeling of competence, which can occur when patients have sufficient knowledge and skill to perform the expected activities.
- *Autonomy*, which can come from feeling that the activities are personally meaningful and valuable.

Critical Thinking Clinical Scenario

Your patient, Mrs. R, had total hip replacement 2 days ago. Your plan is to give her some exercises to perform and to teach her how to get out of bed properly. You read her chart and notice that she is on a high dose of pain medication and has not been out of bed yet. You go in the room, and you notice that the room is rather dark, the curtains are drawn, and Mrs. R is lying down in bed. You introduce yourself, tell her what your plan is, and ask her if she is ready for therapy. Her response is, "No, I can't."

Reflective Questions

1. Given this scenario, what is your assessment of Mrs. R's readiness to participate in the therapy session?
2. What types of questions might you ask to assess her readiness to participate further?
3. Besides pain, what other potential barriers might be affecting her ability to participate in today's session?
4. How might you alter your initial plan?
5. How might you incorporate the factors described by Ryan and Deci into your treatment approach?

Key Points to Remember

- For your educational session to be effective, your patient must be both ready and willing (ie, motivated) to fully participate.
- Readiness means that your patient is both emotionally and physically able to participate in the teaching and learning situation.
- Motivation includes both extrinsic and intrinsic motivation. To optimize long-term adherence, intrinsic motivation is essential.
- Intrinsic motivation can be optimized by providing your patient with a sense of:
  - *Connectedness*, which can come from a sense of being trusted, respected, and cared for by the therapist.
  - *Self-efficacy*, or a feeling of competence, which can occur when patients have sufficient knowledge and skill to perform the expected activities.
  - *Autonomy*, which can come from feeling that the activities are personally meaningful and valuable.

Our role as health care providers goes beyond just telling our patients what to do. Our role is to facilitate the behavior changes needed to maximize their function, prevent future injuries, and optimize their health. Behavior change is more likely to persist if it is internally motivated.

Although our ultimate goal is to help our patients assume responsibility for their own health, we may need to modify this expectation depending on where the patient is in the rehabilitation process and what associated cognitive and/or emotional factors may be present. Early on, there may be significant comorbid physical, cognitive, and/or emotional factors (eg, delirium, confusion, fatigue, medical complications) that can interfere with the patient's readiness to participate.[13] Rather than focusing on your patient's ability to adhere to a given program, your role may be to seek and provide additional external supports that will enable your patient to overcome these barriers to participation.

During the later or more chronic phase of rehabilitation, patients may experience loss of function, changes in their medical condition, or the need for assistive devices, all of which require effective coping skills if they are to complete their rehabilitation successfully. Developing self-efficacy and problem-solving skills to optimize independence and function is an essential component of your patient education at this point. As a physical therapist, it will be important for you to modify your educational approach based on your patient's needs, capabilities, and comorbid factors. Depending on what phase of recovery your patient is in, you may need to assume more or less responsibility for encouraging and managing your patient's abilities to participate in and adhere to the therapeutic plan.[13] Regardless of the phase of the rehabilitation process, obtaining patient cooperation and motivation is critical to optimizing health and function. Remember that just because we tell our patients or their family members/caregivers to do something for the patient's own good, it doesn't necessarily mean that they will do it. Nor can we assume that a patient who is not fully participating in the therapeutic process lacks motivation. Rather, our role is to assess the readiness of our patients to participate on a continuous basis and modify our approach as necessary.

Key Points to Remember

- In assessing your patient's readiness to participate, it is important to consider your patient's needs and abilities, comorbid factors (eg, cognitive, emotional, psychological, physical), and where he or she is along the continuum from the acute to the chronic phase of recovery/rehabilitation.

- Your patient's educational needs may vary significantly depending upon whether he or she is in the acute or post-acute (chronic) phase of rehabilitation.

- Depending on what phase of recovery your patient is in, you may need to assume more or less responsibility for encouraging and managing your patient's abilities to participate in and adhere to the therapeutic plan.

Negotiating Shared Meaning Through Explanatory Models

Stop and Reflect

Think back to a time when you tried to "kick a habit" (eg, smoking) or start a new regimen (eg, an exercise regimen) because you knew it was for your own good.

- What prompted you to want to change?

- How challenging was it for you to initiate the change?

- Were you able to maintain the behavior change? If not, why not? If so, how challenging was it for you to maintain the change?

- What things made it easier for you?

- What was the most challenging aspect of this change process for you?

Our goal is to motivate our patients by influencing their beliefs, attitudes, and ultimately their behaviors. We are more likely to influence behavior if we first take time to understand our patients' and their family members'/caregivers' perceptions of their illnesses. Patients make sense of their illnesses based on their experiences. Their culture, experience, support systems, and social networks shape their beliefs and their view of the illness. As a result, they develop explanations for what happened to them and for the type of medical care they think they need (including home remedies and alternative therapies). Our patients develop explanatory models to help them make sense of their illness experience.[18] These explanatory models guide what our patients will and will not do and how they view therapy itself. These explanatory models may influence their readiness to participate in the therapy session. By taking the time to elicit our patients' explanatory models, we can begin to understand the following:

- What they believe caused their disease or injury

- What their reaction has been to the disease (ie, illness experience)

- What they believe will cure their disease

- Their personal preferences

- Their valued activities

- Their expectations of their role as patient in the recovery process

- Their expectations of your role as a therapist involved in their recovery process

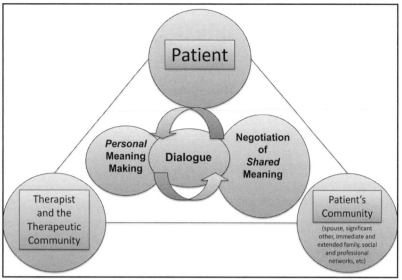

Figure 9-1. The patient's learning triad.

<table>
<tr><td>

Stop and Reflect

- When you were young, what were some of the "old wives tales" you heard? For example, did your grandmother say, "Don't go outside with wet hair or you will get sick"?

- In what ways did this guide what you were and were not able to do?

- Did your grandmother have any favorite remedies that she would use when you were sick?

</td><td>

Stop and Reflect

Think back to the concepts of intention and impact and the development of shared meaning. How do those concepts relate to the following statement from the text? "Unless we consider the patient's and family members'/caregivers' explanatory models and use them in developing the most appropriate plan of care, we may fail to motivate or get 'buy in' from our patient... As a result, despite being best practice, our plan may not be successful."

</td></tr>
</table>

It is important to remember that not only do patients have explanatory models, but health care providers do as well. As a health care provider, you will likely have your own thoughts about the mechanism of your patient's injury and about which interventions will be most effective. You will base your beliefs on what and how you were taught, your own search of current evidence, and your own personal experiences with other patients. As therapists, we think we know the following:

- What caused the impairment or illness
- What the patient needs
- How the disease should be treated
- What the long-term consequences might be

In fact, we often develop a plan of care for our patients based on our own explanatory models. However, unless we consider the patient's and family members/caregivers' explanatory models and use them in developing the most appropriate plan of care, we may fail to motivate or get "buy in" from our patient. It is possible that we may extrinsically motivate our patients during the treatment session; however, unless they value the activity, they will not become intrinsically motivated to maintain a particular activity or behavior change. As a result, despite using best practice, our plan may not be successful.

In a previous chapter, we learned that students must not solely rely on their own personal meaning-making process; rather, they must negotiate shared meaning to optimize their learning in the clinical setting. The same is true for therapists. Therapists must develop shared meaning with their patients. You will remember also that to achieve shared meaning you must engage in dialogue. Your initial dialogue with your patient should be to elicit information about his or her explanatory model. It is important to understand how your patient experiences a particular disease state because that will guide his behaviors and so too must it guide your actions and your plan of care. If your patient's limitations prevent him from being fully involved in this negotiation process, it would be important to engage family members or care providers and seek additional supports to overcome barriers to participation and to ensure that your patient's voice is considered.

Do you remember how a learning triad is developed in the clinical setting (ie, student, clinical instructor, and community) and how each member of that community is essential in the learning process? Similarly, with patients, a triad develops, that includes the patient, the therapist and the therapeutic community, and the patient's own community or network (Figure 9-1). With patients, the community extends beyond the health care setting to include spouses, significant others, immediate family, extended family members, members of their social network, spiritual advisors, and the like. Just as members of the health care community help to facilitate student learning, members of the patient's community may help to facilitate your understanding of your patient and may be equally instrumental in helping you educate, motivate, and facilitate change in your patient. Further, just as barriers and supports can emerge from all aspects of the student's learning triad, similarly, barriers and supports can emerge from all aspects of the patient's learning triad. To be effective in enhancing your patient's adherence to the therapeutic plan, it is important to consider the potential barriers and supports with every patient.

In attempting to understand a patient's explanatory model fully, Kleinman et al[18] developed 8 questions you can ask (Table 9-1). Realize that, in asking these questions, your goal is to understand your patient's beliefs, so it is important to suspend judgment and actively listen. This is not the time to educate your patient; rather, this is a time for you to become educated about your patient. You want to ask the question and be sure to listen to what your patient tells you so you can understand your patient's perspective fully. It is also a good time for you to check your own assumptions and compare your personal explanatory model with your patient's explanatory model.

At one time, the dominant explanatory model for physical therapists was one of a biomedical model. In the biomedical model, the belief is that there is a pathology with resultant impairments and functional limitations; an intervention will "fix" the impairments and possibly the pathology; and the therapist is at the center of the decision-making process. This focus alone can lead to a disconnect between the patient and the practitioner. Practitioners using a biomedical model focus on the physiological state of dysfunction (ie, disease) and may miss how the individual experiences that disease (ie, illness). As practitioners, we may fully understand the pathology but can never fully know how the patient experiences that pathology. We now recognize this disconnect and the important influence that culture and experience have on an individual's attitudes and beliefs toward disease, rehabilitation, and recovery. We no longer simply look at pathology and impairments but rather our focus has changed to one of a biopsychosocial model.[19] As practitioners, we move beyond pathology and impairments (ie, the disease state) to fully consider the patient's illness experience (ie, participation restrictions, environmental factors, and personal factors; Figure 9-2). This places the patient at the core of the decision-making process and makes the negotiation of shared meaning even more critical to effective clinical care.

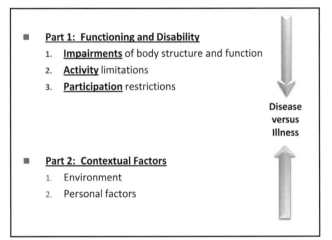

Figure 9-2. The biopsychosocial model.

Only when we understand both our patient's and our own explanatory models fully can we begin to negotiate the plan of care that best meets our patient's personal needs and goals. It is important that our goals are patient centered, and to ensure that they are, we must engage our patients, to the extent possible, in the decision-making process. In the negotiation process, we may need to clarify any misperceptions or misunderstandings our patients might hold regarding the disease process (eg, cause of the problem, length of the course of treatment, etc). Providing complete and accurate information will enable our patients to engage more

Table 9-1. Kleinman's 8 Questions to Elicit Explanatory Models

1. What do you call the problem?
2. What do you think has caused the problem?
3. Why do you think it started when it did?
4. What do you think the illness does? How does it work?
5. How severe do you think your illness is? Do you believe it will have a short or long course?
6. What kind of treatment do you think you need? What results do you expect from the treatment?
7. What major problems has this illness caused for you?
8. What do you fear most about this illness?

Adapted from Kleinman A, Eisenberg L, Good B. Culture, illness, and care: clinical lessons from anthropologic and cross-cultural research. *Ann Intern Med.* 1978;88:251-258.

fully in the therapeutic relationship and in developing an effective plan of care. By engaging our patients, or a family member if the patient has significant limitations, in the process, together we can identify the best plan of care. This plan is not always necessarily the one that will have the greatest impact on the disease process, but rather the one that will have the greatest impact on the illness experience. Recognize also that if our patients are involved in the decision-making process, to the greatest extent possible, it is likely that they will feel more connected and have a greater sense of self-efficacy and autonomy, which may lead to enhanced adherence.

Key Point to Remember

The best plan of care is not always necessarily the one that will have the greatest impact on the **disease process** but rather the one that has the greatest impact on the patient's **illness experience.**

Negotiation of shared meaning is an ongoing process. Just as you learned the importance of asking questions to facilitate reflection and enhance learning, questions are equally if not more important in helping you understand your patients. Kleinman et al's[18] 8 critical questions are a springboard to help you begin to understand your patient's illness experience. However, it is only the beginning. It is helpful to ask questions of your patients and family members throughout the process. For patients with communication or cognitive limitations, family members or caregivers may be able to provide you with important and helpful information.

Critical Thinking Clinical Scenario

A student once shared with me an experience she had in the clinic. She was working with a patient with significant expressive aphasia (ie, difficulty using expressive language) for the first time, and she (the student) was having difficulty understanding anything her patient told her. When her clinical instructor came over to speak with the patient, the clinical instructor seemed to understand everything the student said.

Reflective Questions
1. What do you think may have been going on in this scenario?
2. Why might it have been easier for her clinical instructor to understand the needs of this patient?
3. How might having more knowledge of the patient's likes and dislikes, hobbies, routines, etc, have helped in this situation?
4. Where might the student have obtained more information to help provide context to what her patient was saying? How might the patient's learning triad have helped?

It is also important to remember that as patients learn more and experience therapy longer, their explanatory models may change, as may their goals and motivations. Questions can help ensure that the plan of care initially established remains consistent with your patient's evolving needs. Questions such as the following may be helpful throughout the process:

- What is limiting you most from participating in your usual activities?
- What activity would you most like to do that you currently cannot?
- What do you see as your biggest barrier to following your exercise regimen?
- Who might you call on to help you with your exercises?
- How confident are you in performing your exercises on your own?
- In what ways do you think these exercises will/will not help your recover or return to the activities you want to do?
- What changes have you experienced in your overall health lately?
- What previous experiences have you had related to physical therapy or any physical exercise?

Critical Thinking Clinical Scenario

This is a good time to review your chapter on reflection and consider the variety of questions you might consider asking your patients or family members to facilitate the reflective process. For example, you have a patient you are seeing for her third therapy session. She had been following her home program of exercises but recently has become inconsistent in performing her exercises.

Reflective Question
Using the frameworks described in the chapter on reflection, what questions might you ask your patient to understand her continually evolving illness experience? Consider each of the elements of reflection in formulating your questions:
- Content
- Process
- Premise
- Reflection-in-action
- Reflection-on-action
- Reflection-for-action

Table 9-2. The Health Belief Model

Behavioral change requires the following:

1. The belief that one is *susceptible* to disease.
2. The belief that the disease has significant *consequences*.
3. The belief that making a *change can reduce the threat* of the disease.
4. The belief that the *benefits of change outweigh the cost* or barrier to change.
5. The belief that one has the ability to *change*.

Adapted from Rimer BK, Glanz K. Theory at a glance: a guide for health promotion practice. Available at http://cancer.gov/aboutnci/oc/theory-at-a-glance/page1. Accessed June 21, 2009.

Facilitating Behavior Change by Understanding Health Beliefs

Once you more fully understand how your patient experiences his or her illness, you can begin to facilitate change. However, change will be difficult if your patient does not believe the following:

- There are consequences to continuing his or her current behavior or that the consequences are significant
- The benefits to change outweigh the costs
- He or she has the potential to change[20]

Just as we need to understand our patients' illness experiences through their explanatory model, we also need to understand their beliefs about health, wellness, and therapeutic intervention. We can develop a better understanding of our patients' beliefs by using the Health Belief Model. Psychologists in the United States Public Health Service developed this model in an attempt to understand why a program that provided free access to health promotion and prevention activities failed.[20] Despite the availability of free chest x-rays to detect tuberculosis, few individuals accessed the service. After studying this phenomenon, they identified a number of factors that influenced the decision-making process and motivated individuals to change. They suggested that to facilitate behavior change in our patients we must first engage our patients in conversation about those factors noted in Table 9-2.

What follows is an example of how a patient's health beliefs might influence behavior change. You are working with overweight teens at risk for such health-related issues as obesity, diabetes, and heart disease. It may be important to recognize that teens often do not believe they are susceptible to disease, and if they do, they may not recognize the significance of the potential

consequences of obesity. They may recognize that they are overweight and that it is harder to exercise but not believe that being overweight can lead to heart disease or stroke in the future. They also may not believe that the benefits of exercise outweigh the time, hard work, and energy it takes to engage in a diet and exercise regimen. They may have tried many fad diets that failed and so do not believe they have the potential to lose weight. Finally, if their social network consists of other overweight teens, there may be nothing prompting them to change. Educating these young teens about the consequences of obesity and helping to modify their health beliefs toward obesity is the first step. We must then begin to motivate these young teens to take action in changing their behaviors.

To facilitate change, our patients must first be motivated to change. Lorish and Gale[21] promoted the use of a "behavioral change conversation" to help us begin to understand our patient's motivation. They encourage us to engage our patients in a dialogue to understand their assumptions about their own susceptibility to disease; about whether change is possible and, if so, whether it will make a difference; and about the cost-benefit of the needed change. During this dialogue, as a therapist, you will also provide expert information, resources, and prompts to facilitate action.

We can never really know what will motivate our patients sufficiently to enable behavior change to occur, but determining those motivating factors will be critical to facilitating change. For example, you may think it is sufficient to explain the potential health-related risks of obesity to teens, but if an overweight teen does not believe that he or she is susceptible to heart disease or diabetes, an explanation may not be sufficient to facilitate a change in his or her behavior. Perhaps what will motivate him or her is information about a healthy teen program in his or her neighborhood. He or she may see others exercising and meet individuals who have been successful with their weight loss and exercise programs. He or she may suddenly care more about his or her appearance and his or her physical abilities. He or she may begin to view him- or herself as having the potential to change and view his or her new relationships as important. For this patient, the benefit of fitting in with new peers and maintaining new relationships may outweigh the energy it takes to participate in a weight loss and exercise regimen. It is important to remember that motivating factors may be non-health-related as well as health-related. By engaging your patient in the behavior change conversation, you can begin to determine the factors that will be most effective in facilitating behavior change in that particular patient.

Key Point to Remember

Engaging in a behavioral change conversation is the first step to understanding the factors that may motivate and facilitate change in our patients.[21] The behavior change conversation is to elicit your patient's assumptions about whether:

- He is or is not susceptible to disease
- The disease has significant consequences or not
- Making a change (if even possible) will or will not make a difference (ie, reduce the threat) in the disease process
- The benefits of change outweigh the cost to change

Critical Thinking Clinical Scenario

Your patient is a 42-year-old gentleman who recently had an anterior cruciate ligament reconstruction. He is also obese. As part of your plan of care, you would like to address his weight. In preparation, you have begun to engage your new patient in a behavior change conversation. In doing so, you realize that he does not recognize the potential health risks related to obesity.

Reflective Questions
1. What strategy would you use to facilitate change in your patient?
2. How would your strategies change if your patient told you the following:
   o He believes exercise may help but he does not have the time or energy to engage in a routine exercise regime.
   o He has tried numerous diets in the past but they never worked.

It is also important to recognize that you may not see an immediate change in your patient's behavior; rather, you may only be able to provide the prompts needed to get your patient at least thinking about the need for change. The change process takes time, and you may not see immediate results. However, your patient education may be just the call to action (ie, the prompt) your patient needs to begin the change process, which is why it is important to incorporate patient education and health promotion in every session you have with your patients.

Critical Thinking Clinical Scenario

Your supervisor has asked you to develop an education and health promotion program for senior citizens in a local extended care facility. He wants you to include information on falls prevention and the importance of exercise.

Reflective Questions
1. What types of questions would you use to complete a needs assessment (consider the concepts of explanatory models and health beliefs)?
2. What are some potential barriers to the success of this program?
3. What are some potential supports to the success of this program?
4. What aspects of the community of practice paradigm might you incorporate to make this program most successful?

Think back to the "Stop and Reflect" activity presented earlier when we asked you to consider a time when you wanted to make a change in your behavior. Do you remember how difficult it was to change your behavior or your lifestyle? You may very well work with patients who know that they need to change their behaviors because they are at risk for a disease with significant consequences, who recognize that the benefits outweigh the barriers to change, and who know that they have the ability to change, yet they are not ready to make the change. If a person is not ready to change, then change will not occur. In facilitating change, it is important that we assess our patient's readiness to change so we can match our strategies to our patient's needs.

Facilitating Behavior Change: The Transtheoretical Model and Stages of Change

Stop and Reflect

Again, think back again to that time when you tried to kick a habit (eg, smoking) or start a new regimen (eg, exercise regimen) because you knew it was for your own good.
- This time, think about how that happened; how did you kick a habit?
- Did you simply wake up one morning, decide that you needed to change your behavior, and immediately change it? If not, what steps did you go through to make that change?

Prochaska and DiClemente[22] and Prochaska et al[23] studied addictive behaviors, particularly in smokers in the process of quitting. They described 5 stages that individuals move through as they progress through the change process:

1. *Precontemplative*—No thought of change
2. *Contemplative*—Thinking about changing
3. *Preparation*—Preparing to change
4. *Action*—Implementing the change
5. *Maintenance*—Maintaining the change

These stages, and how individuals experience them, may vary depending on the behavior they are trying to change. For example, there may be differences between those trying to quit smoking and those trying to incorporate exercise into their daily lives. These stages may not occur in a stepwise systematic fashion, either. Individuals may enter the change process at any stage. Furthermore, individuals may experience relapses, or backward movement, at any stage in the change process.

As therapists, we will also select very different strategies for patient education depending on our patient's readiness or stage of change. For example, you are working with a patient who is obese and prediabetic, and he tells you that he is too busy and too tired at the end of his long workday to consider exercise. You would likely consider him in the precontemplative stage. Before you can expect him to adhere to an exercise program, your best strategy might be to discuss the health belief model and possibly work to influence a change in his beliefs by providing information about the consequences of continued inactivity. If you are successful, at the next session, he may tell you that he has given some thought to what you said and would like to consider an exercise plan but just does not have 30 to 45 minutes to fit into his day. At this point, you would consider him to be in the contemplative stage. Your best strategy now might be to brainstorm and problem solve some of his barriers to participation and look for alternative solutions. At the next session, he tells you that he has decided to begin a walking regimen during his lunch hour every day. He has cleared his schedule and is asking your advice on the type of sneakers he should purchase. At this point, you realize that your patient has moved to the preparation stage, and your strategy might be to provide positive reinforcement, information about shoe wear and how to monitor his heart rate, and help him establish realistic goals for the upcoming weeks. Finally, the big day comes, and he starts his exercise regimen during lunch. He has reached the action stage, and now ongoing reinforcement and support are necessary. You also want to continue to problem solve barriers; provide alternatives related to valued activities; identify rewards for adherence (eg, noted weight loss, decreased windedness on stairs); and remind your patient of the benefits of adherence and the risks of nonadherence. Two weeks later, you see your patient again and ask whether he is still walking every day. He tells you that it was impossible to keep up; his lunch hours were busy, and he became frustrated and just quit walking. He indicated that he would really like to continue his walking program but it is

just not working. Your patient has relapsed into the contemplative stage. Your best strategy might be to work with him to develop realistic goals (eg, walking twice per week during lunch and once per week on the weekend) and help him move back into the action stage. This is a cyclic process, with the ultimate goal being to reach the maintenance stage in which your patient is able to follow his exercise regimen routinely and consistently. Even during the maintenance stage, patients/clients need ongoing reinforcement and problem solving to prevent relapse. Table 9-3 provides a list of questions you can ask your patients/clients to determine where they are in the process of change along with potential educational strategies to consider while working with patients and clients during each stage of change.

Critical Thinking Clinical Scenario

You are working with Mr. T, a 42-year-old male patient who recently had a myocardial infarction. You determine that a home program of aerobic exercises would improve his level of fitness and cardiovascular health. Your patient does not think the home exercise program you prescribed will make a difference and indicates that given his busy work and home life, he will have a hard time performing his exercises consistently.

Reflective Questions
1. How might Mr. T's health beliefs impact his level of adherence to the home exercise program you prescribed?
2. What other barriers might be preventing Mr. T from engaging in an exercise program?
3. What is your assessment of Mr. T's readiness to change (ie, what stage of change do you think he is in)?
4. What educational strategies might you consider using with Mr. T?
5. What suggestions might you give Mr. T to address some of the potential barriers present?

Key Points to Remember

- To facilitate change, select the most effective educational strategies and apply them at the most appropriate time.
- Before selecting your educational strategy, it is important to first understand your patient's health beliefs and identify your patient's readiness to change (ie, stage of change).
- It is important for you to match the chosen educational strategy to your patient's physical, cognitive, and emotional capabilities, and stage of readiness to best optimize the potential outcome.
- Patients may not move linearly through the stages of change; rather, there may be episodes of relapse so ongoing assessment of your patient's readiness to change or stage of change is essential to facilitate and maintain change.

Table 9-3. Potential Assessment and Educational Strategies for Each Stage of Change

Stage of Change	Definition	Assessment Question	Potential Educational Strategies
Precontemplative	No intention to change in the near future; may not recognize a problem exists; may resist change	"Are you thinking about changing your behavior?" (eg, "Are you thinking about adding exercise to your daily routine?")	Provide information about the risks and benefits of change and the potential consequences of not changing the behavior; consciousness raising; problem solve barriers to contemplation
Contemplative	Recognize that a problem exists; may seriously be thinking about a change even potentially within the next 6 months but has no definite plans	"Are you thinking about changing your behavior in the near future?" (eg, "Are you thinking about starting an exercise program soon?")	Provide feedback and/or information; raise consciousness; provide positive role models; reinforce the consequences to no change; reinforce the risks and benefits to change; problem solve barriers to change; discuss pros and cons; identify all potential goals and solutions; identify supports from the community; encourage self-assessment
Preparation	The intent to change is present and the individual is actually preparing to change within the next month	"Are you ready to begin to develop a plan to effect a change in your behavior?" (eg, "Would you like to develop a plan that will increase your daily level of exercise?")	Encourage self-assessment; encourage restructuring the environment to enable change; reinforcement; problem solve barriers; provide role models; help to establish realistic goals and action plans
Action	Implementing a change; modifies behavior for at least 1-6 months	"Are you in the process of changing your behavior?" (eg, "Have you begun to increase your daily level of exercise?")	Provide feedback/positive reinforcement; provide measures of accountability (eg, weekly check-in; daily logs); encourage self-assessment; restructure the environment to remove temptations for relapse; re-evaluate goals and modify them as appropriate; identify ongoing community supports
Maintenance	Maintaining the change for at least 6 months	"Are you trying to maintain your change in behavior?" (eg, "Are you continuing to exercise every day?")	Ongoing feedback, reminders, rewards, and measures of accountability; ongoing self-assessment; reinforcement, ongoing problem-solving of barriers and potential causes of relapse; ongoing community supports
Relapse		"Have you attempted to change your behavior in the past year?" (eg, "Have you attempted to increase your daily exercise this past year?")	Provide emotional support; identify the stage to which he or she has relapsed and use the strategies identified

Adapted from Rimer BK, Glanz K. Theory at a glance: a guide for health promotion practice. Available at http://cancer.gov/aboutnci/oc/theory-at-a-glance/page1. Accessed June 21, 2009; Lorish C, Gale J. Facilitating behavior change: strategies for education and practice. *J Phys Ther Educ.* 1999;13:31-37; Prochaska JO, DiClemente CC. Transtheoretical therapy: toward a more integrative model of change. *Psychother Theory Res.* 1982;3:276-288; Prochaska JO, DiClemente CC, Norcross J. In search of how people change: applications to the addictive behaviors. *Am Psychol.* 1992;47:1102-1114.

Factors Influencing Adherence to Home Exercise Programs

Because one of the primary purposes of patient education is to extend the physical therapy session beyond the boundaries of the 30 to 45 minutes you can spend with your patients, a frequent focus of patient education is the home exercise program. We often design exercise programs to increase flexibility, strength, endurance, balance, coordination, and the like. We refer to the degree to which a patient participates in this self-managed aspect of care as *compliance* or *adherence.* In recent years, the term adherence has been preferred because it connotes more of a partnership between patient and health care provider.[24]

Because adherence to medical and exercise regimens has significant health benefits for patients, there is interest in identifying factors that appear to influence adherence. For more than 50 years, researchers have been unable to come to consensus on constructs to define adherence, which has made it difficult to compare adherence across populations. Instead, the literature describes a number of factors that reflect adherence, such as characteristics of the patient and characteristics of care.[13] Some focus on outcome markers, emphasizing medical concepts such as cure rate. Others focus on process markers such as the number of appointments kept or medications taken. Still others use patient self-report on the degree to which they have followed the health care provider's recommendations.[24]

Given the variety of factors chosen to represent adherence, it is not surprising that information on actual rates of adherence for different activities vary considerably. In the rehabilitation literature, home exercise program adherence rates are reportedly in the 40% to 60% range.[25-28] Further, Zinn[13] emphasized the need to recognize that adherence in rehabilitation is a complex phenomenon. It is more complicated than studying adherence to exercise or lifestyle change in otherwise healthy populations because physical therapists see patients for a great variety of reasons, and many may have comorbid cognitive and/or emotional health conditions as well.

For example, depending on the type and severity of a stroke or cerebrovascular accident, the patient may need physical therapy for neuromuscular, balance, and/or strengthening issues. The stroke may also have caused cognitive, language, and emotional difficulties, which will influence participation in the patient education process and adherence to a home exercise program.[13] Despite the recognized difficulties in studying adherence in rehabilitation, our concern is how to enhance adherence in physical therapy.

Management of cognitive and emotional comorbidities is beyond the scope of this book; however, Table 9-4 provides some examples of common comorbid conditions that may serve as barriers to adherence, along with potential strategies you may use to help minimize the impact of these impairments and barriers and optimize adherence.[13]

As you can see from the previous discussion, it is important to consider potential comorbidities that may interfere with our patient's abilty to participate in therapy or adhere to a home program (eg, depression, dementia). You may think that your patient is in the precontemplative stage, and, as a result, you might decide that it is important to give him information about the risks and benefits of change and the potential consequences of not changing his behavior. It is equally important to recognize that it may be your patient's current medical condition that is preventing him from fully engaging in, and adhering to, a particular therapeutic program, not necessarily a function of motivation or readiness to change.

Implementation of the Transtheoretical Model of Change and the Health Belief Model both assume that our patient's cognitive function is intact, which may not be the case with a number of our patients. Rather than focusing on education, motivation, and self-efficacy for patients with cognitive or emotional impairments, it may be more important to focus on providing additional environmental and social supports that will enable these patients to participate in the therapeutic process.

As our patients progress through the rehabilitative process, their needs may change as well. Consider your role in patient education as the equivalent of working with learners along the continuum from dependent to independent. Our goal is always to maximize our patient's/learner's level of independence; however, for patients with significant comorbid factors, this may begin with us being primarily responsible for setting up an environment in which our patients can participate, which may require significant engagement of the patient's entire learning triad.[13]

Key Point to Remember

It is important to consider potential comorbid conditions that may interfere with adherence when planning your patient education and follow-up.

Stop and Reflect

Comorbid factors such as the ones noted in Table 9-4 are not the only factors that you should consider while planning a home program. Lifestyle, occupation, age, and personality are among the many factors that we may need to incorporate in planning a home program. What additional factors might you need to take into consideration in planning a home exercise program for each of the following:

- A pediatric patient?
- An adolescent patient?
- A geriatric patient?
- A highly competitive athlete?
- A new mother of triplets?

Although the factors that influence a patient's likelihood of adherence to a therapeutic program vary tremendously, some factors appear to be more significant than others. A patient's prior experience may influence adherence. Prior experience with physical activities, especially as an adult, may increase the likelihood that your patient will follow a home exercise program.[29] As we also know from the Health Belief Model, a person's beliefs will influence adherence. Your older patient who believes that a balance training/falls prevention program will improve his strength, mobility, and ultimately optimize his independence will more likely adhere to the program than your patient who is in denial about her risk of falling.[30] Both personal and environmental factors can present as barriers to adherence for some of our elderly patients as well. Personal factors can include factors such as poor health, lack of interest, depression, shortness of breath, fatigue. Environmental factors can include factors such as lack of time, poor weather conditions, and lack of social supports.[28,31]

Thoughtful dialogue with our patients allows us to learn about their valued activities, health beliefs, and potential barriers to treatment. Based on this information, we can work with our patients to develop individualized home exercise programs. Despite our efforts to individualize our home exercise programs, however, barriers to adherence may remain for many people.[25,27,32]

Table 9-4. Strategies for Optimizing Adherence in Complex Patient Populations

Common Comorbid Conditions	Potential Barriers to Adherence and Performance	Strategies to Optimize Adherence and Performance
Postsurgical delirium or confusion (eg, a postsurgical repair of a hip fracture)	Patients with postsurgical delirium are confused and may not realize what is going on in the situation, which may result in occasional violent outbursts	Provide external structures and supports as opposed to expecting both full participation and individual responsibility for adherence; set lower-level goals until delirium or confusion clears; repeat instructions; redirect behavior without causing increased agitation; use shorter sessions multiple times per day; adjust sessions to medication levels whenever possible
Emotional lability or irritability (eg, post stroke)	Patients who are emotionally labile may become easily overwhelmed and distracted; they may become irritable and easily frustrated, confused, or uncooperative	Be observant and sensitive to the demands you are placing on your patient; pause to allow your patient to regain composure; acknowledge that this emotional lability is a typical response given the diagnosis; educate the family; allow the patient and family to talk about "tough" issues; be prepared for trigger topics such as kids, finances, home, etc; calmly redirect and keep session moving forward, never minimize your patient's emotion
Expressive or receptive aphasia (eg, post stroke)	Patients with expressive aphasia may become easily frustrated; a patient with receptive aphasia may have more difficulty following your instructions	Increase social supports; rely on information from family members and close friends to help you better understand your patient; use proprioceptive and visual cues to facilitate learning and participation with limited language requirements; schedule your session together with the speech pathologist and/or occupational therapist to learn more about your patient's levels of receptive and expressive language; use demonstration, verbal cues, pictures, etc, consistently to allow for carryover; use simple cues; do not use jargon; choose simple interventions that do not require too much explanation; do not continually change the task just because the patient does not understand; allow additional time for comprehension
Deficits in memory, organization, or planning (eg, secondary to traumatic or acquired brain injury, stroke, delirium following hip fracture surgery)	Patients with memory, planning, or organization problems may have difficulty following directions and following through on exercise programs	Provide external and environmental cues and reminders; provide a structured environment with routines and repetition; provide stepwise, detailed instructions; use planners, journals, written logs, or specialized PDAs, pagers, and other memory aids; schedule joint sessions with the speech pathologist and/or occupational therapist to gain more information on your patient's cognitive level; review any cognitive assessments that may have been completed; identify level and type of memory loss (eg, 1-step command, 2-step command, multiple commands, delayed recall, complex directions, related and unrelated memory topics, interrupted memory tasks, memory while in a quiet environment vs memory during a physical activity and/or in a noisy environment, short-term, long-term); Remember: you as the PT may be "bored" with the repetition, but the patient is not!
Frailty (eg, secondary to aging, osteoporosis)	Patients who are frail may view themselves as less capable than they are (ie, lack self-efficacy); they may show a fear of falling and/or movement	Help patients reframe perceptions about impairments and focus on capabilities; provide verbal encouragement and feedback on any achievements; provide role models; provide social supports; assess environmental factors to optimize safety; focus on patient- and family-identified goals; continually identify abilities and limitations during therapy; refer to the Health Belief Model
Depression* (eg, secondary to chronic pain, spinal cord injury, multiple sclerosis, myocardial infarct)	Patients with depression may view themselves as less capable than they are (ie, lack self-efficacy)	Use a team approach using cognitive behavioral therapy; help patients reframe perceptions about impairments and focus on capabilities rather than disabilities; define goals and provide verbal encouragement and feedback on achievements; identify social supports and support groups
Attention deficits	Patients with attention difficulties may have a limited attention span and may be easily distracted from the task at hand	Use external cues to refocus attention; provide structured therapy sessions; identify goals and possible rewards for focused attention to task; provide choices to maximize relevance and interest in the task; work in a quiet treatment area to minimize distraction; minimize the distraction of other patients, family members, etc; use behavior modification techniques if appropriate
Disinhibition, poor judgment, or impulsivity (eg, secondary to traumatic or acquired brain injury, stroke, traumatic brain injury)	Patients with impulsivity often act before they think and may not recognize the potential danger in their actions	Use a team approach to behavior management, including external cueing systems to help reduce inappropriate behaviors and increase appropriate behaviors; establish limits and clear expectations; provide structure and consistency; provide detailed directions; assess environmental factors to optimize safety

Adapted from Zinn S. Patience adherence in rehabilitation. In: Bosworth H, Oddone E, Weinberger M, eds. *Patient Treatment Adherence.* Mahwah, NJ: Lawrence Erlbaum Associates; 2006:195-236. With input from Heidi Dunfee, PT, DSc, Mayo Clinic, Rochester, MN. PDA indicates personal digital assistants; PT, physical therapist.
*It is important to note that depression may occur during the acute phase of rehabilitation; however, at times, there is a delayed onset.

Given the challenge we face in increasing adherence, it may be helpful to incorporate techniques that others have used successfully to increase physical activity in adults in other settings. Though certain strategies have been shown to enhance adherence, they have been underutilized by physical therapists.[33,34] For example, among the most commonly used strategies is self-monitoring, where individuals record activities in a written log.[35,36] Although it may seem simple to adapt a patient's written home exercise program into a diary or log format, physical therapists use home exercise logs infrequently.[34] Even simply asking your patient to write (or dictate) specific personal goals related to his home exercise may be helpful in having your patient take ownership of his program and may increase the chances of better follow-through.[37,38] Engaging family members and other members of your patient's social network or accessing community resources to expand your patient's social network may increase participation.[4] Using memory aids, cues, and prompts and designing your patient's home program to fit within his daily routine will also enhance adherence.[4] Finally, adding some type of follow-up contact after discharge from physical therapy may encourage longer term adherence and the opportunity to modify exercise prescriptions if a person's health status changes.[28,34]

Critical Thinking Clinical Scenario

Mrs. D is a 62-year-old patient who recently had a stroke. Her right arm is flaccid and has very limited sensation. She is mildly depressed because before she had her stroke, she enjoyed going for daily walks with group of women from her neighborhood, and she can no longer join them. You want Mrs. D to begin a daily routine of passive range of motion for her right arm and hand, and you would like her to walk from the front of her home to the back of her home several times per day. She indicates that she is willing to perform her home exercises but she just forgets. Besides, Mrs. D indicates that she does not really believe the exercises are going to make a difference; her father had a stroke when he was 70, and he never recovered function of his hand.

Reflective Questions

1. What comorbidities may be interfering with Mrs. D's ability to participate fully in the therapeutic process?
2. What potential barriers to adherence and performance are present in this scenario?
3. How might a behavior change conversation help in this situation?
4. What potential supports are available in this scenario?
5. What kind of strategies would you use to optimize Mrs. D's adherence and performance?

Key Points to Remember

Some strategies to facilitate increased patient participation and adherence include the following:

- Incorporating strategies to encourage patient accountability such as written logs or diaries.
- Having your patient develop his or her own personally relevant goals.
- Designing the home program to fit into your patient's daily routine.
- Identifying community resources and social networks.
- Using memory aids such as videos, written instructions, and illustrations.
- Identifying different cues or prompts that can be used as daily reminders.
- Providing follow-up contact after discharge.

Literacy and Patient Education

Literacy is a significant problem in the United States. In 2003, the National Adult Literacy Survey (NALS) revealed that 38% of the adults in the United States are at or below a basic level of literacy.[39] Look at Table 9-5, which provides a description of the literacy levels as described in the NALS; you will see this means that more than one-third of all American adults have difficulty reading and understanding basic instructions and written information.

Literacy is of particular concern in medicine and the health professions because patients are often required to read and understand discharge instructions, prescription labels, nutrition labels, home exercise plans, insurance forms, and the like. The American Medical Association Web site defines health literacy as "the ability to obtain, process, and understand basic health information and services needed to make appropriate health decisions and follow instructions for treatment." It further states, "Over 89 million American adults have limited health literacy skills" (http://www.ama-assn.org/ama/no-index/physician-resources/8115.shtml).

In 1996, Williams et al[40] conducted a study in the emergency department (ED) at an urban hospital to determine (1) the reading level required for the typical discharge instructions given to patients and (2) the reading level of the typical patient in the ED. They found that most instructions were written at the 9.8 grade level (range eighth to 14th grade); yet only 55% of the patients had sufficient reading comprehension skills to understand the plans. At the same time, Davis et al[41] reported that most Americans read 3 to 5 grade levels lower than the highest grade completed in school, which at the time was typically the sixth- through eighth-grade level. An analysis of Web-based pediatric educational materials conducted by D'Alessandro et al[42] in 2001 concluded that all of the educational materials they reviewed were written at or above the 10.6 grade level. This trend has continued, and still more recently, literature indicates that most health care materials are written at the 10th-grade level despite the fact that 80% of adults read at the eighth-grade level and 20% read below the fifth-grade level.[43,44]

In 2004, the Agency for Healthcare Research and Quality reported a link between low literacy and poor health outcomes.[45] The literature is replete with examples supporting this assertion. In 1998, Williams et al[46] found that only 55% of those patients with hypertension with inadequate levels of literacy recognized that a blood pressure reading of 160/100 mmHg was high and potentially problematic; similarly, in patients with diabetes, only 50% of those with inadequate literacy recognized symptoms of hypoglycemia. In 2003, Schillinger et al[47] found that patients with diabetes who had low literacy levels had more difficulty controlling their glycemic levels and were more likely to have retinopathy resulting from uncontrolled diabetes. Still more recently, in 2005, Kennen et al[48] noted that obese patients with low literacy were less likely to understand the potential health risks of obesity or the benefits of weight loss and were therefore less likely to change their behaviors. Studies have shown that patients with low literacy are less likely to use their medications properly, recognize health-related risk factors, and engage in preventative health measures.[46,49-51] Reports show that individuals with low literacy are also more likely to be hospitalized than their counterparts with adequate levels of literacy and incur 4 times more medical costs per year than those with adequate literacy levels, often because of unnecessary medical visits.[51-53]

The evidence provided suggests that health literacy is a strong predictor of health status, and so it is important that we consider this in developing any type of patient education materials. It is our responsibility as health care providers to understand our patient's level of health literacy to ensure optimal outcomes. The question is how do we determine our patient's level of health literacy? Often in health care, we rely on self-reported level of education or self-assessment of reading ability. This is problematic because as noted earlier, individuals often read 3 to 5 grade levels below the last grade they completed in school.[41] In addition, individuals with low literacy are often ashamed and embarrassed to admit when they encounter difficulty. There are some overt signs of low literacy we should consider when assessing our patients. Table 9-6 provides some examples of these overt signs.[54,55]

Even when medical professions are aware of these overt signs of inadequate health literacy, they often fail to identify many patients with inadequate levels of literacy.[56] As therapists, we can use a number of standardized measures to more effectively assess our patient's literacy level. Those most commonly used are the Test of Functional Health Literacy in Adults (TOFHLA), the Rapid Estimate of Adult Literacy in Medicine (REALM), and more recently the Newest Vital Sign (NVS):

- TOFHLA is a comprehensive assessment that takes about 20 minutes to administer. It is a 50-item reading comprehension and 17-item mathematical abilities test.[57] What is nice about this test is that there is a Spanish version as well (TOFHLA-S). Researchers often use this test; however, the length of time it takes to administer makes it somewhat impractical in a clinical setting.

- The REALM, on the other hand, is a valid screening instrument used to assess an adult's ability to read common medical words and lay terms for body parts and illnesses, and the shortened version takes only 2 to 3 minutes to administer (Table 9-7).[58]

Table 9-5. Literacy Levels

Literacy Level	Definition	Tasks	Example
Below basic	Ranges from being non-literate in English to being able to perform the most simple and concrete literacy tasks	Locates information in a short text; follows noncomplex instructions; completes noncomplex math functions	Identifies the date, time, and location of a physical therapy appointment; signs name; adds noncomplex numbers
Basic	Performs simple everyday literacy tasks	Reads and understands simple texts; completes simple math problems	Reads and understands a basic explanation of what physical therapy is; compares the cost of 2 grocery items
Intermediate	Performs moderately challenging literacy tasks	Reads and understands moderately dense text; summarizes material; draws inferences; determines cause and effect; solves simple math problems	Understands references that describe the vitamin content of various foods; uses a noncomplex map
Proficient	Performs complex and challenging literacy skills	Reads and understands lengthy texts; integrates and synthesizes information from multiple sources; completes multi-step math problems	Compares 2 differing points of view; interprets tables related to blood pressure and physical activity; computes cost per ounce of food

Adapted from White S. Assessing the nation's health literacy: key concepts and findings of the National Assessment of Adult Literacy (NAAL). Available at http://prospectus.lsbu.ac.uk/lluplus/docs/Reports/hl_report_2008.pdf. Accessed July 21, 2009.

Table 9-6. Overt Behaviors That May Suggest Inadequate Health Literacy

Patients with inadequate health literacy may be observed to:

- Say, "I forgot my glasses, I will read it when I get home."
- Wait until the illness is advanced before seeking help.
- Have difficulty providing a complete history or explaining the problem.
- Identify medication by color and shape rather than name.
- Ask staff for help.
- Bring along friends to help them read and interpret written material or understand instructions.

- Lack follow-up.
- Lack adherence to recommendations or instructions (eg, medication, home exercise prescriptions).
- Ask for time to go home and think about it before making any decisions.
- Copy the behaviors of those around them.
- Rarely have questions.

Adapted from Baker DW, Parker RM, Williams MV, et al. The health care experience of patients with low literacy. *Arch Fam Med.* 1996;5:329-334; Meade C, McKinney W, Barnas G. Educating patients with limited literacy skills: the effectiveness of printed and videotaped materials about colon cancer. *Am J Public Health.* 1994;84:119-121.

- The NVS is a screening tool that includes 21 questions on 5 scenarios related to health issues such as medication instructions, informed consent, self-care instructions, and nutrition labels. This, too, comes in a Spanish version. The short form includes 1 scenario (ie, a nutrition label from an ice cream container) and 6 related questions. It takes about 3 minutes to administer and has been shown to be a valid screening tool for adult health literacy levels (Figures 9-3A and 9-3B).[59]

Health literacy has significant implications for the development of patient education materials. Writing all patient-related information at the fifth- to sixth-grade level will help optimize readability. You can use a number of methods to determine the readability of the material you are preparing. Three commonly used measures are the Simple Measure of Gobbledygook (SMOG), the Flesch-Kincaid Index, and the Gunning FOG Index.

McLaughlin[60] developed the SMOG grade to determine the educational level an individual would need to understand a given text. Instructions for calculating the SMOG grade are as follows:

1. Count 10 consecutive sentences at the beginning, middle, and end of a passage, for a total of 30 sentences.
2. Count every word with 3 or more syllables.
3. Estimate the square root of the number of polysyllabic words counted.
4. Add 3 to the approximate square root.
5. This number represents the SMOG grade or the level of education that the reader needs to fully understand the text.

As a gross estimate, you can count the number of words in a 3- to 10-sentence sample, estimate the square root of that number, and add 3. However, the simplest way to calculate the SMOG grade is to use the SMOG calculator on the Internet at http://www.word-scount.info/hw/smog.jsp.

The Flesch-Kincaid Index is a readability index that rates the degree of difficulty of reading passages on US school grade levels. It is only valid for materials written at grade levels 3 through 12.[42] The formula uses the length of sentences and the number of polysyllabic words used to determine level of difficulty. The formula used to calculate the Flesch-Kincaid Index is as follows:

$$(0.39 \times ASL) + (11.8 \times ASW) - 15.59$$

ASL = Average sentence length (ie, number of words divided by the number of sentences).

ASW = Average number of syllables per word (ie, the number of syllables divided by the number of words).

You can calculate the Flesch-Kincaid Index and Flesch Reading Ease Score automatically using the Spelling and Grammar tools on Microsoft Word. The Flesch Reading Ease ranges from 0 to 100; the higher the score, the easier it is to read.

- Scores of 70 or above are considered easily readable at the grade school level.
- Scores of 60 to 70 are considered to be written at the high school level.
- Scores below 60 are considered difficult to read.

Finally, the Fog Index is a readability test designed to determine the level of difficulty of a given reading passage. This one has the simplest formula to remember and calculate. The Fog Index uses the following formula:

$$ASL + PPSW \times 0.4$$

ASL = Average sentence length (ie, number of words divided by the number of sentences).

PPSW = Percent of polysyllabic words (ie, divide the number of words with more than 2 syllables by the total number of words in the passage). This does not include simple polysyllabic words that combine simple words such as *butterfly, bookkeeper,* nor does it include words with suffixes such as -ed or -es (eg, assumed, sentences).

Table 9-7. Rapid Estimate of Adult Literacy in Medicine

Patient name _____ Date of birth _____ Reading level _____

Date of Clinic _____ Examiner _____ Grade completed _____

List 1		List 2		List 3	
Fat	☐	Fatigue	☐	Allergic	☐
Flu	☐	Pelvic	☐	Menstrual	☐
Pill	☐	Jaundice	☐	Testicle	☐
Dose	☐	Infection	☐	Colitis	☐
Eye	☐	Exercise	☐	Emergency	☐
Stress	☐	Behavior	☐	Medication	☐
Smear	☐	Prescription	☐	Occupation	☐
Nerves	☐	Notify	☐	Sexuality	☐
Germs	☐	Gallbladder	☐	Alcoholism	☐
Meals	☐	Calories	☐	Irritation	☐
Disease	☐	Depression	☐	Constipation	☐
Cancer	☐	Miscarriage	☐	Gonorrhea	☐
Caffeine	☐	Pregnancy	☐	Inflammatory	☐
Attack	☐	Arthritis	☐	Diabetes	☐
Kidney	☐	Nutrition	☐	Hepatitis	☐
Hormones	☐	Menopause	☐	Antibiotics	☐
Herpes	☐	Appendix	☐	Diagnosis	☐
Seizure	☐	Abnormal	☐	Potassium	☐
Bowel	☐	Syphilis	☐	Anemia	☐
Asthma	☐	Hemorrhoids	☐	Obesity	☐
Rectal	☐	Nausea	☐	Osteoporosis	☐
Incest	☐	Directed	☐	Impetigo	☐
List 1 score	_____	List 2 score	_____	List 3 score	_____
				Raw score _____	

Directions:

1. Give the patient a laminated copy of the REALM form, and score answers on an unlaminated copy that is attached to a clipboard. Hold the clipboard at an angle so that the patient is not distracted by your scoring. Say, "I want to hear you read as many words as you can from this list. Begin with the first word in List 1 and read aloud. When you come to a word you cannot read, do the best you can or say, 'blank' and go on to the next word."
2. If the patient takes more than 5 seconds on a word, say "blank" and point to the next word, if necessary, to move the patient along. If the patient begins to miss every word, have him or her pronounce only known words.
3. Count as an error any word not attempted or mispronounced. Score by marking a plus (+) after each correct word, a check (✓) after each mispronounced word, and a minus (–) after words not attempted. Count as correct any self-corrected words.
4. Count the number of correct words for each list, and record the numbers on the "Score" line. Total the numbers, and match the score with its grade equivalent in the table below.

Scores and Grade Equivalents for the REALM Questionnaire	
Raw score	Grade range
0 to 18	Third grade and below; will not be able to read most low-literacy materials; will need repeated oral instructions, materials composed primarily of illustrations, or audio- or videotapes
19 to 44	Fourth to sixth grade; will need low-literacy materials, may not be able to read prescription labels
45 to 60	Seventh to eighth grade; will struggle with most patient education materials; will not be offended by low-literacy materials
61 to 66	High school; will be able to read most patient education materials

A. The newest vital sign–English	
Nutrition Facts	
Serving Size	½ cup
Servings per container	4
Amount per serving	
Calories 250	Fat Cal 120
	%DV
Total Fat 13 g	20%
Sat Fat 9 g	40%
Cholesterol 28 mg	12%
Sodium 55 mg	2%
Total Carbohydrate 30 g	12%
Dietary Fiber 2 g	
Sugars 23 g	
Protein 4 g	8%

*Percent Daily Values (DV) are based on a 2,000 calorie diet. Your daily values may be higher or lower depending on your calorie needs.

Ingredients: Cream, Skim Milk, Liquid Sugar, Water, Egg Yolks, Brown Sugar, Milkfat, Peanut Oil, Sugar, Butter, Carrageenan, Vanilla Extract.

Note: This single scenario is the final English version of the newest vital sign. The type size should be 14-point (as shown above) or larger. Patients are presented with the above scenario and asked then questions shown in Figure 9-3B.

B. Questions and answers score sheet for the newest vital sign–English		
ANSWER	**CORRECT?**	
READ TO SUBJECT: This information is on the back of a container of a pint of ice cream.	**YES**	**NO**
QUESTIONS:	_____	_____
1. If you eat the entire container, how many calories will you eat?		
Answer ❏1,000 is the only correct answer	_____	_____
2. If you are allowed to eat 60 g of carbohydrates as a snack, how much ice cream could you have?	_____	_____
Answer ❏ Any of the following is correct:	_____	_____
1 cup (or any amount up to 1 cup)	_____	_____
Half the container		
Note: If patients answers "2 servings" ask "How much ice cream would that be if you were to measure it into a bowl?"	_____	_____
3. Your doctor advises you to reduce the amount of saturated fat in your diet. You usually have 42 g of saturated fat each day, which includes 1 serving of ice cream. If you stop eating ice cream, how many grams of saturated fat would you be consuming each day?	_____	_____
Answer ❏33 is the only correct answer	_____	_____
4. If you usually eat 2,500 calories in a day, what percentage of your daily value of calories will you be eating if you eat 1 serving?	_____	_____
Answer ❏10% is the only correct answer	_____	_____
Pretend that you are allergic to the following substances: Penicillin, peanuts, latex gloves, and bee stings.	_____	_____
5. Is it safe for you to eat this ice cream?	_____	_____
Answer ❏No	_____	_____
6. (Ask only if the patient responds "no" to question #5): Why not?	_____	_____
Answer ❏Because it has peanut oil.	_____	_____
Total Correct	_____	_____

Figure 9-3. (A) The Newest Vital Sign short form—English. (B) Questions and answers score sheet for the Newest Vital Sign—English. (Adapted with permission from "Quick Assessment of Literacy in Primary Care: The Newest Vital Sign," December 2005, Annals of Family Medicine. Copyright © 2005 American Academy of Family Physicians. All Rights Reserved.)

These formulas are merely estimates of readability. It is important to remember that given the typical layperson's lack of familiarity with medial information these readability scores may likely underestimate the difficulty of readability.[42] Furthermore, because each of these readability formulas uses a slightly different method, the resulting reading levels may vary. The Flesch-Kincaid and other computer-generated scores generally underestimate level of difficulty, whereas the Flesch Reading Ease Index more closely estimates the hand-calculated SMOG score, which appears to be a better estimate of readability. Though it may be easiest for many to calculate the Flesch-Kincaid Index or Flesch Reading Ease Score on your computer, to ensure readability, it is recommended that written materials be analyzed using the SMOG method.[42,61]

Key Points to Remember

- To optimize readability of your patient education materials, be sure that they are written at or below the sixth-grade reading level.
- Several methods are available to compute the ease of readability:
  - Simple Measure of Gobbledygook (SMOG)
  - Flesch-Kincaid Index
  - Flesch Reading Ease Score
  - Gunning FOG Index
- The SMOG method appears to be most accurate.
- These readability analysis methods are based on the
  - Length of sentences
  - The number of polysyllabic words

Critical Thinking Clinical Scenario

Mr. T is a 52-year-old male retired firefighter who just recently underwent an anterior fusion of his cervical spine (C3-5). He is a high school graduate and does not report having difficulty with reading complex texts. You are developing a home exercise program for him, which includes isometric cervical exercises, and you have written the following: "Complete 3 sets of 10 isometric cervical flexion, lateral flexion, and extension twice per day."

Reflective Questions
1. Calculate the grade level required to read this passage using the Flesch-Kincaid Index.
2. Is this consistent with the grade level that was computed using the Fog Index?
3. How might you modify this text to conform to a fifth- to sixth-grade level?

These formulas are gross estimates and provide information about the readability of the passages; they are based on the assumption that the more 3-syllable words and the longer the sentences, the more difficult the material is to read. However, simply writing shorter sentences with less complex words is not enough. Content, organization, and design are critical elements of well-written patient information.[62]

Designing and Evaluating Effective Patient Education Materials

In developing any patient education information, it is critical to consider the content that needs to be included. Remembering the concept from Chapter 4, less is more; you want to be sure to include only that information that the patient needs to know versus what you think might be nice to know. Excessive information about the pathophysiology of the disease may only serve to cloud your important message.

Consider some of the concepts we discussed in developing presentations (ie, systematic effective instruction). In your patient education/information pamphlet, it is helpful to include the following:

- A motivational hook (eg, why should your patient read any further?)
- Objectives (eg, bulleted major points you want them to learn and will expand upon in the pamphlet)
- Content boosters (eg, pictures, mnemonics to remember the exercises or frequency of performance)
- Formative assessment (eg, a few questions for them to ponder or to test their understanding)

- Summary (eg, reinforce major points; a few bulleted take-home points or things to remember)

Patient education materials should always be jargon free and culturally appropriate, and it is helpful to use the active voice as if you were speaking directly with your patient. For example, rather than writing, "Complete cervical isometric exercises twice per day," you might say, "It is important that you do your neck bending exercises in the morning and again in the evening. Put the palm of your hand on your head. Push against it with your head but do not let your head move. Do this twice in all directions, front, back, and each side." If you need to use medical jargon, be sure to explain it in the text. For example, "You will be doing neck flexion (bring your chin toward your chest) and neck side-bending (bring your ear down toward your shoulder) exercises." Make sure that your directions are simple and concise. If you want them to follow a specific step-wise progression, be sure to number each step and describe it simply but fully.

Drawings and illustrations can enhance your patient's comprehension and recall of health education information.[63] They may be particularly helpful for your patients with inadequate literacy skills. No commercial product can take the place of you sitting with your patient and making your instructions clear and precise. Including well-drawn stick figures can help clarify the text and enhance recall. It is often helpful to make this a collaborative effort in which your patient helps you draw the exercise in a way that it will make the most sense to him. If the picture makes sense to your patient, he is more likely to remember what it means. Make sure that your patient can follow and understand exactly what you are trying to explain. When drawing stick figures, be sure to include major body parts and the direction of movement (Figure 9-4). Drawing stick figures is a critical skill, particularly given the low literacy rate and the percentage of the US population that speaks English as a second language. Stick figures allow you to get your point across without words. We encourage you to invest in a stick figure drawing book and practice your drawing skills!

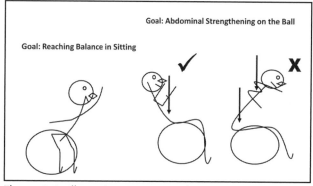

Figure 9-4. Illustrating 2 activities for a patient to perform using stick figures.

Table 9-8. Additional Guidelines for Designing Written Patient Education Materials

- Check readability (fifth- to sixth-grade level)
- Jargon free
- Use black lettering on white paper
- Use clear font, 12 point or larger
- Do not use all capital letters
- To minimize distractions, use no more than 2 types of fonts
- Left justify your words
- Short paragraphs
- Bulleted lists, key points, and take-home messages
- Use bolded headers to separate topics
- Lots of white space
- Active voice (ie, as if you were talking to your patient)
- Content boosters (eg, pictures, pneumonic)
- Formative assessments (eg, questions, problem-solving scenarios, teach-back strategies)

Adapted from D'Alessandro DM, Kingsley P, Johnson-West J. The readability of pediatric patient education materials on the world wide web. *Arch Pediatr Adolesc Med.* 2001;155:807-812; Dreeben O. *Patient Education in Rehabilitation.* Sudbury, MA: Jones and Bartlett Publishers; 2010.

Table 9-8 provides additional factors to consider when designing patient education materials.[4,6]

Doak et al[64] developed a useful guide for evaluating written educational materials, the *Suitability Assessment of Materials Instrument* (SAMI). The SAMI addresses 6 factors that affect the reader's ability to understand the material presented:

1. Content, including purpose, topics, summary, and review.

2. Literacy demand, including reading level, writing style (active voice), sentence construction, vocabulary, advanced organizers (eg, headings and subheadings).

3. Graphics, including cover picture, clarity of illustrations, relevance of illustration, clear instructions, and captions for all graphics.

4. Layout and type, including type and font size, organization of the layout, chunk information using headers.

5. Learning stimulation and motivation, including interactive application of the content through questions or problem-solving activities; content includes concrete examples not abstract principles; tasks are doable.

6. Cultural appropriateness, including materials that are culturally relevant and specific for the targeted audience.

Each of the factors is rated on a 3-point scale (ie, Superior = 2; Adequate = 1; Not Suitable = 0) to allow for comparisons across categories and across materials.

Though initially designed to assess written materials, the SAMI has since been used to evaluate the suitability of videos, audiotapes, and computer-based patient education materials.

Patient handouts, brochures, and line drawings are used routinely in today's health care environment. However, there is an increased interest in the use of more technologically sophisticated educational materials.[65] Exercise videos are used commonly in the general population. It is not surprising that researchers have examined the effectiveness of videos and other computer-assisted technology for teaching home exercises and for increasing adherence to home exercise programs in physical therapy practice.[65-68] Some studies have reported benefits of video or computer-based approaches over written instructional materials,[68,69] whereas others found no differences in adherence between groups who received traditional versus more technologically sophisticated instructions.[65]

The key is to provide the most appropriate instructional materials for each patient. The availability of a variety of formats, including digital videos of the physical therapist demonstrating specific exercises taken by a patient's camera phone or individualized computer-based videos, may make it easier to customize patient education strategies. Based on your needs assessment and problem-solving conversations with your patients, you may determine that one patient is less comfortable with the newer technologies and another really enjoys anything related to computers. These findings will influence how you develop and modify your educational approach with each patient.

Maintaining Behavior Change

Once your patients move beyond the preparation phase to the action phase of behavior change, you are not done! You will want to continue to work with them to help them maintain their healthy lifestyles. One way you can help them do this is through the "5 A's of Behavior Counseling."[21]

- *Address.* Each time your patient returns for therapy, you will want to be sure to address any issues that may have arisen for your patient. This includes issues related to knowledge, motivation, and resources. Using adult learning principles, you want to be sure they realize (1) what they need to do, (2) why they need to do it, (3) when they need to do it, and (4) how they need to do it. You also will want to be sure they recognize the risks of nonadherence and the benefits of adherence to their program.

- *Assess.* It is important to remember that patients have a tendency to do either too much or too little; either one can be harmful. Just as we do formative and summative assessments in our classroom or in our presentations, it is important that we continually monitor/reassess the understanding and adherence of our patients. You also will want to ask your patient about his level of adherence in performing his exercises. You will want to ask what changes he may have noticed, what progress he may have made, and what problems he may have encountered. You will want to assess his level of confidence in performing his home exercises because the more confident your patient feels in performing his exercises, the more likely he will be to continue to perform them. You will want to assess whether and to what degree he is following the exercise prescription you provided. By assessing his level of adherence, you are keeping your patient accountable. Your patient knows that you will ask, and by asking, you send a message to your patient that the program or exercise is important and that you care about his continued improvement. Remember also that the desire to please you, the therapist, can be very motivating and just what the patient needs to maintain his behavior change. On the other hand, if through your assessment you find that your patient is nonadherent, it might be a good time to explore his health beliefs, problem solve barriers to progress, and suggest alternatives that are more suitable.

- *Advise.* Once you have assessed your patient's level of adherence, you will want to provide advice on any changes you recommend based on his current level of activity. Depending on the stage of change or your patient's readiness to participate, your advice may differ. For example, if you note that your patient has relapsed, you may remind him of the risks and benefits to nonadherence. If your patient is in the preparation stage of change, you may help him problem solve any perceived barriers to adherence.

- *Assist.* Once you have given advice, you want to assist your patient in developing realistic goals tied to personally relevant and valued activities. You will want to help your patient develop strategies for accomplishing those goals and again problem solve any perceived barriers. You will want to do a formative assessment to ensure that your patient is confident in performing his home exercises and provide strategies to help reinforce adherence (eg, weekly log of activities). You will want to provide information about community resources.

- *Arrange.* Finally, you will want to be sure to arrange for some type of follow-up. Ensuring follow-up reinforces accountability on the part of the patient, reinforces the importance of adherence, and, again, demonstrates that you care.

Keys Points Remember

The 5 A's of Behavioral Counseling, Change, and a Healthy Lifestyle:
- Address
- Assess
- Advise
- Assist
- Arrange

Summary

Just as preparing to teach is a complex process, so too is preparing to educate your patient. Telling your patient what to do is not sufficient to ensure adherence to any program. Patient education is a valued activity in all of the health professions. The ultimate goal of patient education is to empower our patients to take full responsibility for their own health and wellness. Adherence is a complex problem, which is compounded in physical therapy because of the comorbidities our patients often experience. To increase levels of adherence, it is important that we select appropriate patient education strategies. Understanding our patients' illness experiences through their explanatory models and health beliefs as well as recognizing their readiness to change and learning preferences, in the context of the task and their environment, will help us select the most appropriate strategy for each patient. Written materials may also encourage follow-through and adherence at home. However, we must take care in designing written materials to ensure ease of readability. Finally, follow-up and ongoing monitoring is essential for facilitating long-term adherence to behavior change and a healthy lifestyle. Building on concepts from previous chapters, Table 9-9 synthesizes the major concepts presented in this chapter and provides a framework for developing a mutually agreeable plan of care designed to optimize patient adherence and long-term behavior change.

Key Points to Remember

- Understanding your patient's illness experience is as important as understanding the disease process.
- Patient education is more than telling; it is influencing behavior change in your patient and to do so requires a systematic approach.
- Influencing adherence requires us to:
  - Consider health beliefs and explanatory models
  - Recognize the many variables that influence adherence, including comorbid conditions
  - Recognize our patients' readiness to change
  - Negotiate mutually agreeable goals
  - Provide ongoing behavior counseling
- We can optimize our educational intervention by selecting educational approaches and learning strategies that match our patient's literacy level, learning preferences, health beliefs, phase of recovery, and readiness to change.
- To optimize the potential for long-term adherence we can use the 5 A's of Behavioral Counseling:
  - Addressing the issues
  - Assessing
  - Advising
  - Assisting
  - Arranging for follow-up

Table 9-9. Negotiation of Shared Meaning: Steps to Developing a Mutually Agreeable Plan of Care That Optimizes Patient Adherence

Step 1: Develop Shared Meaning through Dialogue
• Identify your patient's explanatory model and health beliefs
• Identify your own explanatory model and what you believe to be the best treatment
• Identify activity limitations and participation restrictions
• Negotiate a shared understanding of the disease state and the illness experience
Step 2: Develop a Plan of Care
• Link interventions to valued activities
• Identify your patient's priorities
• Design a mutually agreeable plan of care
Step 3: Assess Readiness
• Assess readiness to change (ie, stage of change)
• Assess self-efficacy (ie, confidence in performing)
• Identify potential barriers and supports to adherence including comorbid conditions
• Identify patient and community resources
• Assess literacy level
• Assess learning preferences
Step 4: Provide Intervention and Education
• Provide background knowledge (including rationale for the intervention or home exercise program)
• Teach appropriate home exercises using appropriate learning strategies
• Provide instructions that consider appropriate literacy levels and learning preferences
Step 5: Check for Understanding
• Incorporate formative assessments throughout your session as well as in written materials
Step 6: Check for Adherence
• Address issues
• Assess/ask
• Advise
• Assist
• Arrange for follow-up
Step 7: Reinforce Adherence
• Problem solve any new barriers to adherence
• Identify additional community resources for support
• Modify goals and plan of care to ensure continued compliance and to ensure that the patient's goals are being met
• Develop learning contracts, reflective journals, or weekly logs to reinforce accountability

Integrative Patient Case Scenario

Therapist

You have been assigned a new patient with a diagnosis of cervical strain as a result of a car accident. Having completed your evaluation, your plan of care consists of hot packs, soft tissue mobilization, ultrasound, and a home exercise program (HEP). Your plan is to teach a HEP consisting of isometric cervical exercises, and you want to provide your patient with the following HEP: "Complete 3 sets of 10 isometric cervical flexion, lateral flexion, and axial extension exercises twice per day."

1. What questions will you ask to get a sense of the patient's explanatory model?

2. What questions will you ask to help determine her learning style?

3. What is the literacy level of the HEP described above? How would you enhance readability?

4. What type of stick figure diagram would you include to illustrate the activities you want your patient to perform?

Integrative Patient Case Scenario

Patient

You are a 29-year-old mother of 4 children, ages 8, 7, 4, and 10 months. You dropped out of high school as a junior to go to work to help with the family finances. You work part-time as a clerk typist, and your job requires a great deal of typing and desk work. You were in a car accident 5 days ago and suffered whiplash. You are in pain, especially at the end of the day (8 on a scale of 1 to 10). You have been to therapy twice and received massages, hot packs, and an ultrasound. Therapy provides short-term relief but you are concerned that you still have pain at the end of the day when you can feel that your muscles are in spasm. You are so busy at home that you have little time to do your exercises, and you figure that because you are receiving therapy twice per week, they are not really necessary. You believe that the only things that will really help are massages, painkillers, and muscle relaxants but do not like to take any medication because it makes you groggy. You believe that your muscles became spasmed as a result of the car accident, and so you cannot really understand how a strengthening exercise will help decrease your pain. You learn best by working with others and are motivated to do your exercises when you have someone there to guide you and let you know you are doing them correctly. You are concerned about the pain because it limits you from taking care of the baby as you need to, and it limits your concentration at work.

1. What type of learner is this patient?

2. Given her learning style, what precautions might you consider? What strategies might you use in therapy?

3. How might you address her health beliefs to facilitate a change in behaviors?

4. Where is she along the readiness to change scale? Given her readiness to change, what change strategies might you consider?

5. What are some of the factors that may lead to patient nonadherence?

6. What are her valued activities?

7. What goal might you establish with your patient?

8. After 3 sessions, your patient returns and indicates that she has been following the exercises you recommended. What steps will you use to ensure that she continues to maintain this behavior change?

References

1. Dewey J. *Experience and education.* New York, NY: Simon & Schuster; 1938.

2. Dewey J. *How we think.* Amherst, NY: Prometheus Books; 1991.

3. American Physical Therapist Association. *Guide to Physical Therapist Practice.* 2nd ed. Alexandria, VA: American Physical Therapist Association; 2003.

4. Dreeben O. *Patient Education in Rehabilitation.* Sudbury, MA: Jones and Bartlett Publishers; 2010.

5. American Hospital Association. The patient care partnership: Understanding rights and responsibilities. http://www.aha.org/aha/issues/Communicating-With-Patients/pt-care-partnership.html. Published 2003. Accessed June 21, 2009.

6. May BJ. Patient education: past and present. *J Phys Ther Educ.* 1999;13:3-7.

7. *CARF: Medical Rehabilitation Standards Manual.* Tucson, AZ: CARF International; 2009.

8. *A Normative Model of Physical Therapist Professional Education: Version 2000.* Alexandria, VA: American Physical Therapy Association; 2000.

9. *Evaluative Criteria for Accreditation of Education Programs for the Preparation of Physical Therapists.* Alexandria, VA: Commission on Accreditation of Physical Therapy Education; 2006.

10. Elias JL, Merriam SB. *Philosophical Foundations of Adult Education.* 2nd ed. Malabar, FL: Krieger Publishing Company; 1995.

11. Todd J, Loewy J, Kelly G. Managing challenging behaviours: getting interventions to work in nonspecialized community settings. *Brain Impair.* 2004;5:42-52.

12. Pierson FM, Fairchild SL. *Principles and Techniques of Patient Care.* 4th ed. St. Louis, MO: Saunders Elsevier; 2008.

13. Zinn S. Patience adherence in rehabilitation. In: Bosworth H, Oddone E, Weinberger M, eds. *Patient Treatment Adherence.* Mahwah, NJ: Lawrence Erlbaum Associates; 2006:195-236.

14. Peters M, Gluck M, McCormick M. Behaviour rehabilitation of the challenging client in less restrictive settings. *Brain Inj.* 1992;6:299-314.

15. Candy P. *Self-Direction for Lifelong Learning.* San Francisco, CA: Jossey-Bass; 1991.

16. Wilson AL, Hayes ER, eds. *Handbook of Adult and Continuing Education.* San Francisco, CA: Jossey-Bass; 2000.

17. Ryan RM, Deci EL. Intrinsic and extrinsic motivations: classic definitions and new directions. *Contemp Educ Psychol.* 2000;25:54-67.

18. Kleinman A, Eisenberg L, Good B. Culture, illness, and care: clinical lessons from anthropologic and cross-cultural research. *Ann Intern Med.* 1978;88:251-258.

19. Steiner WA, Ryser L, Huber E, Uebelhart D, Aeschlimann A, Stucki G. Use of the ICF model as a clinical problem-solving tool in physical therapy and rehabilitation medicine. *Phys Ther.* 2002;82:1098-1107.

20. Rimer BK, Glanz K. Theory at a glance: a guide for health promotion practice. Available at http://cancer.gov/aboutnci/oc/theory-at-a-glance/page1. Accessed June 21, 2009.

21. Lorish C, Gale J. Facilitating behavior change: strategies for education and practice. *J Phys Ther Educ.* 1999;13:31-37.

22. Prochaska JO, DiClemente CC. Transtheoretical therapy: toward a more integrative model of change. *Psychother Theory Res.* 1982;3:276-288.

23. Prochaska JO, DiClemente CC, Norcross J. In search of how people change: applications to the addictive behaviors. *Am Psychol.* 1992;47:1102-1114.

24. Bosworth H, Weinberger M, Oddone E. Introduction. In: Bosworth H, Weinberger M, Oddone E, eds. *Patient Treatment Adherence.* Mahwah, NJ: Lawrence Erlbaum Associates; 2006.

25. Sluijs EM, Kok GJ, van der Zee J. Correlates of exercise compliance in physical therapy. *Phys Ther.* 1993;73:771-786.

26. Minor M, Reid J, Griffin J, Pittman C, Patrick T, Cutts J. Development and validation of an exercise performance support system for people with lower extremity impairment. *Arthritis Care Res.* 1998;11:3-8.

27. Resnick B, Magaziner J, Orwig D, Zimmerman S. Evaluating the components of the exercise plus program: rationale, theory and implementation. *Health Educ Res.* 2002;17:648-658.

28. Forkan R, Pumper B, Smythe N, Wirkalla N, Ciol M, Shumway-Cook A. Exercise adherence following physical therapy intervention in older adults with impaired balance. *Phys Ther.* 2006;86:401-410.

29. Trost SG, Woen N, Bauman AE, Sallis JF, Brown W. Correlates of adults' participation in physical activity: review and update. *Med Sci Sports Exerc.* 2002;34:1996-2001.

30. Yardley L, Bishop FL, Beyer N, et al. Older people's views of falls–prevention interventions in six European countries. *Gerontologist.* 2006;46:650-660.

31. O'Shea SD, Taylor NF, Paratz J. But watch out for the weather: factors affecting adherence to progressive resistive exercises for persons with COPD. *J Cardiopulm Rehabil Prev.* 2007;27:166-174.

32. Friederich M, Gittler G, Haberstadt Y, Cermak T, Heiller I. Combined exercise and motivation program: effect on the compliance and level of disability of patients with chronic low backpain: a randomized controlled trial. *Arch Phys Med Rehabil.* 1998;79:475-487.

33. Kahn E, Ramsey L, Brownson R, et al. The effectiveness of interventions to increase physical activity: a systematic review. *Am J Prev Med.* 2002;22:73-107.

34. Holden MA, Nicholls EE, Hay EM, Foster NE. Physical therapists' use of therapeutic exercise for patients with clinical knee osteoarthritis in the United Kingdom: In line with current recommendations? *Phys Ther.* 2008;88:1109-1122.

35. Meichenbaum D, Turk D. *Facilitating Treatment Adherence.* New York, NY: Plenum Press; 1987.

36. King A, Castro C, Wilcox S, Eyler A, Sallis J, Brownson R. Personal and environmental factors associated with physical activity among different racial-ethnic groups of US middle-aged and older adults. *Health Psychol.* 2000;19:354-364.

37. Heesch K, Masse L, Dunn A, Frankowski R, Mullen D. Does adherence to a lifestyle physical activity intervention predict changes in physical activity? *J Behav Med.* 2003;26:333-348.

38. Simons-Morton DG. Effects of physical activity counseling in primary care: the activity counseling trial. *JAMA.* 2001;286:677-687.

39. White S. Assessing the nation's health literacy: key concepts and findings of the National Assessment of Adult Literacy (NAAL). Available at http://prospectus.lsbu.ac.uk/lluplus/docs/Reports/hl_report_2008.pdf. Accessed July 21, 2009.

40. Williams DM, Counselman FL, Caggiano CD. Emergency department discharge instructions and patient literacy: a problem of disparity. *Am J Emerg Med.* 1996;14:19-22.

41. Davis TC, Arnold C, Berkel HJ, Nancy I, Jackson RH, Glass J. Knowledge and attitude on screening mammography among low-literate, low-income women. *Cancer.* 1996;78:1912-1920.

42. D'Alessandro DM, Kingsley P, Johnson-West J. The readability of pediatric patient education materials on the world wide web. *Arch Pediatr Adolesc Med.* 2001;155:807-812.

43. Safeer R, Keenan J. The gap between physicians and patients. *Am Fam Physician.* 2005;72:463-468.

44. Wallace LS, Lennon ES. American Academy of Family Physicians patient education materials: can patients read them? *Fam Med.* 2004;36:571-574.

45. Berkman ND, DeWalt DA, Pignone MP, et al. Literacy and health outcomes. Evidence Report/Technology Assessment Number 87. Available at http://www.ahrq.gov/clinic/epcsums/litsum.pdf. Accessed July 5, 2009.

46. Williams MV, Baker DW, Parker RM, Nurss JR. Relationship of functional health literacy to patients' knowledge of their chronic disease. A study of patients with hypertension and diabetes. *Arch Intern Med.* 1998;158:166-172.

47. Schillinger D, Piette J, Grumbach K, et al. Closing the loop: physician communication with diabetic patients who have low health literacy. *Arch Intern Med.* 2003;163:83-90.

48. Kennen EM, Davis TC, Huang J, et al. Tipping the scales: the effect of literacy on obese patients' knowledge and readiness to lose weight. *South Med J.* 2005;98:15-18.

49. Williams MV, Baker DW, Honig EG, Lee TM, Nowlan A. Inadequate literacy is a barrier to asthma knowledge and self-care. *Chest.* 1998;114:1008-1015.

50. Scott TL, Gazmararian JA, Williams MV, Baker DW. Health literacy and preventive health care use among Medicare enrollees in a managed care organization. *Med Care.* 2002;40:395-404.

51. Baker D, Gazmararian J, Williams M, et al. Functional health literacy and the risk of hospital admission among Medicare managed care enrollees. *Am J Public Health.* 2002;92:1278-1283.

52. Howard DH, Gazmararian J, Parker RM. The impact of low health literacy on the medical costs of Medicare managed care enrollees. *Am J Med.* 2005;118:371-377.

53. Weiss BD, Palmer R. Relationship between health care costs and very low literacy skills in medically needy and indigent Medicaid population. *J Am Board Fam Pract.* 2004;17:44-47.

54. Baker DW, Parker RM, Williams MV, et al. The health care experience of patients with low literacy. *Arch Fam Med.* 1996;5:329-334.

55. Meade C, McKinney W, Barnas G. Educating patients with limited literacy skills: the effectiveness of printed and videotaped materials about colon cancer. *Am J Public Health.* 1994;84:119-121.

56. Bass PF, Wilson JF, Griffith CH, Barnett DR. Residents' ability to identify patients with poor literacy skills. *Acad Med.* 2002;77:1039-1041.

57. Parker RM, Baker DW, Williams MV, Nurss JR. The test of functional health literacy in adults: a new instrument for measuring patients' literacy skills. *J Gen Intern Med.* 1995;10:537-541.

58. Davis TC, Long SW, Jackson RH, et al. Rapid estimate of adult literacy in medicine: a shortened screening instrument. *Fam Med.* 1993;25:391-395.

59. Weiss BD, Mays MZ, Martz W, et al. Quick assessment of literacy in primary care: the newest vital sign. *Ann Fam Med.* 2005;3:514-522.

60. McLaughlin GH. SMOG grading: a new readability formula. *J Read.* 1969;12:639-646.

61. Mailloux SL, Johnson ME, Fisher DG, Pettibone TJ. How reliable is computerized assessment of readability? *Comput Nurs.* 1995;13:221-225.

62. Ivnik M, Jett MY. Creating written patient education materials. *Chest.* 2008;133:1038-1040.

63. Houts PS, Doak CC, Doak LG, Loscalzo MJ. The role of pictures in improving health communication: a review of research on attention, comprehension, recall, and adherence. *Patient Educ Couns.* 2006;61:173-190.

64. Doak CC, Doak LG, Root JH. Teaching patients with low literacy skills. *Am J Nurs.* 1996;96:16.

65. Lysack C, Dama M, Neufeld S, Andreassi E. Compliance and satisfaction with home exercise: a comparison of computer-assisted video instruction and routine rehabilitation practice. *J Allied Health.* 2005;34:76-82.

66. Maller C, Twitty V, Sauve A. A video approach to interactive patient education. *J Perianesth Nurs.* 1997;12:82-88.

67. Weeks DL, Brubacker J, Byrt J, Davis M, Hamann L, Reagan J. Video tape instruction versus illustrations for influencing quality of performance, motivation, and confidence to perform simple and complex exercises in healthy subjects. *Physiother Theory Pract.* 2002;18:65-73.

68. Reo JA, Mercer VM. Effects of live, videotaped, or written instruction on learning an upper-extremity exercise program. *Phys Ther.* 2004;84:622-633.

69. Jenny NY, Fai TS. Evaluating the effectiveness of an interactive multimedia computer-based patient education program in cardiac rehabilitation. *Occup Ther J Res.* 2001;21:260-275.

Harnessing Technology
Tools to Enhance Learning in the Clinic and the Classroom

Laurie J. Posey, EdD

Chapter Objectives

After reading this chapter, you will be prepared to:

- Plan effective technology-based educational experiences (ie, e-Learning) for your patients and other audiences.
- Engage diverse audiences with multisensory e-Learning.
- Ensure clear and accessible Web-based learning materials for people with special needs.
- Use "just in time" information and resources to support patient compliance and decision making.
- Transform perceptions and understanding through simulated or problem-based experiences.
- Foster online social interaction to support the healing process.

In this chapter, many of the concepts presented earlier are reinforced as they are applied to the design, development, implementation, and assessment of e-Learning products. From needs assessments and goal setting to the development of storyboards, strategies and resources are offered to help you design effective educational offerings. This chapter provides the basics of developing and incorporating digital images, audio, video, text, and interactivity into your e-Learning products to capture a diverse audience, which includes individuals with special needs. Examples of Web material including patient education, digital repositories, and clinical decision support tools are provided along with criteria to evaluate online resources. The concepts of social networking and other Web 2.0 technologies are also explored as possible sources of patient education and support strategies.

Critical Thinking Clinical Scenario

Martin Banks is a 55-year-old man who experienced a moderate brain injury after falling off a ladder. After 2 months of physical therapy, Martin is now able to carry out most activities of daily living with minimal assistance from his 50-year-old wife, Marian. During a follow-up appointment, Marian takes you aside and confides that her husband has been refusing to do the exercises you have prescribed. Whenever she mentions the exercises, Martin becomes angry and oppositional. She suspects that he is embarrassed to admit that he is having difficulty remembering how to do them.

Reflective Question

How might you use technology to help the Banks family?

The Banks family has a personal computer, so you decide to create a narrated PowerPoint presentation that describes and demonstrates the sequence and steps for the exercise regimen you have prescribed. The presentation is organized around a checklist that you provide as a laminated quick reference sheet. You also provide Marian with a short video that includes personal stories and expert advice related to brain injury symptoms and coping strategies along with a link to the Web site of a nonprofit organization dedicated to helping individuals who have experienced brain injury. The Web site includes a wealth of educational materials to help those impacted by brain injury cope with its complex outcomes, including mood swings and irritability. Through the Web site, Marian subscribes to a brain injury blog where she is able to get many of her questions answered. She also discovers and joins an online support group for family members of individuals with brain injuries.

Plack M, Driscoll M. *Teaching and Learning in Physical Therapy:
From Classroom to Clinic* (pp 225-248).
© 2011 SLACK Incorporated

As this simple example illustrates, technology can be a helpful adjunct to your therapy. You can use it to inform, teach, empower, motivate, and connect patients, students, and colleagues in educational, clinical, and professional settings. Most everyone has access to a computer and the Internet, whether in the home, at work, or at a public library. These basic technologies put a host of interactive multimedia and online educational opportunities at your fingertips. Even individuals from the Silent Generation, who may not be as technologically savvy as individuals from the Xer or Millennial generations, are getting used to using search engines such as Google to find out more about their own health issues. Yet, they may not be aware of the readily available social networking tools that allow them to more actively engage with others around a particular topic of interest or concern. Add to this the ever-expanding world of portable media devices, such as MP3 players, smart phones, and netbooks, and today's learner can access education anytime, anywhere. These are just a few of the concepts that we will explore in this chapter.

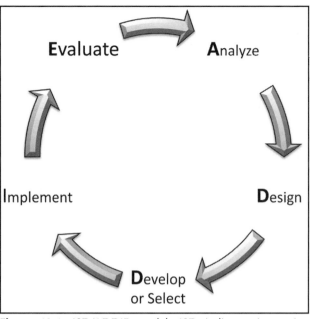

Figure 10-1. ISD/ADDIE model. ISD indicates instruction systems design; ADDIE, analysis, design, development, implementation, and evaluation.

A Systematic Approach to Design and Delivery

With so many options to choose from, where do you begin? What technologies should you consider? When should you consider using them? Why bother? Should you look for existing materials or create something new? What is the best way to present your message? How can you be sure that your time and money are well invested?

If you have limited experience with educational technologies, the prospect of developing or even selecting computer- or media-based educational materials may at first seem overwhelming. Fortunately, as a health care practitioner, you are better equipped than many to tackle this new challenge. Your diagnostic abilities will serve you well.

Educational technologists follow a systematic process to ensure optimal outcomes of e-Learning experiences analogous to the framework we provided in the previous chapter on systematic effective instruction. As illustrated in Figure 10-1, the instructional systems design (ISD) process includes 5 phases, sometimes referred to as ADDIE: Analysis, Design, Development, Implementation, and Evaluation.

The ISD/ADDIE model is intended to guide the development of new training products and is equally applicable to both face-to-face training and e-Learning projects. By replacing *Development* with *Selection*, the process can also be applied to instructional projects that make use of existing, "off-the-shelf" e-Learning products.

ISD begins with an analysis of the educational challenge, audience, and setting. As in systematic effective instruction, this means asking the right questions (ie, completing a needs assessment) of your audience and other stakeholders as well as yourself so that you have the information you need to make good decisions as you start to plan the educational experience. This information provides the foundation for the design and development stages.

Consider this example. You work with an elderly population for whom falls are a significant risk, and you would like to develop an educational program about fall prevention. Think about your audience. What factors would you need to consider in planning an educational program that best meets their needs? What, if anything, do they already know about fall prevention? What is the most common cause of falls in this population? Are there particular behaviors you are trying to correct? What educational formats are likely to be most appealing and usable for this audience? These are some of the questions you would need to answer in planning an effective program, and you would probably need to do a good bit of research to answer them. What does the literature say about falls and fall prevention in this population? What types of educational interventions have been most effective in the past? In addition to reviewing existing evidence, it would be useful to conduct a survey or focus groups with representative members of your specific target audience to learn more about their learning needs. You can see how the information you gather through this analysis process would help to guide your educational approach.

The design phase of ISD includes defining goals, learning objectives, and instructional strategies. Just as in designing other teaching-learning experiences, learning objectives are the backbone of instructional design and provide the framework for everything that follows, so it is important to define them carefully. Typically, a summary of the analysis, the learning objectives, a content outline, the planned instructional approach, and a description of the materials to be developed are documented in an instructional design plan that is reviewed by all members of the project team (ie, stakeholders, subject matter experts, instructional designers, media production staff, and programmers).

An instructional design plan for the falls prevention program would begin with a summary of the analysis, describing the problem, the audience, and how the proposed educational program will help to reduce falls in this population. This would be followed by a statement of educational goal(s); for example:

- The goal of this program is to reduce incidences of falls in the elderly by increasing their awareness of common causes of falls and strategies to prevent them.

Next, you would write learning objectives designed to enable learners to achieve the stated goal. For example:

- After participating in this educational experience, learners will be able to:
  o Recognize common causes of falls.
  o Apply fall prevention strategies in their daily lives.

These objectives would provide a framework for developing a more detailed content outline.

With the objectives stated and content outlined—and having a good idea of the types of educational experiences that would be most appealing and effective for your target audience—you are ready to begin thinking about instructional strategies. Continuing with our falls prevention example, imagine that you decide to create a self-paced, interactive e-Learning program that would be set up in a waiting room and also available on CD for patients' use at home. To engage learners, you might begin the program with a montage of video clips showing different types of falls. To teach your first objective, you might present the learner with a list of common fall incidents that they could click on to learn about common causes of falls in the elderly, through case examples. To teach the second objective, you might present a list of fall prevention strategies and challenge learners to identify a strategy that could have prevented the fall in each case. You might wrap up the program with a summary of common causes of falls and fall prevention strategies, presented using a combination of narration, still or video images of active, healthy seniors, and text to highlight key points. The instructional design plan would include

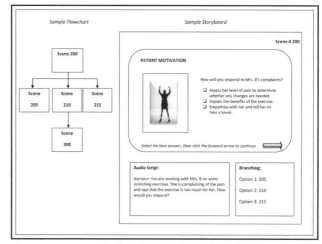

Figure 10-2. Sample flowchart and storyboard.

a high-level description of the e-Learning format, instructional strategies, and delivery media in narrative form.

Creating e-Learning products such as the example described above requires careful up-front planning of media elements and navigational flow. For these kinds of programs, the high-level design is followed by a more detailed design that includes a flowchart illustrating the structure of the different scenes in the program and how a learner can navigate through them and a storyboard that details the visuals, audio, and navigational options available for each scene (Figure 10-2). Storyboards for the fall prevention program would detail the narration, images, text, and interactivity for each scene in the program. When working in a team setting, all of the flowcharts and storyboards are reviewed, revised, and agreed upon by all stakeholders. Given the expense that may be associated with developing e-Learning products, this review is critical.

In the development stage, digital media artists and audiovisual producers compile all of the graphics, photos, audio, and/or video that are defined in the storyboards. These program "assets" may be created new for the project or obtained from a stock media library. To produce the opening montage for the fall prevention program, for example, you might be able to find and edit together existing footage of real falls; if not, you would need to hire actors, actresses, and a professional video crew and stage and record a series of fall incidents. You can see how a simple idea can quickly become costly, and you might need to revisit your instructional approach.

Using one of many available development platforms, a programmer or author assembles the media according to the flowchart and storyboard specifications. The product is tested and any programming "bugs" corrected, and then it is reviewed by the project team. Alternatively, for projects that make use of existing e-Learning products, the development stage includes selecting materials that meet the goals and objectives defined during the design phase and creating any printed learner and instructor materials needed to guide the use of these materials.

Once developed, the e-Learning program is implemented, and, as with any educational presentation, outcomes must be evaluated. For the fall program, you might ask some of your elderly patients, your grandparents, or an elderly neighbor to review the program, report any problems they encounter, and provide feedback about its usability and content. Based on this evaluative process, materials may be revised or new materials selected. Notably, the process is cyclical, inferring an ongoing continuous improvement process.

The ISD process has been used for many years to provide training development teams with a common, systematic framework that results in efficient design and production of high-quality instructional products. The process has been detailed by many authors and is the foundation for a professional discipline called *instructional design*. An expanded model and good, thorough explanation of the process is provided in *The Systematic Design of Instruction*,[1] and an Internet search using the key words *instructional design* will yield many, many more resources. If you are working on a small e-Learning project independently, you may not need to delve too deeply into this area; just follow the basic steps outlined above. If you decide to tackle a more complex e-Learning project, however, it may be in your best interest to become familiar with the process and to consider hiring a professional instructional design and development team.

In addition to making the process manageable, following this systematic approach will help ensure that the technology solutions you create or choose are appropriate and meet the learning needs of your target audience. Educational technologies can be dangerously alluring—it is all too easy to be swept away by a flashy presentation or the latest gadget. Remember, even the most fabulous e-Learning program will be useless to a patient who does not own, know how, or want to use a computer.

Stop and Reflect

Think about some of the learning needs of your patients or your coworkers.
- Can you translate these needs into measurable learning goals and objectives?
- What types of educational experiences would best support these goals and objectives?
- How, if at all, might technology enhance these learning experiences?

You are the architect of your patient's educational technology experience, and as every architect knows, form always follows function. For an architect, this means that the form (ie, structure and features) of a building must be based on its function (ie, intended purposes). For example, consider the differences between a residential and commercial kitchen. To plan its features effectively, an architect would need to know the function of the kitchen—who will use it, how it will be used, and with what desired outcomes. Similarly, when designing e-Learning, you must be clear about the purpose of the application before determining what form it will take. To ensure that form follows function, again, a thorough needs assessment is critical. Ask yourself: Who is my audience? What do I want them to know or do? Where and when will they be learning? Thinking through and answering these questions thoroughly will prepare you to determine how to use technology to deliver an effective educational message.

Key Points to Remember

ISD is a process that:
- Provides a systematic approach for managing the selection or developing technology-based learning products.
- Ensures consistency among learner needs, learning objectives, and technology-based learning solutions.
- Fosters continuous improvement through ongoing evaluation.

Form follows function—Effective technology solutions must address real learning needs.

Motivating Diverse Learners

If you have practiced physical therapy for any length of time or have worked in other people-oriented professions, you know that people come in many shapes and sizes. From earlier chapters, you will recall the importance of knowing your audience and recognizing the influence that individual filters have on learning. Differences in culture, language, attitude, disposition, motivation, expertise, experience, learning style, literacy, and comorbid conditions can all impact how an educational message is received. How can you create messages that are appealing and effective for such diverse audiences? How can technology help you meet this challenge?

As we have discussed before, the best way to appeal to a diverse audience is to provide a variety of learning options. The more you can vary the teaching-learning strategies, media, and modes of delivery you use, the more likely you are to meet the needs of everyone in your audience—whether that audience is live or sitting behind some electronic medium. Meeting the needs of your audience in a virtual community becomes even more challenging and may be limited by the time and resources you have available. You may not be able to please all of the people all of the time, but as in systematic effective instruction, it is important that you make an effort to include a number of strategies to appeal to a variety of individuals with differing learning preferences.

Keeping diversity in mind during the planning process can help you maximize your investment in technology-based education. For example, if you were planning to produce an exercise DVD, developing complementary materials based on the content you are already developing would require little additional time and money. You might decide to create a spiral-bound, laminated booklet including exercise plans and instructions for each exercise along with illustrative photos taken during the DVD production. You might even be able to take the same script you created to support your exercise DVD and create an audio recording or podcast that patients can listen to using a portable MP3 player while exercising in the gym, rather than when they are at home in front of the television. The key point here is to think about delivery options early in the process so that you can streamline the design and development of different media formats.

In addition to maximizing the use of different media formats, embracing a learner-centered approach to teaching will help ensure that the educational experiences you create or facilitate will meet the unique needs of diverse learners. Learner-centered education requires learners to take ownership over their own learning. By reflecting on their individual learning needs, relating instructional objectives to personal goals, and taking an active role in the learning process, learners become co-authors of the educational experience. This makes it possible for diverse individuals to come away from a common educational experience having met the established objectives yet having connected differently with the material, allowing it to become more personally relevant. For example, if you were facilitating an online support group for teens with spinal cord injuries, rather than simply presenting general information about community resources and support, you might ask participants to find and share resources from their own communities. In addition to providing participants with meaningful, useful connections, this experience would also be more empowering than a "spoon-fed" approach (ie, providing all the information). As an added benefit, others in the group would be exposed to a richer array of examples that may relate to their own needs and setting.

Simply considering different modes of delivery may not be sufficient to motivate and meet the needs of diverse learners. Keller[2] developed a useful framework for planning educational experiences based on research related to human motivation. The ARCS model includes 4 categories: Attention, Relevance, Confidence, and Satisfaction. As illustrated in Table 10-1, each of these categories includes 3 components that can be used to guide the selection of instructional strategies that engage and motivate learners.

The ARCS model can be applied to the design of any instructional project and is particularly useful when thinking through the different types of learning experiences you may wish to include in an e-Learning program. For example, to build confidence, designers of an e-Learning program may decide to organize practice activities from simple to complex and allow learners to repeat the activities as many times as needed to succeed.

The ARCS model is intended to complement, rather than replace, the instructional design process previously described. Like instructional strategies, the selection of motivational strategies is based on a thorough understanding of your audience and the instructional objectives you are trying to achieve. Armed with an analysis of audience characteristics, knowledge of what motivates people to learn, and insight into instructional strategies that enhance motivation, we are well positioned to plan learning activities and experiences that are both motivational and instructionally effective. There is no prescribed formula for using the model, and the sample strategies provided are not intended to be comprehensive. The ARCS model simply provides additional factors to consider and possible strategies you can use to enhance your learner's motivation to learn.

Though you do not need to address every component of ARCS in every e-Learning project, it is worthwhile to consider each one within the context of your audience and project goals. The third column of Table 10-1 illustrates how one e-Learning project might integrate all of the different components of ARCS. Keller[2] provides more information about designing instruction using ARCS, along with additional resources, on the ARCS Web site.[3]

Critical Thinking Clinical Scenario

You have been asked to create an online workplace wellness program for the physical therapy aides in your department. You just learned about the ARCS model and would like to use it to ensure that you have optimized learner motivation.

Reflective Question

What strategies would you use to address each of the 4 components of the ARCS model?
1. Attention
2. Relevance
3. Confidence
4. Satisfaction

Table 10-1. ARCS Model*

	Components	Strategies	Example
Attention	Perceptual arousal	Stimulate interest through novelty, surprise, incongruence, conflict, or uncertainty.	An online learning program on customer service for medical office professionals opens with several video clips of challenging client situations.
	Inquiry arousal	Pose questions, challenges, or problems for learners to solve.	The learner is challenged to select appropriate responses or actions to mediate challenging client situations.
	Variability	Vary instructional methods and formats.	The online learning program includes a mix of media and interactivity types.
Relevance	Goal orientation	Connect education to learner goals; demonstrate its value and future usefulness.	The introduction explains how the strategies presented in the online learning program will help learners manage challenging client situations in the future.
	Motive matching	Match instruction to learner interests and learning style; provide choice.	The program includes a variety of situations and settings and encourages learners to choose those that are most relevant to them.
	Familiarity	Create links or hooks to prior knowledge and experience.	Scenarios and challenges explicitly build upon basic customer service skills that learners already possess.
Confidence	Learning requirements	Present learning objectives and criteria for success.	Learning objectives are stated at the beginning of the program. The introduction explains that learners will need to complete 5 scenarios successfully to "pass" the course.
	Success opportunities	Provide incremental challenge and feedback to foster meaningful success.	Scenarios are organized from simple to complex. Immediate remedial feedback or reinforcement is provided at every decision point.
	Personal control	Demonstrate the link between success and learner effort.	Learners can complete the scenarios as many times as needed to succeed.
Satisfaction	Intrinsic reinforcement	Demonstrate benefit by providing opportunity to use new knowledge and skills in a real setting.	Learners are encouraged to practice their newly acquired customer service skills on the job and make note of their effects.
	Extrinsic rewards	Provide praise, positive feedback, reinforcement, and/or tokens of achievement.	Learners are congratulated and receive a printable certificate after successfully completing the program.
	Equity	Ensure that learning assessments are fair (eg, participants are evaluated in a consistent manner; assessment is consistent with stated requirements and learning experiences).	Scenarios are consistent with stated objectives and instructional content.

*Keller's[2] ARCS model of motivational design: components, strategies, and examples. ARCS indicates attention, relevance, confidence, and satisfaction.

Key Points to Remember

To meet the needs of diverse learners, provide diverse learning options.

- A learner-centered approach enables diverse individuals to come away from a common educational experience having met the established objectives yet having connected differently with the material, allowing it to become more personally relevant.
- Follow the ARCS model to motivate learners:
  - Gain **A**ttention
  - Demonstrate **R**elevance
  - Build **C**onfidence
  - Ensure **S**atisfaction

Multisensory Approach to Teaching and Learning

Stop and Reflect

Think about a time when you have been completely engaged in some type of learning experience. Perhaps you were immersed in an IMAX film with surround sound, participating in a workshop presented by a gifted facilitator, working through a collaborative simulation, or just walking through an art museum.

- What was it about the experience that captured and held your attention?
- How did your mind and senses interact to create a memorable learning experience?

Table 10-2. VARK Perceptual Preferences*

Perceptual Preference	Description
Visual (V)	Visual learners prefer to learn by viewing information presented in graphical form. To appeal to visual learners, integrate illustrations, diagrams, charts, symbols, and other visual devices into the instructional presentation.
Aural/auditory (A)	Aural learners prefer to learn by listening or speaking. To appeal to auditory learners, integrate lecture, audio recordings, and opportunities for discussion into the educational experience.
Read/write (R)	Read/write learners prefer to learn by reading. To appeal to these learners, integrate text explanations, readings, Web sites, and writing assignments into the educational experience.
Kinesthetic (K)	Kinesthetic learners prefer to learn by doing. To appeal to kinesthetic learners, integrate real-world experience, opportunities to touch and feel, and simulated or real practice activities into the educational experience.
Multimodal	Multimodal learners fall into 2 categories: those who choose a mode based on the situation and those who use all modes in all situations. Most learners have some preference for each of the learning modes. To appeal to multimodal learners, integrate diverse media and activities into the educational experience.

*For more information on the VARK model, see http://www.vark-learn.com/english/page.asp?p=categories. VARK indicates visual, aural, read/write, and kinesthetic.

Something as simple as text on a page can provide an engaging and effective educational experience, particularly if it makes readers think. It is likely, however, that your most memorable experiences have involved something more than the written word. A summer evening spent in a hammock with a great novel would not be complete without the feeling of a soft breeze and the sounds of owls and crickets. Our senses work together to create our experiences—whether or not we are conscious of them.

In the first chapter of this text, we discussed how learners have different learning styles or preferences. In addition to learning styles presented earlier, Fleming and Mills[4] observed that learners have different perceptual preferences as well, which is particularly important when considering the use of technology in a teaching-learning situation. The acronym VARK categorizes learner perceptual preferences as visual, aural/auditory, read/write, and kinesthetic.

The authors also describe a fifth category, multimodal (MM), noting that most learners prefer some combination of the VARK categories, with some having a preference for all. Multimodal learners may either base their preference on the learning context or use all 4 learning modes in every learning situation (Table 10-2).

How does this relate to the learning process and the design of technology-based instruction? We know that multisensory experiences are engaging, whether online or in-person. We also know that most learners prefer some combination of visual, auditory, read/write, and kinesthetic stimuli. The challenge is to engage the senses in a way that most effectively facilitates learning. Visual elements most engage the visual learner; audio elements, the auditory learner; text elements, the read/write learner; and interactive elements, the kinesthetic learner. As we just said, however, most learners prefer a multimodal approach, so it is important for us to think about how visuals, audio, text, and interactivity work together to stimulate the thinking and learning processes.

To design and develop a multisensory e-Learning experience, you must know a bit about different multimedia elements. Digital images, audio, video, and text can be combined in an unlimited number of ways to engage different types of learners.

Digital Images

Images can be used to illustrate concepts or procedures, augment text or audio communications, display data, or communicate a mood or metaphor. Images are also foundational to the look, feel, and functionality of an online or computer-based learning program. A program's graphical user interface (GUI) is made up of clickable buttons, menu items, and other screen elements that have been programmed to act in a certain way when you click on them or run your cursor across them.

Graphic elements, illustrations and photos are all are digital images made up of tiny bits of information called *pixels*. The number of pixels in a digital image determines its resolution. High resolution images have more pixels and are generally better quality than low resolution images.

Digital images may be saved in one of several electronic file types. When creating interactive multimedia, you should save your images in 1 of the 3 formats shown in Table 10-3.

The .gif format is primarily used for graphics. This format allows you to save images with a transparent background, which is important if you plan to overlay one image on top of another. For example, if you pasted a graphic of a sun on top of another graphic of the sky, you would not want a white box around it. Because .gif files are limited to 256 colors, they are not suitable for photo-real images. A better choice for digital photographs is

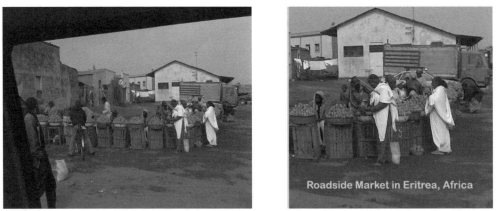

Figure 10-3. Sample unedited (left) and edited (right) photos.

Table 10-3. Digital Image File Types

Image Formats	Use
.gif Graphics Interchange Format	Best for solid colors Supports transparency
.jpeg Joint Photographic Experts Group	Best for photos and continuous tone images Supports millions of colors (24 bit)
.png Portable Network Graphics	Most flexible Supports different color depths Supports transparency

the .jpeg format, which supports millions of colors. Even more flexible is the .png format, which supports transparency and any range of colors. Software, such as Adobe Photoshop or the GNU Image Manipulation Program (GIMP),[5] available as a free download, can be used to help you edit digital images based on the needs of the educational program. Editing may involve adding labels or captions to a graphic, adding a consistent border to a series of photographs, changing colors, resizing an image, or other types of manipulation (Figure 10-3).

Audio

Audio may include narration, music, or sound effects. The spoken word is essential to many e-Learning programs. Simply adding narration to a PowerPoint presentation can engage the senses further, motivate the learner, and enhance memory and learning. Sound effects can be used to enhance or add realism to a story or other communication. Music can convey emotion and is often used to introduce and close a program or to transition between sections. Like images, digital audio files are made up of bits of digital information, can be edited using computer software, and can be saved in a variety of digital file formats. Because of the amount of digital data stored when a sound is captured in a digital format, audio files are relatively large. MP3 is a digital audio file that has been compressed to create a smaller file that can be stored efficiently on a portable digital audio player

such as an iPod or downloaded for quick playback on the Internet. Web-based audio broadcasts, or podcasts, are saved as MP3 files. Other common formats used when developing professional e-Learning products are .wav (for Windows) and .aiff (for Macintosh). You can use sound editing software, such as Sound Forge by Sony, Adobe Audition, or Audacity,[6] which is available as a free download, to record audio using a microphone plugged into your computer, edit the recorded files, and save the recording in different digital audio formats.

Video

Digital video can be used to tell a story, demonstrate a process, document real events, or whenever both audio and action are important. Like audio and images, digital videos are made up of bits of digital information and are much larger than an audio file of the same length. If you imagine a motion video as a series of changing images or "frames" accompanied by the audio, it may help you to understand why. The number of frames per second—the number of times the computer redraws the screen each second—impacts the file size and also the video quality. The smooth motion video that we are used to seeing on television is recorded at 30 frames per second. Another factor that impacts file size is the size of the video window that displays on the computer screen; the smaller the video window, the smaller the file size. Common video file formats used in e-Learning include MPEG, Windows

Audio Video Interleaved (.avi), Windows Media Video (.wmv), Flash video (.flv), and Quicktime (.mov). There are a variety of digital video cameras available, from consumer to professional grade. Many digital cameras and smart phones also have video recording capability. You can edit digital video files using software such as Windows Media Maker, Apple's iMovie, or Adobe Premiere.

Text

The written word is essential to most educational communications. Though some e-Learning makes appropriate use of long text passages, as a general rule, text used in e-Learning should be succinct. Short phrases, paragraphs, or bulleted lists may be used to highlight key points. Labels or captions may be used to add meaning to images. Text-based interface elements, such as menu items on a Web page, hyperlinks, or labels on a button, provide navigational aids. It is good practice to provide text prompts to guide learners through an interactive experience.

Interactivity

Self-paced e-Learning programs depend upon interactivity between learner and computer. Interactive educational programs require the learner to click on active screen elements such as menu items, text links or hyperlinks, or navigational buttons to navigate through the learning experience. Images or parts of images may be programmed to display text or other images or to link the learner to new information. Interactive learning assessments may ask learners to click to enter data in response to a question or indicate a choice within a simulation. Learners may also enter text to communicate with the educational program. There are a variety of e-Learning authoring tools available to enable nonprogrammers to assemble a mix of digital media to create interactive e-Learning. Popular programs include Adobe Captivate, Articulate, and Camtasia.

How can images, audiovisuals, text and interactivity be combined most effectively to facilitate learning? As we discussed in an earlier chapter, the most effective educators connect learning to emotion and personal meaning to arouse attention and use multiple pathways to enhance memory. Combining multimedia and interactivity can stimulate cognition and critical thinking and foster deeper, more memorable learning.

It should always be remembered that technology should be selected to enhance the learning experience. Take a minute to think about some of the educational presentations you have attended in the past. Does the

phrase "death by PowerPoint" come to mind? Although there are certainly exceptions, at many professional conferences and meetings, the bulleted list is the star of the day. Though bulleted lists can help organize a presentation or highlight key points, unfortunately these benefits have been abused. If we hear something spoken, do we really need to see the same words written on the PowerPoint slide? A better use of our visual capacity might be to interpret an illustration or diagram that reinforces the speaker's message. For example, consider Figure 10-4; in a presentation on designing a clinic, a diagram of a floor plan can provide important visual information and is much more interesting than a list of suggestions that duplicate what the speaker is saying.

Critical Thinking Clinical Scenario

You are developing an e-Learning experience for first-year DPT students. Consider the picture below.

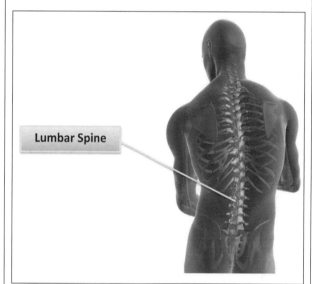

©iStockphoto.com/comotion_design

By adding highlights and labels, you have made the image more meaningful. Now imagine this image as an e-Learning program in which the learner can click on the label to learn more about the anatomy of the lumbar spine or common malalignments or pathologies associated with the lumbar spine. Or perhaps an audio narration could present learners with a description of the pathology and challenge them to select appropriate tests and measures or interventions. Finally, hyperlinks could provide connections to evidence-based resources.

Reflective Question

1. What other types of interactive media might you use to enrich the experience for your learners?

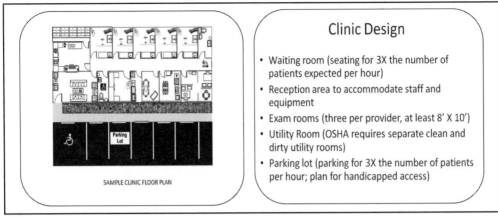

Figure 10-4. Which slide would best complement a discussion of clinic design?

Because it requires the audience to use their senses to attend to multiple stimuli simultaneously, this kind of audiovisual approach is naturally more engaging. Of course, it is important to remember, as with motivational hooks and content boosters, that multisensory stimuli must complement rather than overwhelm or compete with each other or with the content. Keeping this caveat in mind, don't be afraid to challenge your audience to see, hear, think, and do.

Key Point to Remember

- Multisensory learning experiences are naturally engaging. Consider combining the following sensory preferences:
  - o Visual
  - o Auditory
  - o Read/write
  - o Kinesthetic
- Most learners prefer some combination of sensory input. Consider incorporating technology-based teaching strategies:
  - o Visual
  - o Audio
  - o Text
  - o Interactivity
- Optimal education uses multiple pathways to enhance memory.
- Connecting learning to emotion and personal meaning arouses attention.
- Combining media and interactivity fosters deeper more memorable learning.
- Motivational hooks, content boosters, and multisensory stimuli must complement rather than overwhelm or compete with each other or with the content.

Critical Thinking Clinical Scenario

Mr. E is a 62-year-old patient with diabetes. You want to develop some instructional aids on exercise and proper skin care for him and his caregiver. You have a series of exercises you want Mr. E to perform daily. You also want him to be able to properly check his skin, identify potential problem areas, and determine what to do once they are identified.

Reflective Questions

1. What questions might you ask to assess the perceptual preferences (VARK) of both Mr. E and his caregiver?

2. What types of technology-based teaching might you use to promote retention in both the patient and caregiver after they leave your office?

3. How might you combine different media and interactivity to create an engaging, multisensory experience?

Adapting Technology-Based Teaching for Individuals With Special Needs

Diverse audiences include individuals with special needs. This is especially true in a field focused on helping people overcome physical challenges. According to the US Census Bureau, approximately 41 million (15%) people living in the United States have at least 1 type of disability.[7] A wide range of assistive technology products can help to bridge the learning divide for these learners such as TDD (telecommunications device for the deaf), computer screen readers, and voice recognition software. Microsoft provides a useful description of the different types of assistive technologies in the Accessibility section of its Web site.[8] Technology may also provide a means of accessing education that some people could not otherwise utilize.

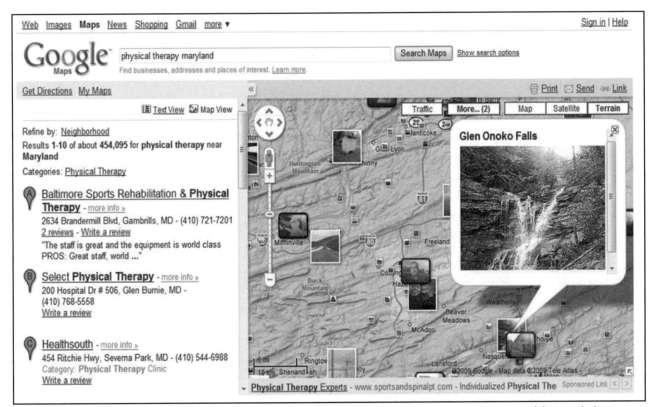

Figure 10-5. Consistent with universal design for learning principles, multiple presentation strategies and formats help to meet the needs of a diverse audience. (Reprinted with permission from Google. © 2009 Google, Map Data © 2009 Tele Atlas.)

From a planning and design perspective, it is important to consider the special needs of your audience—known and unknown. This means making sure that education is both effective and accessible for those with disabilities or other special needs. *Effective* and *accessible* are related but distinct considerations. Providing education that is effective for all requires attention to instructional content and teaching strategies as they relate to limitations, disabilities, and differences that may impact an individual's ability to learn. These may include cognitive, sensory, or physical disabilities; language barriers; emotional problems; or lack of interest and motivation. Providing education that is accessible involves ensuring that people with physical or cognitive impairments can successfully use a technology-based educational offering. Thus, accessibility is a subset of effectiveness—in order for an e-Learning program to be effective, it must be accessible to all learners.

Researchers at the Center for Applied Special Technology (CAST) have developed a framework called *universal design for learning* (UDL) to guide the design of educational experiences that are effective for all learners. UDL principles focus on providing learners with multiple options for achieving educational goals; representing information and knowledge; expressing or demonstrating what the learner knows; and engaging learners' interest and motivation (Figure 10-5). These principles are consistent with the concept of providing diverse learning options to meet the needs of diverse learners. Technology is widely used in UDL because it offers an alternative to traditional instruction. The UDL Web site is rich with guidelines, strategies, and examples of how UDL principles can be applied in different educational settings.[9] One example is the Improving Comprehension OnLine (ICON) project.[10] This is a project to help individuals with limited reading comprehension or who speak English as a second language. Researchers are embedding such items as pictures, vocabulary, language translation, and text-to-speech translation to digital texts. This enables the reader to access other forms of representation (eg, pictures, spoken word) to help them better understand the written text. Given what you now know about the prevalence of low literacy in the United States, this may have some significant implications for you as you design patient education materials.

Though UDL's primary focus has been to equalize traditional education for students with diverse learning styles, its principles are also applicable to Web site and e-Learning design. Well-designed user interfaces incorporate principles of universal design by integrating options for different kinds of learners.

Critical Thinking Clinical Scenario

On the Web site of your physical therapy practice, you have a link to Google Maps (http://maps.google.com), which you encourage prospective patients to use to help them locate your facility. Take a moment to access Google Maps via the Internet.

Reflective Questions

1. How do the designers of Google Maps integrate multiple modes of exploration to provide flexibility for diverse users?

2. How do the designers of Google Maps use the principles of UDL to make it both effective and accessible for all users?

3. How do you see using similar principles in your business practices?

4. How else might you envision using UDL principles in your practice?

Technologies intended for use by the general population should also include options to address the accessibility needs of the disabled. Interestingly, innovations designed to help those with special needs overcome barriers often provide serendipitous benefits for all. For example, the ability to adjust screen resolution and text size on a computer may be essential for people with vision impairments, but it is a useful feature for everyone.

In the United States, section 508 of the Americans with Disabilities Act (ADA) defines standards for the design and programming of accessible learning technologies. Section 508 requires that any electronic and information technology products procured, developed, maintained, or used by a federal agency must comply with ADA technical specifications and performance requirements. These requirements delineate specific criteria for accessible Internet and multimedia products, such as providing subtitles for audio content and a text alternative for other visual elements. Although it is not illegal to produce nonaccessible e-Learning products for nongovernment applications, it is important to understand the overarching intent of the standards, and good practice mandates that we make every effort to accommodate those with special needs. To learn more and review the specific requirements, visit the Section 508 Web site.[11]

Stop and Reflect

Take a moment to browse the Internet. Search for Web sites that provide health care information for patients.

- What elements of UDL did you observe?
- Did you see some sites where (UDL) was not used?
- How might this limit accessibility? How might this limit the effectiveness?
- What recommendations would you make to the designers?

Key Points to Remember

- UDL provides multiple options to ensure that education is effective for all learners, including those with special needs.
- Section 508 of the Americans with Disabilities Act specifies technical standards to ensure the accessibility of Web and computer-based learning.
- Providing options to accommodate those with special needs often benefits all learners.

Accessing, Assessing, and Managing Health-Related Information on the Internet

The How Much Information (HMI) project at the University of Berkeley reported that businesses and consumers worldwide produced 5 EB (exabytes) of new information in 2002—comparable to 37000 new libraries the size of the Library of Congress.[12] Futurists estimate that the amount of technical information is doubling every 2 years and will be doubling every 72 hours by 2014.[13] There is little doubt that health care research is contributing significantly to this information explosion. With this kind of exponential growth in information and knowledge—some of which may be vital to practitioners and patients—how can anyone possibly keep up?

Stop and Reflect

How do you keep up with ongoing research and advances in physical therapy practice? Is it practical or even possible to know it all?

As the amount of information grows, the ability to manage it becomes increasingly important. The ability to store and catalogue information and deliver it on demand is a key benefit of computer, database, and Internet technologies. The pervasive influence of Google, Yahoo, Bing, Wikipedia, Scholarpedia, and other quick-search applications are evidence of just how much we have come to value—even take for granted—easy access to information and resources. Need a quick answer? Just Google it! Yet despite filtering improvements, "Googling" remains an imperfect science that often yields too many results to sift through efficiently. And though Wikipedia may provide convenient access to educational information, that information may or may not be accurate or evidence based.

In a world of constant change, learning is a continuous process. Surviving and thriving in this environment requires us to become lifelong learners with the ability to find, critically evaluate, and apply knowledge and information in response to situational demands. As health care providers, we are well schooled in evidence-based practice. We know how to find, critically evaluate, and apply knowledge and information to effectively diagnose and manage patient dysfunctions. However, we cannot assume that our patients have the same ability.

In today's information age, patients have a wealth of health information at their fingertips. It can be disconcerting when patients start to use this information, assuming that it is accurate when in fact it might not be. As practitioners, we must be prepared to search and screen not only the scientific literature but also patient-related and popular literature to provide effective information for our patients, and we must take the initiative to find and refer patients to reliable, credible health information resources.

When searching the Internet, whether to find resources for a patient or information to guide clinical practice, evaluating the quality and credibility of the source is essential. To be effective educators, it is not only important for us to know what resources are available for our patients but perhaps more important is knowing whether those resources are accurate or not. In *The Good, The Bad & The Ugly: Or, Why It's a Good Idea to Evaluate Web Sources*, Susan Beck[14] provides 5 major criteria to consider when evaluating online resources. These criteria are summarized in Table 10-4.

Stop, Do, and Reflect

Access a Web site that has up-to-date patient information. Assess the site for the following:

- Authority
- Accuracy
- Objectivity
- Currency
- Coverage

What did you find? Is this a Web site you would recommend to your patient?

These criteria are not intended to diminish the value of the Internet as an information resource but to empower you to evaluate and use Web-based information and resources wisely. Depending on the topic and the potential consequences of misinformation, consider seeking additional sources, such as peer-reviewed studies or advice from experts, to validate your Internet findings. In some cases, the Internet may simply provide you with a jump start and foundation for additional research.

Table 10-4. Criteria to Consider When Evaluating Online Resources

Authority	Who created the site?	Anyone can publish anything on the Web, so in judging the value of the information on a given Web site, it is important to identify and assess the credibility of the source. Often, it is hard to determine the author of the Web page. Even if a page is signed, the author's qualifications are rarely provided, and sponsorship is not always indicated.
Accuracy	How credible is the information that is being presented? (Again, who is the source?)	Even if you can determine the author of the Web site, you still need to determine the accuracy of the information provided. Unlike traditional print resources, Web resources rarely have editors or fact-checkers, and, currently, no Web standards exist to ensure accuracy.
Objectivity	Is the information objective or is the author presenting his or her own perspective?	Determining the motives or the objectives of the Web site author(s) is often difficult. Without knowing the goal or purpose of the Web site and perhaps a bit about the author, it is difficult to determine whether the information has been provided in an objective manner. Sometimes, Web information is "just for fun," a hoax, someone's personal expression or opinion, or even outright silliness.
Currency	Is the information current?	As noted earlier, information is changing on an ongoing basis, so equally important in judging the credibility of the information provided on a given Web site is the publication or revision date. Many Web sites do not provide publication dates; when they do, the dates may have various meanings. For example, it may indicate when the material was first written, when it was first placed on the Web, or when it was last revised. Again, without this information, it is difficult to determine the currency and accuracy of the information provided.
Coverage	How comprehensive is the information provided?	Web coverage often differs from print coverage. It is often difficult to determine the extent of coverage of a topic from a Web page. The page may or may not include links to other Web pages or print references or provide other resources for the reader to check facts or delve more deeply into the topic.

Table 10-5. Examples of Credible Patient Education Web Sites

- The WebMD Consumer Network. WebMD owns and operates 4 different consumer health information Web sites: www.WebMD.com, www.MedicineNet.com, www.eMedicineHealth.com, and www.RxList.com. Visitors to these sites can search for information on diseases or conditions, check symptoms, locate physicians, assess their personal health status, receive e-newsletters and alerts, participate in online communities with peers and medical experts, and view slide shows and videos on different health topics.

- Mayoclinic.com (http://www.mayoclinic.com/). This comprehensive consumer health site provides information about diseases and conditions, drugs and supplements, treatment decisions, and healthy living. The site features an array of interactive tools, slideshows, videos, blogs, and podcasts related to various health topics.

- Medline Plus (http://medlineplus.gov/). This National Library of Medicine Web site provides information on an array of health topics, drugs, and supplements; a medical encyclopedia and dictionary; health-related news; practitioner directories and links to other health resources; surgical videos; and interactive tutorials.

- Healthwise Knowledgebase (http://healthwise.net/). This site provides decision aids to guide patients in choosing among health care options (see Figure 10-7).

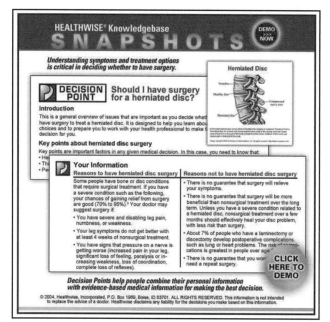

Figure 10-6. Sample patient education Web site. (© 2009 Healthwise, Incorporated. www.healthwise.org. Reprinted with permission. This information does not replace the advice of a doctor. Healthwise disclaims any warranty or liability for your use of this information.)

Just-in-Time Learning

Effective learning requires access to credible, appropriate information as new challenges present themselves. Educators use the term *just-in-time learning* to refer to educational experiences that take place at the moment of need. Just-in-time learning moves away from the traditional approach of obtaining knowledge and skills in advance of performance providing customized education based on the situation or decision at hand, in the context of daily or work tasks—when it is most relevant. Rather than attempting to store up knowledge for the future, learners access and use knowledge where and when they need to use it—in the "teachable moment."

A variety of just-in-time learning applications are available to support you both as a clinician and educator, including patient education Web sites, digital repositories, and clinical informatics and decision support Web sites. At the heart of these systems is a database that enables the structured collection, organization, and retrieval of informational or educational content. Software applications that provide access to database content range in complexity, from basic search applications that enable users to browse or query the content to intelligent systems that present tailored information based on user interactions and/or learning context.

Patient Education Web Sites

There are a number of searchable health education Web sites to support patients in learning about health conditions, making decisions about care options, or complying with prescribed health regimens. Table 10-5 and Figure 10-6 provide examples of credible patient education Web sites.

Digital Repositories

A digital repository is an online system designed to store and manage digital content.[15] Digital content may include documents, images, audio files, or more complete e-Learning units called *learning objects*. Conceptually, a learning object is a stand-alone chunk of e-Learning content that does the following:

- Includes activities and context to teach one or more instructional objectives.
- Can be used and reused for different educational purposes.
- Can be retrieved by search engines.

This broad definition can be applied to any self-contained e-Learning package, from simple demonstrations to more elaborate e-Learning modules or even online courses. For example, a 30-second, narrated animation explaining hip-flexor motion and a 6-hour online course on therapeutic exercise could both be considered learning objects *if* they are made available as self-contained learning units and are discoverable by a search engine.

Table 10-6. Examples of Health-Related Digital Repositories

- Health Education Assets Library (www.healcentral.org). An online library of freely accessible digital teaching resources for health sciences education. HEAL includes digital assets, such as sonographic images, as well as more complete learning experiences.

- Med-Ed Portal (www.aamc.org/mededportal). Developed and maintained by the American Association of Medical Colleges (AAMC), Med-Ed Portal is a peer-reviewed, open-access learning object repository. Med-Ed Portal includes a variety of educational resources, including tutorials, cases, lab manuals, assessment tools, simulations, faculty development materials, board review questions, and others.

- Intute (www.intute.ac.uk/healthandlifesciences/). Intute provides a searchable online database of health and life science Internet resources for education and research, evaluated and selected by a network of subject specialists. Intute includes descriptions and links to a wide range of online resources, including Web sites, scholarly works, databases, online education, and others.

- Multimedia Educational Resource for Teaching and Learning (MERLOT). An online database of peer-reviewed teaching materials to support a broad array of subject areas. Merlot's Health Sciences Community page (http://healthsciences.merlot.org/) includes a direct link to the Health Sciences collection and providesinformation about teaching in the health sciences with technology and other resources.

Learning objects may be used by individuals to explore a subject of interest or by educators who wish to enhance their courses with existing e-Learning content. Searchable online learning object libraries, also referred to as *repositories*, facilitate the discovery and use of e-Learning content by diverse audiences. For example, the National Library of Medicine has produced a collection of 165 interactive tutorials covering an array of diseases and conditions, diagnostic tests, surgery and treatment procedures, and health and wellness topics. The tutorials are available on the Medline Plus Web site[16] and have also been catalogued and included in an open-access health education learning object repository, the Health Education Assets Library (HEAL).[17] Visitors to either site can view the tutorials for their own education. If an educator would like to include one of the tutorials in a course he or she is teaching, he or she can either provide students with a link to the Web site or download the learning object from the HEAL repository (Figure 10-7).

To enable their retrieval, digital repository resources and learning objects are tagged with metadata; that is, descriptive information such as title, author, keyword(s), etc. Standardized metadata systems and vocabularies have been developed to facilitate the sharing of digital resources across different types of repositories. Two widely adopted metadata standards are the Dublin Core Metadata Initiative[18] and the Learning Object Metadata (LOM).[19]

Some repositories physically store digital resources and make them available both online and as downloadable digital files. Others simply provide a search engine with links to online content located on external Web sites. Though less commonly used, a more accurate term for these types of sites is *referatory* because they actually refer visitors to the original location of the resource on the Internet. Table 10-6 and Figure 10-7 provide examples of health-related digital repositories.

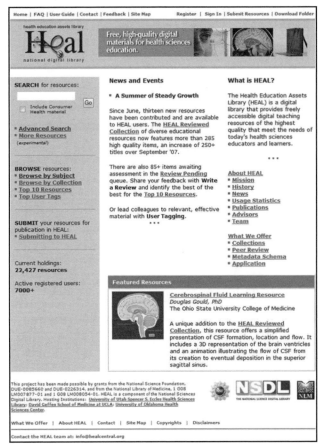

Figure 10-7. Sample health-related digital repository. (Reprinted with permission from the Health Education Assets Library.)

Table 10-7. Sample Clinical Decision Support Sites/Tools

- The Cochrane Collaboration. A searchable database of up-to-date evidence-based medical information to support clinical decision making.

- Clin-eguide. An online clinical decision support tool that integrates content from scientific literature such as Ovid, Facts & Comparisons, and Lippincott Williams and Wilkins, as well as other publishers to provide evidence-based information for health care providers (see Figure 10-8).

- First Consult. First Consult is an evidence-based, continuously updated clinical information resource designed for use at the point of care. It includes 3 complementary components: medical topics (information on evaluation, diagnosis, clinical management, prognosis, and prevention), differential diagnoses (rapid evaluation of patient complaints with interactive access to potential diagnoses ordered by age and prevalence), and procedures (systematic guidance, including videos and medical animations, of procedures integral to the practice of medicine across many specialties).

- 5-Minute Clinical Consult (5MCC) Online provides instant access to essential information about 700+ medical conditions. Resources include dermatology images, videos of medical procedures, AAFP patient handouts, and more. 5MCC is updated regularly for quick reference at the point of care.

- McGraw-Hill's Diagnosaurus 2.0 on AccessMedicine is a differential diagnosis tool that allows users to search 1000+ differential diagnosis for common diseases and disorders. Users can search by symptoms, diseases, and/or organ system.

Clin-eguide and Facts & Comparisons are registered trademarks of Wolters Kluwer Health, Inc., Conshohocken, PA. Ovid is a registered trademark of Ovid Technologies, Inc., New York, NY.

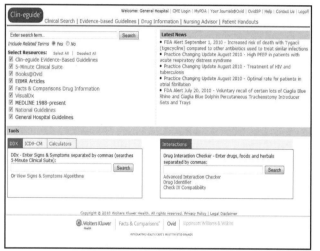

Figure 10-8. Sample clinical decision support site. (Reprinted with permission from Wolters Kluwer Health Clinical Solutions.)

Clinical Informatics and Decision Support

In recent years, concerns about health care quality and patient safety have sparked significant investment in information systems to improve health care processes and outcomes. Electronic medical records (EMRs) and computerized provider order entry (CPOE) systems help to automate and manage patient information. Clinical decision support (CDS) systems augment these systems by providing clinical knowledge and best practices at the moment of need to inform decision making and enhance patient care.[20] Table 10-7 and Figure 10-8 provide examples of clinical decision support sites.

Critical Thinking Clinical Scenario

Your patient has come to you with a complaint of low back pain after playing ice hockey this weekend. After a thorough evaluation, you develop a plan of care that includes a series of back extension exercises for your patient to start with at home. He returns the next session with information from the Internet that provided a series of flexion exercises for patients with low back pain. He appears concerned and wants to know why you decided to give him the wrong exercises.

Reflective Questions

1. How might you approach your patient's question?

2. How might you use what you have learned about sources of online information and evaluating those sources to validate your recommendations and reassure your patient?

3. What other resources might you recommend for your patient?

Key Point to Remember

- Lifelong learning is a must in today's information/knowledge society.

- It is not enough to be able to find information when we need it; we must also be able to critically evaluate it and use it effectively.

- Examples of just-in-time learning applications that support performance and decision making include the following:

  o Patient education Web sites

  o Health-related digital learning object repositories

  o Clinical informatics and decision support systems.

Transforming Minds: Promoting Critical Thinking With Technology

As discussed in previous chapters, active learning experiences that engage participants in inquiry, problem solving, collaboration, or other types of critical thinking are more likely than passive modes of instruction to create deep, meaningful, transformative learning. The interactivity and rich media capabilities of e-Learning environments offer a unique opportunity to provide learners with experiences that require, and thereby actively build, critical thinking skills.

Teaching strategies intended to promote critical thinking in face-to-face settings can be efficiently and effectively implemented using e-Learning modalities. For example, a common strategy used in physical therapy education is to present learners with a case study; ask them to make decisions about assessment, diagnosis, or management; and then provide feedback about their choices. This strategy can be easily replicated in a self-directed, e-Learning format wherein the computer becomes the instructor, presenting the case study, asking questions, assessing the learner's responses, and providing feedback based on the learner's choices (Figure 10-9). Videotaped scenarios, or a series of photos accompanied by a story presented using audio or text, can engage learners as participants in real-world experiences. As the story evolves, learners can be challenged to make appropriate decisions or diagnose problems, with feedback presented in the context of the story. Varied outcomes may be presented based on the learner's choices, or a narrator (instructor voice) can simply provide feedback along the way, correcting the learner when they make mistakes and explaining and reinforcing why the correct choices are appropriate.

The ability to simulate real-world experience is a key benefit of e-Learning technologies. Online or computer-based simulations can provide learners with an opportunity to practice high-risk skills or high-stakes decision making in a safe setting and experience the consequences of their choices without the risk of real harm. In their truest form, simulations model real-world phenomena such that the simulated environment responds in a realistic way to varied inputs from the user. When a physical therapy student interacts with a patient simulator in a classroom, the simulator responds to their actions as a real patient would. For example, a patient simulator may be programmed to present with signs of a heart attack, and the student must be prepared to react. If the student reacts appropriately, the simulator would indicate that the patient recovered nicely; if not, the simulator may indicate that the patient died. The higher the accuracy or fidelity of the simulator, the more variable and realistic will be the simulated responses.

Immersive e-Learning environments, sometimes referred to as *microworlds* or *virtual worlds*, use graphic

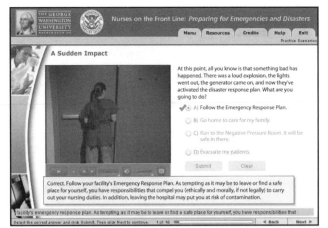

Figure10-9. In this course, learners make decisions and receive feedback after viewing a video scenario. (Reprinted with permission from The George Washington University School of Nursing.)

imagery and media to situate learners in highly realistic contexts for learning. Like simulators, immersive e-Learning environments vary in their degree of realism. Creating highly realistic learning environments using 3-D graphics, professional video, or other kinds of high-end digital media is a painstaking and expensive process; programming multiple learner paths to simulate real-world options and outcomes can be equally complicated. Designers of immersive e-Learning must analyze the potential benefits of highly realistic media and technology—sometimes thinking outside of the box—to ensure that the educational value of an immersive e-Learning is balanced appropriately with their investment. Fortunately for those of us who do not have large budgets for high-end e-Learning production, with a little imagination and creativity, it is possible to immerse learners in realistic learning experiences using relatively simple combinations of digital media.

Stop and Reflect

Imagine yourself in the seat of a learner engaged in the following e-Learning experience. Sounds of sirens and screaming are heard over a black screen. A clap of thunder accompanies a flash of light, and the screen returns to black. As the black screen dissolves to a photo showing the aftermath of a serious car accident, a narrator tells the story of a family that has been struck by a drunk driver. You were driving to the grocery store when you witnessed the accident and stopped to help. You hear the sound of a child crying, and the scene transitions to an image of a toddler inside of the vehicle, still strapped in her car seat. The narrator asks, "What are you going to do first?" and presents you with several viable options.

- How would this relatively simple presentation pull the learner into the story?

- Can you think of another teaching scenario that could be adapted for a self-directed e-Learning program?

- How you might use digital images and sound effects to create an immersive e-Learning experience?

Key Points to Remember

- The interactivity and rich media capabilities of e-Learning provide a unique opportunity to immerse learners in active, simulative learning experiences.
- By requiring critical thinking, active learning strategies build critical thinking.
- Teaching strategies intended to promote critical thinking in face-to-face settings can be efficiently and effectively implemented using e-Learning modalities.
- Examples of active e-Learning strategies include the following:
  - Web- or computer-based simulations
  - Virtual worlds or microworlds
  - Case- or scenario-based learning
  - Virtual patients
  - Educational games
  - Mind mapping

Critical Thinking Clinical Scenario

In classroom or clinical settings, case studies are often presented by an instructor or facilitator as a basis for interactive group discussion. Cases are typically presented verbally or in text format, with visuals such as radiographs provided as appropriate.

Reflective Questions

1. Given what you have learned about active e-Learning strategies, how might you enhance a case study presented in a classroom or clinical setting?
2. What kinds of media and interactivity could you use to tell a patient's story and enrich the experience for your learners?

A variety of active e-Learning strategies take advantage of the simulative and immersive capabilities of e-Learning. Table 10-8 provides a few examples of these strategies. Though each strategy has a unique intent, note that different strategies may use similar media and interactive activities to engage learners in inquiry, problem solving, or exploration. For example, a case-based learning experience may include a virtual patient. The list is not comprehensive, and the strategies are not mutually exclusive. They can be modified, mixed, and matched—with other active strategies or more traditional approaches—based on your instructional objective(s) and the motivational and learning needs of your audience.

Creating Connections

As was emphasized in Chapter 7, social learning theorists believe that all learning takes place through interaction with other human beings; all knowledge is shared knowledge; and knowledge evolves through critical dialogue and the resolution of tensions between individual beliefs or the personal meaning that individuals make. Particularly in physical therapy and the other health professions, there is little doubt that social interaction—whether facilitator to learner or learner to learner—plays a key role in the learning process. We learn through our experiences and by sharing those experiences.

The term *community* refers to a unified group of people with common characteristics or interests living together within a larger society. Communities may share a culture, values, knowledge, skills, experiences, perspectives, or any combination of these or other things. Members of a community may contribute and benefit from this exchange to more or lesser degrees.

Table 10-8. Examples of e-Learning Strategies

Strategy	Description
Case- or scenario-based learning	Learners are presented with a real-world situation and then challenged to answer questions or make decisions based on the facts presented. This can be as simple as a multiple-choice question introduced by a paragraph of text or as elaborate as a series of video scenarios with different paths that move learners through varied story outcomes based on their decisions.
Virtual patients	Learners interact with electronic representations of patients, asking questions and viewing histories, test results, and other indicators of health status. Patient information may be presented using text, perhaps accompanied by a photo of the patient, or using richer combinations of media such as videos of patient answers, x-ray images, etc.
Educational gaming	Sometimes referred to as edutainment, educational games integrate the fun and challenge of a computer game with an educational experience. Games may be as simple as an online version of hangman or as complex as a commercial computer game. Some interesting examples of educational games have been highlighted through the Robert Wood Johnson Foundation's Games for Health initiative (http://www.gamesforhealth.org/). This project promotes the development of games intended to improve health rather than just learn about it.
Mind or concept mapping	Working independently or with others, learners interact with computer software to build a flowchart or diagram that represents their thinking process around a concept or problem. Mind-mapping software tools such as Inspiration and Gliffy facilitate learners' individual or collaborative brainstorming and exploration of concepts or topics. These tools can also be used by designers of e-Learning to create flowcharts of a learning experience.

On his Community of Practice Web site, Etienne Wenger defines *communities of practice* as "groups of people who share a concern or a passion for something they do and learn how to do it better as they interact regularly."[21] This definition could easily be applied to the term *learning community*, a term educators use to describe groups of learners engaged in shared learning experiences. Whether in a community of practice or a community of learners, participants share knowledge, goals, experiences, and interests as they learn with and from one another.

Learning communities may be large or small, broadly or narrowly focused. In a university setting, for example, a cohort of students enrolled in a particular degree program, who socialize, learn together, and help each other over time, are members of a learning community. The same students (or a subset) enrolled in a particular course are members of a more focused learning community. If these students work together in small groups on a problem or project, they become members of smaller, even more focused learning communities. In other settings, such as professional or patient education, a learning community might consist of a group of practitioners sharing knowledge and resources related to a topic of interest, such as alternative medicine, or a support group of patients who share a particular illness or disability.

Online learning research and practice provides useful insight to guide the design and facilitation of targeted learning communities. Once viewed as a significant challenge to delivering effective education at a distance, social interaction through discussion boards, Webinars, and collaborative activity is now a cornerstone of quality online learning. Many experienced online educators and even classroom educators integrate frequent and diverse opportunities for online social interaction into their courses. The educator's role is to set the stage and then facilitate (rather than direct) the dialogue by probing for information, connecting and synthesizing ideas, providing feedback related to accuracy and relevance, and prompting deeper critical thinking related to emerging questions. A good facilitator allows participants to carry the conversation while moving it toward appropriate shared conclusions.

Online learning theory, research, and lessons learned can be applied to the design, development, and facilitation of learning communities in other settings. Researchers at the University of Calgary have developed the community of inquiry model to guide the design and facilitation of shared, critical dialogue in online learning environments.[22] This model involves complementary and overlapping relationships among a number of the concepts we have already discussed: self-reflection through metacognitive processes; social interaction through dialogue; and teaching through content, structure, and facilitation. Garrison described how participants in an online community of inquiry move between dialogue and personal reflection when engaged in shared, purposeful learning and how the additional time for individual reflection afforded by asynchronous communication can result in deeper levels of critical discussion.[23] By providing an appropriate mix of social, reflective, and teacher-facilitated experiences, along with sufficient time for reflection and critical dialogue, online educators can achieve optimal outcomes.

The strategies noted above, along with the action learning strategies we discussed in the chapter on reflection, can be effective means for developing virtual learning communities and engaging students in critical inquiry when they are off-site. The clinical internship or rotation is a critical component of the education of most health professionals. These clinical education experiences often occur off campus and at distant sites. Using virtual action learning sets can enhance students' reflective processes and critical thinking while simultaneously establishing a community of inquiry. It enables students to engage in the virtual dialogue and self-reflection processes as they help each other solve real-world problems and conflicts.[24,25]

By removing barriers of time and place, technology can foster and facilitate the development and sustainability of learning and practice communities. Though some argue that technology isolates, others note the ongoing conversation taking place through text messages, instant messaging, blogs, e-mail, and other technology tools.

We have seen the evolution of the Internet from Web 1.0—a primarily passive space where most of us were consumers of content—to Web 2.0—a much more active, social space where many of us have joined social networks, created personal Web pages, sent e-Cards, and posted videos on YouTube. Some envision Web 3.0—a virtual world where we interact through our avatars (ie, 3-D computerized representation of a person) rather than the keyboard, talking to friends at a virtual coffee shop rather than instant messages and choosing products from a shelf rather than a list on Amazon (Figure 10-10).

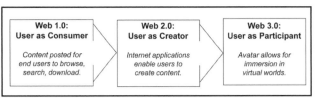

Figure 10-10. The social *Webolution*.

Table 10-9. Web 2.0 Applications

Application	Description
Social networks	Social networking tools enable users to create and share personal profiles to build a community of friends or others around an activity or interest area. Common features include e-mail; text, voice, or video chat; discussion forums; and file sharing. Popular social networking tools include MySpace (http://www.myspace.com) and Facebook (http://www.facebook.com).
Blogs	Blogging tools enable nonprogrammers to create Web pages and facilitate conversations around topic(s) of interest. Users can create posts and upload pictures and multimedia. Popular blogging tools include Blogger by Google (http://www.blogspot.com), WordPress (http://wordpress.org), and Typepad (http://www.typepad.com). Notably, social networking and blogging tools provide similar features. Tools such as Ning (http://www.ning.com) and LiveJournal (http://www.livejournal.com) are intended to be used for either purpose.
Instant messaging	Instant messaging tools enable users to conduct text chats in real time with a network of friends. Instant messaging has traditionally been conducted via text; however, most tools now provide voice and video capability. Popular instant messaging tools include AIM (http://www.aol.com) and Yahoo Messenger (http://messenger.yahoo.com), Skype (http://www.skype.com), and Google Talk (www.google.com/talk).
Wikis	Wikis enable users to contribute to a shared online document. The most popular wiki is MediaWiki, the free, server-based software application used by Wikipedia (http://www.mediawiki.org/wiki/Download). Another example is Google Docs (http://docs.google.com), which operates completely online with no download required.
Webcasting	Webcasting sites enable users to broadcast digital content, which can be audio and/or video, over the Internet. Popular examples include iTunes for podcasting (http://www.apple.com/itunes/) and YouTube for videocasting (http://www.youtube.com).
Web conferencing	Web conferencing tools enable users to convene group meetings and conduct presentations online in real time. Common Web conferencing features include a whiteboard, screen sharing, and text, voice, and/or video chat. Popular Web conferencing tools include GoToMeeting (http://www.GoToMeeting.com) and WebEx (http://ww.webex.com). Some Web conferencing tools include additional features to support online seminars, such as hand raising, polling, and group breakout rooms. Examples include Adobe Connect (www.adobe.com/products/acrobatconnect/) and Elluminate (www.elluminate.com).

Table 10-10. Social Networking Tools in Action

Tools	How This Tool Might Be Used With Students in the Classroom or Clinic	How This Tool Might Be Used With Patients
Social network or blog	Physical therapy students share their clinical experiences with their teacher and fellow students. Participants share ideas and learn and mentor from each other. The site is also used to help new students find appropriate clinical placements.	A practice establishes a blogging site with separate areas for common physical therapy problems. Patients can explore links to appropriate online resources and talk with others sharing their condition. Practitioners facilitate and participate in the discussions; respond to patient questions; and share the responsibility for weekly real-time "office hours."
Instant messaging	Students in a computer-enabled classroom explore ideas and ask questions of each other without interrupting an instructional presentation.	Patients attending a virtual support group retreat meet and talk with other participants.
Wikis	Students in a classroom or clinic work together on a case-based collaborative activity to create a treatment plan.	Patients contribute to an annotated bibliography and list of Web site resources related to a common condition.
Webcasting or Web conferencing	Members of a physical therapy association provide and participate in monthly presentations on various educational and/or research topics.	A practice broadcasts virtual exercise classes for seniors and others who have difficulty coming to the clinic.

Web 2.0 applications have opened new doors for educators, and Table 10-9 summarizes some of your options.

As with active e-Learning strategies, there is overlap in the features and functions of these Web 2.0 technologies. For example, you can post digital videos on a blog or use instant messaging on a social networking site. So it is important to be clear about your educational goals and objectives so you can choose the tool or combination of tools that will best facilitate their achievement. Table 10-10 provides a few examples of how Web 2.0 applications can be used in clinical, classroom, or patient education settings.

Stop and Reflect

- How can you tap into the educational opportunities available through Web 2.0 applications?
- How can you harness the power of these technologies to build new learning communities and foster targeted, educational dialogue?

Key Points to Remember

- We learn through our experiences and by sharing those experiences.
- Learning communities engage participants in the sharing of knowledge, goals, experiences, and interests as they learn with and from one another.
- By removing barriers of time and place, technology can foster and facilitate the development and sustainability of learning and practice communities.
- Web 2.0 applications, which enable users to create and share Web content, provide diverse opportunities for online community building to support educational goals.

Disseminating the Message

Once you have designed and developed a technology-based learning experience, you will need to make it available to your learners. As you have learned in this chapter, there are many options. The best choice depends upon the nature of your message and the learning and technology preferences of your target audience.

When determining the best way to disseminate e-Learning, think about the best time, place, and means of (a) reaching your audience and (b) facilitating learner access.

- On-site. What e-Learning opportunities exist at your professional practice? Perhaps you could set up a computer learning station for waiting patients, family, and friends, or provide continuing education for physical therapists, physical therapist assistants, and office staff, or provide training for new aides.

- Online. What audiences would you like to reach outside of your daily practice? Can you add value to your practice's Web site by integrating some e-Learning modules? Perhaps you would like to create a blog for your patients or produce a podcast or videocast for referring physicians. You and your colleagues may also want to take advantage of the many online continuing education opportunities offered by professional organizations and universities.

- On the go. Portable media devices such as MP3 players, smart phones, and netbooks let users download digital media content to play back at their convenience. e-Learning for these devices that includes text and visuals must be designed for effective presentation on a small screen and must be provided in the appropriate format. Consult the vendor Web sites for information about supported media formats.

Key Points to Remember

- Digital e-Learning is flexible e-Learning.
- Consider the following ways to reach learning audiences:
  - On-site
  - Online
  - On the go

Summary

Whether delivered on-site, online, or on the go, e-Learning is one of many options available to help you provide effective education to students, colleagues, patients, and the public. e-Learning materials can stand alone as complete, self-directed learning experiences or can complement other types of educational materials you may be using. As you approach new educational challenges, think about how you can best support your learners by doing the following:

- Creatively combining digital media to create multisensory e-Learning that motivates and engages diverse learners.
- Applying UDL principles along with accessibility standards to meet the educational needs of all learners, including those with special needs.
- Harnessing the wealth of just-in-time information and resources available on the Internet to support patient compliance and decision making.
- Immersing learners in critical thinking scenarios and simulated real-world experience.
- Building and facilitating social interactions and collaborative educational networks.
- Disseminating e-Learning materials in convenient, accessible formats.

This chapter introduced some basic concepts and strategies to guide the design, selection, and use of e-Learning materials. You have learned that designing an e-Learning program involves determining who your audience is, what your goals are, and planning how learners will interact with diverse media elements in order to achieve learning objectives. Bringing this design to fruition involves creating digital media and using appropriate software to assemble and produce the e-Learning product. Depending upon the level of sophistication you are looking for, both of these tasks may require substantial investment and collaboration with an interdisciplinary team of subject matter experts, instructional designers, media developers, graphic artists, and/or programmers.

We have also described some of the software that can empower you to create effective, professional e-Learning products on your own. You have seen how the emergence of blogs, wikis, social networks, and other tools has made Web publishing accessible to all. An Internet search or visit to your local library or bookstore will likely yield many more useful resources. Many community colleges offer introductory courses in instructional technology, Web design, and digital media production as well. If you have the desire to create your own e-Learning materials, we encourage you to give it a try. With the right tools and a little ingenuity, you may be surprised at how much you can do to enrich your teaching with technology.

Key Points to Remember

- Instructional Systems Design provides a structure and systematic process to facilitate and guide the development of effective e-Learning products.

- e-Learning technologies provide a rich array of media and interactive possibilities to engage and motivate diverse learners, including those with special needs.

- The most engaging e-Learning experiences will provide opportunities for learners to see, hear, think, and do.

- Educational Web sites, digital learning object repositories, clinical informatics, and decision support systems are a rich resource of just-in-time learning for both patients and practitioners.

- By requiring critical thinking, active e-Learning strategies such as simulations, virtual worlds, case-based learning, virtual patients, and educational games foster deep and memorable learning.

- Web 2.0 technologies such as wikis, blogs, social networks, and virtual worlds enable collaborative learning as well as community building.

- e-Learning can be distributed in multiple formats to meet the needs of diverse audiences and settings.

References

1. Dick WO, Carey L, Carey JO. *The Systematic Design of Instruction.* Boston, MA: Allyn & Bacon; 2004.

2. Keller JM. Development and use of the ARCS model of motivational design. *J Instr Devel.* 1987;10:2-10.

3. Keller J. Keller's ARCS model of motivational design: attention, relevance, confidence, satisfaction. Available at http://www.arcsmodel.com. Accessed August 18, 2009.

4. Fleming ND, Mills C. Not another inventory, rather a catalyst for reflection. In Wulff DH, Nyquist JD, eds. *To Improve the Academy.* Fort Collins, CO: The POD Network; 1992:137.

5. GIMP. GNU image manipulation software. Available at http://www.gimp.org/. Accessed August 18, 2009.

6. Mazzoni D. Audacity. Available at http://audacity.sourceforge.net/. Accessed August 18, 2009.

7. US Census Bureau. 2006 American Community Survey. Available at http://www.census.gov/acs/www/. Accessed July 19, 2009.

8. Microsoft. Types of assistive technology products. Available at http://www.microsoft.com/enable/at/types.aspx. Accessed August 18, 2009.

9. CAST. CAST: transforming education through universal design for learning. Available at http://www.cast.org/. Accessed August 18, 2009.

10. Dalton B, Snow C. Improving comprehension online (ICON). Available at http://www.cast.org/research/projects/icon.html. Accessed August 18, 2009.

11. US General Services Administration. Section 508. Available at http://www.section508.gov/. Accessed August 18, 2009.

12. Regents of the University of California. How much information? 2003. Available at http://www2.sims.berkeley.edu/research/projects/how-much-info-2003/execsum.htm. Accessed August 6, 2009.

13. Jukes I, McCain T. Windows on the world: thinking about the future today. Available at http://web.mac.com/iajukes/thecommittedsardine/Handouts_files/wof.pdf. Accessed August 6, 2009.

14. Beck S. *The Good, the Bad & the Ugly: Or, Why It's a Good Idea to Evaluate Web Sources.* Available at http://lib.nmsu.edu/instruction/eval.html. Accessed August 17, 2009.

15. Henderson S, Johnson E. OnCoRe blueprint: the art & science of repository creation. Paper presented at the 14th Sloan-C International Conference on Online Learning; November 5-7, 2008; Orlando, FL.

16. US Library of Medicine, National Institutes of Health. MedlinePlus: health information tutorials. Available at http://www.nlm.nih.gov/medlineplus/tutorial.html. Accessed August 18, 2009.

17. Dennis S, Uijtdehaage S. The Health Education Assets Library. Available at http://www.healcentral.org. Accessed August 18, 2009.

18. Dublin Core Metadata Initiative. Available at http://dublincore.org. Accessed August 18, 2009.

19. Institute of Electrical and Electronics Engineers. Draft standard for learning object metadata from the learning technology standards committee. IEEE Standard 1484.12.1. Available at http://ltsc.ieee.org/wg12/files/LOM_1484_12_1_v1_Final_Draft.pdf. Accessed August 6, 2009.

20. Osheroff JA, Pifer EA, Teich JM, Sittig DF, Jenders RA. *Improving Outcomes with Clinical Decision Support: An Implementer's Guide.* Chicago, Ill: Health Information Management Systems Society; 2005.

21. Wenger E. Communities of practice: a brief introduction. Available at http://www.ewenger.com/theory/index.htm. Accessed August 18, 2009.

22. Garrison DR, Anderson T, Archer W. Critical thinking, cognitive presence and computer conferencing in distance education. *Am J Dist Educ.* 2001;15:7-23.

23. Garrison DR. Cognitive presence for asynchronous online learning: the role of refletive inquiry, self-direction and metacognition. In: Bourne J, Moore JC, eds. *Elements of Quality in Online Education: Practice and Direction.* Needham, MA: The Sloan Consortium; 2003:47-58.

24. Dunfee H, Plack MM, Driscoll M, Rindflesch A, Hollman J. Assessing reflection and higher order thinking in electronic discussion threads in the clinical setting. *J Phys Ther Educ.* 2008;22:60-66.

25. Plack MM, Dunfee H, Driscoll M, Rindflesch A, Hollman J. Virtual action learning sets: a model for facilitating reflection in the clinical setting. *J Phys Ther Educ.* 2008;22:33-41.

Financial Disclosures

Maryanne M. Driscoll has no financial or proprietary interest in the materials presented herein.

Joyce R. Maring has no financial or proprietary interest in the materials presented herein.

Margaret Plack has no financial or proprietary interest in the materials presented herein.

Laurie J. Posey has no financial or proprietary interest in the materials presented herein.

Index

Wait...There's More!

SLACK Incorporated's Health Care Books and Journals offers a wide selection of books in the field of Physical Therapy. We are dedicated to providing important works that educate, inform and improve the knowledge of our customers. Don't miss out on our other informative titles that will enhance your collection.

Patient Practitioner Interaction:
An Experiential Manual for Developing the Art of Health Care, Fourth Edition
Carol M. Davis DPT, EdD, MS, FAPTA

304 pp., Soft Cover, 2006, ISBN 13 978-1-55642-720-6,
Order# 47204, **$47.95**

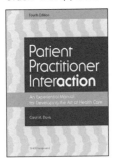

Patient Practitioner Interaction, Fourth Edition is filled with information designed to help improve personal interaction and communication skills, specifically when dealing with difficult circumstances.

Physical Therapy in Acute Care:
A Clinician's Guide
Daniel J. Malone MPT, CCS; Kathy Lee Bishop Lindsay MS, PT, CCS

704 pp., Soft Cover, 2006, ISBN 13 978-1-55642-534-9,
Order# 45341, **$59.95**

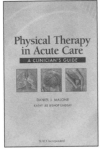

This is a user-friendly, pocket-sized, evidence-based text that guides and reinforces successful acute care patient management. *Physical Therapy in Acute Care* provides clinicians with an understanding of the basic physiological mechanisms underlying normal function of all major organ systems, contrasted with the pathophysiology of the disease and disorders that physical therapists will most often encounter in an acute care environment.

Teaching and Learning in Physical Therapy:
From Classroom to Clinic
Margaret Plack PT, EdD; Maryanne Driscoll PhD

250 pp., Soft Cover, 2010, ISBN 13 978-1-55642-872-2,
Order# 48722, **$43.95**

Cardiovascular/Pulmonary Essentials:
Applying the Preferred Physical Therapist Practice Patterns(SM)
Marilyn Moffat PT, DPT, PhD, FAPTA, CSCS; Donna Frownfelter DPT, MA, CCS, FCCP, RRT

328 pp., Soft Cover, 2007, ISBN 13 978-1-55642-668-1,
Order# 46682, **$58.95**

Integumentary Essentials:
Applying the Preferred Physical Therapist Practice Patterns(SM)
Marilyn Moffat PT, DPT, PhD, FAPTA, CSCS; Katherine Biggs Harris PT, MS

160 pp., Soft Cover, 2006, ISBN 13 978-1-55642-670-4,
Order# 46704, **$50.95**

Musculoskeletal Essentials:
Applying the Preferred Physical Therapist Practice Patterns(SM)
Marilyn Moffat PT, DPT, PhD, FAPTA, CSCS; Elaine Rosen PT, DHSc, OCS, FAAOMPT; Sandra Rusnak-Smith PT, DHSc, OCS

448 pp., Soft Cover, 2007, ISBN 13 978-1-55642-667-4,
Order# 46674, **$58.95**

Neuromuscular Essentials:
Applying the Preferred Physical Therapist Practice Patterns(SM)
Marilyn Moffat PT, DPT, PhD, FAPTA, CSCS; Joanell Bohmert PT, MS; Janice Hulme MS, PT, DHSc

320 pp., Soft Cover, 2008, ISBN 13 978-1-55642-669-8,
Order# 46690, **$58.95**

Gait Analysis: Normal and Pathological Function, Second Edition
Jacquelin Perry MD, ScD; Judith M. Burnfield PhD, PT

576 pp., Hard Cover, 2010, ISBN 13 978-1-55642-766-4,
Order# 47662, **$92.95**

Please visit **www.slackbooks.com** to order any of the above titles!

24 Hours a Day...7 Days a Week!

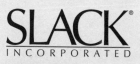